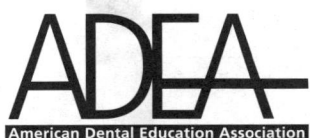

OFFICIAL GUIDE TO
Dental Schools

2007

For Students Entering Fall 2008

American Dental Education Association

1400 K Street, NW, Suite 1100
Washington, DC 20005

Phone: 202-289-7201
Fax: 202-289-7204

publications@adea.org

www.adea.org

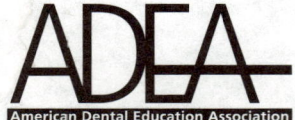

Copyright ©2007 by the American Dental Education Association. All rights reserved. No part of this book may be reproduced in any form or by any electronic or mechanical means, including information storage and retrieval systems, without permission in writing from the publisher.
ISBN 978-0-9709669-9-5
Printed in the United States of America.

Disclaimer
ADEA has made every effort to ensure that the information in this publication is correct, but makes no warranty, either express or implied, of its accuracy or completeness. ADEA intends the reader to use this publication as a guide only and does not intend that the reader rely on the information herein as a basis for advice for personal or financial decisions. The school-specific information was supplied to ADEA by each dental school in the fall of 2006; however, ADEA reminds the reader that authoritative, up-to-date information about a school's admissions policies and practices is issued directly by the school itself.

Contributors: W. David Brunson, D.D.S.
Gina Luke
Richard Weaver, D.D.S.
Anne Wells, Ed.D.
Designer: Judy Myers
Cover Designer: Gustavo A. Mendoza

Photo credits
Page 8: Dr. William Dahlke. Used with permission.
Page 17: Fourth-year dental student Gina Betita. Used with permission.
Page 22: Third-year dental student Kelli Jobman. Used with permission.
Page 46: Third-year dental student Summer Totonchi. Used with permission.

To Readers of the *ADEA Official Guide to Dental Schools*,

At the American Dental Education Association (ADEA) we know that the *Official Guide to Dental Schools* is used largely by two sets of people—those who are exploring the possibility of a career in dentistry and those who are advising the explorers. Both groups are very important to the profession of dentistry, and I am pleased that ADEA can be of service to you through this guide.

To those of you who are exploring the possibility of a career in dentistry, I offer heartfelt encouragement. For me, the practice of dentistry has stimulated my scientific inquisitiveness and my desire to be of use to others. Having also been a dental educator, I know first-hand that dental students are bright lights of enthusiasm, intelligence, and talent. They quickly learn that dental school offers more than just an academic challenge—it stretches their intellect beyond their imaginations, increases their ability to help others less fortunate, and enlarges their interest in discovery and research. Graduates of dental schools are valued oral health-care providers and vital citizens of their communities; their degrees prepare them for great accomplishments in a wide variety of dental-related careers. Best wishes in your application process!

To those of you who are guiding advisees interested in the health professions, I hope this book is a useful tool. First, as reference for the person who already is interested in a career in dentistry. And second as a means for "turning someone on" to dentistry. Dental practitioners are women and men from all backgrounds, cultures, races, and ethnicities who have the motivation and brain power to do well in dental school. I appreciate that you will keep dentistry in mind for the wide range of those who value your counsel.

As you may have noted from the ad on the inside front cover of this book, membership in ADEA is open at no charge to every student in U. S. and Canadian dental schools. I invite entering dental students to join. ADEA is committed to improving the already outstanding quality of dental education—and glad to have each entering class be a part.

Best wishes,

Richard W. Valachovic, D.M.D., M.P.H.
ADEA Executive Director

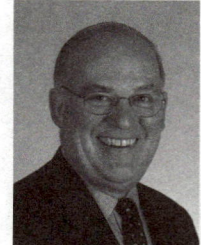

ORDERS

Orders for this book should be addressed to
Publications Department
American Dental Education Association
1400 K Street, NW, Suite 1100
Washington, DC 20005
www.adea.org
202-289-7201

Price: $35 per copy, $29 per copy for orders of ten or more.
Price includes applicable sales tax. Additional charges apply to express delivery.

CONTENTS

Introduction 1

PART I. BECOMING A DENTIST 3

Chapter 1. Exploring a World of Opportunities 5
An Introduction to Dentistry 5
Opportunities in Dentistry 6
Rewards of Practicing Dentistry 6
Career Options 7

Chapter 2. Applying to Dental School 11
The Dental School Program 11
Qualifying for Dental School 12
The Application Process 14
Special Admissions Topics 19

Chapter 3. Deciding Where to Apply 21

Chapter 4. Financing Your Dental Education 39
Types of Financial Aid 40
Applying for Financial Aid 40
An Overview of Student Loan Programs 44
Other Aid 47
Sources of Aid for Canadian and International Students 48
Federally Funded Scholarships 48
Privately Funded Scholarships and Other Helpful Resources 50
The Importance of Building and Keeping Good Credit 53
Other Helpful Resources 54
A Glossary of Terms Every Student Borrower Should Know 55

Chapter 5. Getting More Information 59
Individuals Who Can Help 59
Organizations That Can Help 60
Other Resources 65

PART II. LEARNING ABOUT DENTAL SCHOOLS 67

Introduction 69
How to Use Part II 69

Alabama
University of Alabama at Birmingham 70

Arizona
Arizona School of Dentistry & Oral Health 72
Midwestern University 74

California
Loma Linda University 76
University of California, Los Angeles 78
University of California, San Francisco ... 80
University of the Pacific 82
University of Southern California 84

Colorado
University of Colorado at Denver 86

Connecticut
University of Connecticut 88

District of Columbia
Howard University 90

Florida
Nova Southeastern University 92
University of Florida 94

Georgia
Medical College of Georgia 96

Illinois
University of Illinois at Chicago 98
Southern Illinois University 100

iii

Indiana
Indiana University 102

Iowa
The University of Iowa 104

Kentucky
University of Kentucky 106
University of Louisville 108

Louisiana
Louisiana State University 110

Maryland
University of Maryland 112

Massachusetts
Boston University 114
Harvard School of Dental Medicine 116
Tufts University 118

Michigan
University of Detroit Mercy 120
University of Michigan 122

Minnesota
University of Minnesota 124

Mississippi
University of Mississippi 126

Missouri
University of Missouri-Kansas City 128

Nebraska
Creighton University 130
University of Nebraska Medical Center 132

Nevada
University of Nevada, Las Vegas 134

New Jersey
University of Medicine and Dentistry of New Jersey 136

New York
Columbia University 138
New York University 140
Stony Brook University 142
University at Buffalo 144

North Carolina
University of North Carolina at Chapel Hill 146

Ohio
Case School of Dental Medicine 148
The Ohio State University 150

Oklahoma
University of Oklahoma 152

Oregon
Oregon Health & Science University 154

Pennsylvania
University of Pennsylvania 156
University of Pittsburgh 158
Temple University 160

Puerto Rico
University of Puerto Rico 162

South Carolina
Medical University of South Carolina 164

Tennessee
Meharry Medical College 166
University of Tennessee 168

Texas
Baylor College of Dentistry 170
University of Texas Health Science Center at Houston 172
University of Texas Health Science Center at San Antonio 174

Virginia
Virginia Commonwealth University 176

Washington
University of Washington 178

West Virginia
West Virginia University 180

Wisconsin
Marquette University 182

CANADIAN DENTAL SCHOOLS

Alberta
University of Alberta 184

British Columbia
University of British Columbia 186

Manitoba
University of Manitoba 188

Nova Scotia
Dalhousie University 190

Ontario
University of Toronto 192
University of Western Ontario 194

Québec
Université Laval 196
McGill University 198
Université de Montréal 200

Saskatchewan
University of Saskatchewan 202

LIST OF TABLES

Table 2-1. Total U.S. dental school applicants and first-year enrollees, 2005-06 12

Table 2-2. Undergraduate majors of dental school applicants and enrollees, 2004-05 13

Table 2-3. Dental schools participating in AADSAS 16

Table 3-1. Dental schools' applicants and enrollees by gender, race, and ethnicity—class entering fall 2006 24

Table 3-2. Dental schools' applicants and enrollees, in state versus out of state—class entering fall 2006 26

Table 3-3. Admission requirements by dental school 28

Table 3-4. Characteristics of the class entering fall 2006 by dental school 33

Table 3-5. The class entering fall 2006 at dental schools by state of residence 35

Table 3-6. Combined and other degree programs by dental school 37

Table 4-1. Forms of financial aid 41

Table 4-2. Example of a student's log of outstanding debt on entering dental school 42

Table 4-3. Example of a student's budget worksheet 43

Table 4-4. Quick reference guide to loan programs 44

Table 4-5. Example of first-year dental student's loan log 52

INTRODUCTION

Welcome to the *ADEA Official Guide to Dental Schools*! Whether you're seeking specific information about becoming a dentist or you're just beginning to wonder if dental school might be a career path for you, this book will be of value. And if you're in a position to advise and mentor students considering and preparing for the dental profession, this book will help you give them the information they need.

The *ADEA Official Guide to Dental Schools* is the only authoritative guide to dental education on the market. This comprehensive, annually updated resource guide has been edited and published for more than four decades by the American Dental Education Association (ADEA). The only national organization dedicated to serving the needs of the dental education community, ADEA has since 1923 worked to promote the value and improve the quality of dental education as well as to expand the role of dentistry among other health professions. As such, ADEA is perfectly positioned to provide you with both the most up-to-date information about the dental schools in the United States and Canada and the most useful insights into how to prepare for, apply to, and finance your dental education.

The *ADEA Official Guide to Dental Schools* has two parts:

PART I, BECOMING A DENTIST contains five chapters that will familiarize you with the dental profession and guide you through all the steps toward becoming a dental student.

Chapter 1, Exploring a World of Opportunities explains the wide range of careers in dentistry.

Chapter 2, Applying to Dental School describes the academic background generally necessary for admission to dental school and prepares you for the application process.

Chapter 3, Deciding Where to Apply defines important factors to help you decide which schools are the best match for your educational and professional goals.

Chapter 4, Financing Your Dental Education is an in-depth look at financing options to pay for dental school.

Chapter 5, Getting More Information lists other sources of information about topics covered in the previous chapters.

Part I also contains tables of information about dental schools and dental students across a wide range of categories. These data were collected from ADEA, the American Dental Association (ADA), and the dental schools themselves.

PART II, LEARNING ABOUT DENTAL SCHOOLS introduces each of the U.S. and Canadian dental schools. The information on each school is designed to help you decide which will best suit your academic and personal needs.

The entry for each school includes the following:

- general information;
- admission requirements;
- selection factors;
- timetable for submitting application materials;
- degrees granted and characteristics of the dental program;
- estimated expenses;
- financial aid awards to first-year students;
- academic and other assistance; and
- websites, addresses, and telephone numbers for further information.

The *ADEA Official Guide to Dental Schools* gives you everything you need to increase the likelihood of success in planning for and entering dental school and the dental profession. We wish you well!

PART I
BECOMING A DENTIST

CHAPTER 1
EXPLORING A WORLD OF OPPORTUNITIES

People like you who choose dentistry as a career open up a world of opportunities that will lead to success and satisfaction for the rest of your lives. This is because:

- dentistry is a dynamic health profession;
- dentists are financially successful health professionals and highly respected members of their communities; and
- the demand for dental care will continue to be strong in the future, ensuring the stability and security of the profession.

The opportunities that exist for dentists now and in the future make oral health one of the most exciting, challenging, and rewarding professions. Individuals who choose to pursue dental careers are motivated, scientifically curious, intelligent, ambitious, and socially conscious health professionals. They are men and women from diverse backgrounds and cultures, all of whom want to do work that makes a difference.

This chapter provides an overview of the field of dentistry and its many facets. If you are exploring career alternatives and want to know more about dentistry, this information will be useful for you. And if you have already decided to become a dentist, this information will help you summarize the range of specialties and practice options.

The first section, **An Introduction to Dentistry**, briefly explains what dentistry is and what dentists do; **Opportunities in Dentistry** shows that there is a growing demand for dentists; **Rewards of Practicing Dentistry** describes the professional and personal satisfactions of being a dentist; and, finally, **Career Options** surveys the various fields and practice options in dentistry.

AN INTRODUCTION TO DENTISTRY

Dentistry is the branch of the healing arts and sciences devoted to maintaining the health of the teeth, gums, and other hard and soft tissues of the oral cavity and adjacent structures. A dentist is a scientist and clinician dedicated to the highest standards of health through prevention, diagnosis, and treatment of oral diseases and conditions.

The notion of dentists as those who merely "fill teeth" is completely out of date. Today, dentists are highly sophisticated health professionals who provide a wide range of care that contributes enormously to the quality of their patients' day-to-day lives by preventing tooth decay, periodontal disease, malocclusion, and oral-facial anomalies. These and other oral disorders can cause significant pain, improper chewing or digestion, dry mouth, abnormal speech, and altered facial appearance. Dentists are also instrumental in early detection of oral cancer and systemic conditions of the body that manifest themselves in the mouth, and they are at the forefront of a range of new developments in cosmetic and aesthetic practices.

Furthermore, the dental profession includes not only those who provide direct patient care, but those who teach, conduct research, and work in public and international health.

All of these individuals are vital links in the health care delivery system, necessary to promote social and economic change as well as individual well-being. Dentists understand the importance of and have made contributions to serving both disadvantaged populations and populations with limited access to dental care. It is not surprising, then, that the dental profession is very involved in influencing current health care reform efforts to ensure that the importance of oral health is understood and that oral health care is available to everyone.

Faculty members in schools of dental medicine play an especially critical role because they influence an entire field of study and contribute to shaping the profession in the United States and around the world. Dental school faculty are responsible for bringing new discoveries into the classroom; they stimulate students' intellect and help determine the future of oral health care through dental medicine.

OPPORTUNITIES IN DENTISTRY

The American Dental Association (ADA) reports that as of 2003, there were more than 173,000 professionally active dentists in the United States. On average, that is one dentist for every 1,698 people. Current dental workforce projections indicate a decreasing number of dentists. With continuing population growth and the upcoming retirement of a large group of dentists educated during the 1960s and 70s, the need for new dentists will escalate over the next decades.

It is also important to note that dentists tend to be unevenly distributed across the nation. Rural and inner-city communities are often seriously underserved. Consequently, practicing dentist-to-population ratios are significantly different from state to state and range from one dentist for every 1,200 people to one for every 2,500 or more. These data clearly demonstrate the importance of maintaining an adequate supply of dentists in the years ahead, accompanied by more efficient practice methods, better use of allied personnel, and improved prevention programs that will enable future dentists to extend professional care to more patients.

Opportunities for all individuals interested in becoming dentists are growing because of the intense national need to improve access to general health and oral care and the continuously increasing demand for dental services. Although at this point women and minorities remain underrepresented in dentistry, the profession is strongly committed to increasing its diversity. Consequently, in response to the clear need for dentists to serve all citizens, dental schools are strengthening their efforts to recruit and retain all highly qualified students, including intensively recruiting women and underrepresented minorities.

REWARDS OF PRACTICING DENTISTRY

The rewards of being a dentist are many, starting with the personal satisfaction dentists obtain from their daily professional accomplishments. Highly regarded by the community for their contributions to the well-being of citizens, dentists are often called upon to provide community consultation and services.

In addition, dentists are well compensated. The average income for a dentist is in the upper five percent of family incomes in the United States. Though incomes vary across the country and depend on the type of practice, the ADA reports that in 2003 the average net income of solo, full-time, private general practitioners was $198,100; it was $287,190 for dental specialists. The net hourly income of dentists now exceeds that of family physicians, general internists, and pediatricians.

The public's need and respect for dentists continue to grow with the increasing popular recognition of the importance of health in general and oral health in particular. Approximately 56 percent of the U.S. population is now covered by dental insurance plans, making it easier for many to pay for dental care. Increases in preventive dental care, geriatric

With continuing population growth and the upcoming retirement of a large group of dentists educated during the 1960s and 70s, the need for new dentists is expected to escalate over the next decades.

CHAPTER 1 **EXPLORING A WORLD OF OPPORTUNITIES**

dental care, and cosmetic treatments also have contributed to growth in the demand for dental care that is expected to continue.

CAREER OPTIONS

A career in dentistry has two key components: what the dentist does and how he or she does it. The "what" refers to the specific field of dentistry in which he or she practices; the "how" refers to the type of practice itself. These components offer many options for fulfilling one's professional and personal goals. If you choose to become a dentist, making decisions about these components will allow you to develop a career that suits your professional interests and fits your choice of lifestyle. The following overviews of clinical fields and professional and research opportunities should help you decide.

■ Clinical Fields

There are many clinical fields in dentistry. While most dentists in private practice (80 percent) are general practitioners, others choose to specialize in one particular field. Following is a brief description of the procedures dentists perform in each field, whether education beyond dental school (that is, postdoctoral or specialty education) is required, the length of programs, and the current number of postdoctoral programs and first-year students in those programs nationwide.

1. General Dentistry

General dentists use their oral diagnostic, preventive, surgical, and rehabilitative skills to restore damaged or missing tooth structure and treat diseases of the bone and soft tissue in the mouth and adjacent structures. They also provide patients with programs of preventive oral health care. Currently, there are 56 dental schools in the United States, including one in Puerto Rico. These schools enroll approximately 5,081 students in their first-year classes. Postdoctoral education is not required to practice as a general dentist. However, general practice residencies (GPR) and advanced education in general dentistry (AEGD) are available and can expand the general dentist's career options and scope of practice. The length of these general dentistry postdoctoral programs varies, but most are 12 months long. In the United States, there are 191 GPR programs with 894 first-year students and 94 AEGD programs with 558 first-year students.

2. Dental Public Health

Individuals who enter the dental public health field are involved in developing policies and programs, such as health care reform, that affect the community at large. Advanced dental education is required. The types of programs available vary widely from certificate programs to master's (M.P.H.) and doctoral (D.P.H.) programs. The length of programs varies, but most are between 12 and 24 months long. There are 13 programs and 21 first-year students in the United States.

3. Endodontics

Endodontists diagnose and treat diseases and injuries that are specific to the dental nerves and pulp (the matter inside the tooth) and tissues that affect the vitality of the teeth. Advanced dental education is required. Some programs offer certificates; others are degree programs at the master's (M.S.D.) level. Students interested in academic dentistry generally prefer degree

---

Why consider a dental career?

Not only are dentists part of a dynamic, stimulating field that offers a variety of professional opportunities, but

- dentistry is not generally subject to the effects of managed care and reductions in federal funding that have affected other health care professions;
- net average incomes for dentists in private practice have increased by over 96 percent since 1990; the net hourly income of dentists now exceeds that of family physicians, general internists, and pediatricians;
- dentists are generally able to enter practice directly upon completion of the four years of dental school;
- the lifestyle of a private practice dentist is typically predictable and self-determined;
- dentists enjoy unusual loyalty among their patients;
- the entire dental profession is at the forefront of important new research substantiating the relationship between oral health and systemic health; and
- while most graduates of dental schools eventually choose to set up private practices, the profession offers a wide range of clinical, research, and academic opportunities to both new graduates and dentists at later stages of their careers.

programs. The length of programs varies, but most are 24 to 36 months long. There are 52 programs and 202 first-year students in the United States.

4. Oral and Maxillofacial Pathology

Oral pathologists are dental scientists who study and research the causes, processes, and effects of diseases with oral manifestations. These diseases may be confined to the mouth and oral cavity, or they may affect other parts of the body. Most oral pathologists do not treat patients directly. However, they provide critical diagnostic and consultative biopsy services to dentists and physicians in the treatment of their patients. Advanced dental education is required. Some programs offer certificates; others are degree programs at the master's (M.S.D.) or doctoral (Ph.D.) level. Students interested in academic dentistry generally prefer degree programs. The length of programs varies, but most are 36 months long. There are 14 programs and 14 first-year students in the United States.

5. Oral and Maxillofacial Radiology

Oral radiologists have advanced education and experience in radiation physics, biology, safety, and hygiene related to the taking and interpretation of conventional, digital, CT, MRI, and allied imaging modalities of oral-facial structures and disease. Programs are of 24 to 36 months in length, depending on the certificate or degree offered. This recently designated specialty currently has five programs with 10 first-year students in the United States.

6. Oral and Maxillofacial Surgery

This specialty requires practitioners to provide a broad range of diagnostic services and treatments for diseases, injuries, and defects of the neck, head, jaw, and associated structures. Advanced dental education is required. Programs vary in length from four to

---

STUDENT PROFILE

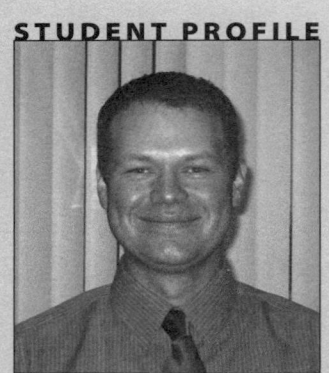

BILL DAHLKE
UNIVERSITY OF NEVADA, LAS VEGAS

Why dentistry?
Dentistry was a conscious choice for me, although it's not often presented as a career choice when you excel in math and sciences. I was a biochemistry major at the University of Nevada, Reno, and I sort of felt like I was shunted toward medicine. For a couple years after graduation, I did research at the medical school there, and then my wife and I moved to Las Vegas and I managed a chemistry stockroom for the state of Nevada. I saw what the lifestyle of my friends who were medical students was like, and I decided it was time to look at other health care fields.

I shadowed my family dentist, and I realized dentistry was the greatest profession. I even pulled the application that I had submitted to medical school before I started the dental school application process. It was great for my family that the dental school had just opened in Las Vegas and I was able to stay in state. I graduated in May 2006.

What are you doing now?
When I was starting dental school, I thought for sure I would go into private practice. But I'd always had some interest in education, and during my fourth year, there was a vertical mentorship program where I worked with second- and third-years in clinic, explaining things to them. I really enjoyed that, so I decided to look into the option of going into dental education. I picked the brains of a lot of the faculty, and I realized that teaching and faculty practice would be the best of both worlds. Now I'm an Assistant Professor of Clinical Sciences at UNLV, and I work with the dentists of the future.

On Mondays, I work in our outreach clinic with Medicaid patients, which is great since I'm still developing some of my own skills. My job is the perfect mix.

Where do you see yourself in five years?
I think about that all the time. I'll be pursuing further education, but I don't know whether it will be in a dental specialty or another field. I'd like to eventually go into dental education administration, and there are some degrees that would prepare me for that, maybe a master's in public administration, a master's in education, or a master's in business administration. If it is specialty training that I pursue, oral and maxillofacial surgery is the one area that I have always found the most challenging and fascinating, and it would cedrtainly be what I choose.

Advice to applicants and first-year students
If you're thinking about going into dentistry … do it! It's a wonderful field with a lot of options in research and education that you can look into. You don't have to be in private practice, doing crowns and bridges all day, and you can still have lots of patient interaction. That's something I love. When I'm supervising six or seven students in clinic, I interact with all of their patients. It takes a lot of trust for a patient to allow you to provide oral health care, and you develop very special relationships. I hope anyone considering dentistry is drawn to this part of the profession.

What do you do for balance in your life?
I spend a lot of time with my family. My children are so young that I don't want to miss anything. We had our first child during dental school. UNLV has many married students, and there were about 30 children among my classmates when we started and about 60 by the time we finished. We had some adult oriented events, and some family oriented ones, like picnics on Saturday, and of course the weather in Las Vegas is always great for things like that.

That's a good example of how, if you're organized and efficient, you can still have quite a bit of time during dental school for a normal life. The training is rigorous, but the material is not that difficult. After all, people graduate from dental school every year! It's the volume and managing it all that can be tough. Just focus in on how you learn best and enjoy the experience – the four years go by quickly.

What is the last book you read?
I haven't read for pleasure much since my second son was born, which was only a few months ago! But at a conference I read *Fingerprints of the Gods* by Graham Hancock, which is an alternative history that looks at whether Earth's civilizations are older than we think.

Are you married/partnered/single? Any children?
I'm married, and my wife is from the Las Vegas area originally. We have two sons, three years and four months.

six years; some programs offer certificates and others include the awarding of an M.D. degree within the residency program. There are 107 programs and 214 first-year students in the United States.

7. Orthodontics and Dentofacial Orthopedics
Orthodontists treat problems related to irregular dental development, missing teeth, and other abnormalities. Beyond "straightening teeth," orthodontists establish normal functioning and appearance for their patients. Advanced dental education is required. Some programs offer certificates; others are degree programs at the master's (M.S.D.) level. Students interested in academic dentistry generally prefer degree programs. The length of programs varies, but most are 24 to 36 months long. There are 60 programs and 322 first-year students in the United States.

8. Pediatric Dentistry
Pediatric dentists specialize in treating children from birth to adolescence. They also treat disabled patients beyond the age of adolescence. Postdoctoral education is required. Some programs offer certificates; others are degree programs at the master's (M.S.D.) or doctoral (Ph.D.) level. Students interested in academic dentistry generally prefer degree programs. The length of programs varies, but most are 24 to 36 months long. There are 65 programs and 272 first-year students in the United States.

9. Periodontics
Periodontists diagnose and treat diseases of the gingival tissue and bone supporting the teeth. Gingival tissue includes the gum, the oral mucous membranes, and other tissue that surrounds and supports the teeth. Advanced dental education is required. Some programs offer certificates; others are degree programs at the master's (M.S.D.) or doctoral (Ph.D.) level. Students interested in academic dentistry generally prefer degree programs. The length of programs varies, but most are 36 months long. There are 53 programs and 157 first-year students in the United States.

10. Prosthodontics
Prosthodontists replace missing natural teeth with fixed or removable appliances, such as dentures, bridges, and implants. Advanced dental education is required. Some programs offer certificates; others are degree programs at the master's (M.S.D.) level. Students interested in academic dentistry generally prefer degree programs. The length of programs varies, with training lasting between 12 and 36 months. There are 59 programs and 155 first-year students in the United States.

As a potential dental student, you are not ready at this time to apply for a position in an advanced dental education program. However, you should know that ADEA's Postdoctoral Application Support Service (PASS) simplifies the process of applying to many postdoctoral programs, such as general practice residencies, oral and maxillofacial surgery, and pediatric dentistry. You will learn more about PASS once you are in dental school and begin to consider dental career options that require additional education and training.

■ Practice Options and Other Professional Opportunities
Dentistry offers an array of professional opportunities from which individuals can choose to best suit their interests and lifestyle goals. These opportunities include the following:

Self-Employed in Private Practice
Traditionally, most dentists engage in private practice either by themselves in solo practice or in partnership with other dentists. Ninety percent of private practice dentists own their own practices, either individually or in partnership with other dentists. Although many recent dental school graduates begin their careers in salaried/associate positions in private practice, most choose to move to practice ownership within several years. Most practitioners provide care on a fee for service basis, and/or participate in preferred provider plans. Fewer than 15% of dentists participate in dental health maintenance organizations.

Practice as a Salaried Employee or Associate

Dentists who are not self-employed may work as salaried employees/associates for dentists who are in private practice. Other salaried situations include working for a corporation that provides dental care. Additional salaried opportunities are in managed health care organizations, such as health maintenance organizations (HMOs).

Academic Dentistry and Dental Education

Once you are in dental school you will see firsthand some of the opportunities that are open to dentists who choose a career in dental education and academic dentistry. Becoming a faculty member allows a dental professional the chance to pass knowledge on to students and mold the future of the profession. Teaching, administration, research, clinical practice, and community service—and being a part of a stimulating university environment—are important to dental educators. Many dental school faculty members combine their love for teaching and research with private practice. ADEA has excellent information on careers in academic dentistry at https://www2.adea.org/adcn.

Dental Research

Dentists trained as researchers are scientists who contribute significantly to improving health care nationally and internationally. Many researchers are faculty members at universities; others work in federal facilities such as the National Institute of Dental and Craniofacial Research (NIDCR) and National Institutes of Health (NIH) or in private industry. In addition, some dental students and practicing dentists, at various points in their careers, may decide that they would benefit from participation in a research experience. For those individuals, postdoctoral fellowships and research opportunities are available in a variety of areas and are sponsored by public and private organizations. Support is given to individuals who are still dental students as well as those who have graduated from dental school. For more information, contact the American Association for Dental Research (AADR), 1619 Duke St., Alexandria, VA 22314-3406; 703-548-0066; www.dentalresearch.org.

Service in the Federal Government

Dentists in the federal government may serve in varied capacities. Research has been described briefly above. In addition, the military enlists dentists to serve the oral health needs of military personnel and their families. The U.S. Public Health Service hires dentists to serve disadvantaged populations that do not have adequate access to proper dental care, and the Indian Heath Service hires dentists to provide oral healthcare for American Indians and Alaskan Natives.

Public Health Care Policy

Dentists who become experts in public policy may work at universities, or they may be employed in government agencies such as the U.S. Department of Health and Human Services or in a state's department of health. Other dentists who are experts in public policy work with associations, such as the ADA or ADEA, or are employed by state and national elected officials to help them develop laws dealing with health care issues.

International Health Care

Dentists engaged in international health care provide services to developing populations abroad. They may work for agencies such as the World Health Organization (WHO).

Final Thoughts

You should note that some of these options overlap. Dentists who work in private practice, for instance, are often self-employed, but some are salaried employees in group practices. Dental researchers, on the other hand, often work in university settings, but may be employed by the federal government or private industry.

This list of practice options is not exhaustive because the horizons of dentistry are expanding every year, especially at this dynamic time in health care. New areas in dental service are being created with opportunities for dental health care providers in practice, industry, government, dental societies, national scientific organizations, and educational institutions.

For additional sources of information on all of these opportunities, see chapter 5 of this guide.

CHAPTER 2
APPLYING TO DENTAL SCHOOL

As you prepare to apply to dental school, you will find it helpful to become acquainted with the usual educational curriculum, typical admission requirements, and the application process. This chapter offers essential information about these topics, organized into four sections: **The Dental School Program** provides an overview of the basic educational curriculum at most schools, recognizing that each dental school has its own mission and distinguishing features; **Qualifying for Dental School** reviews the typical numbers of students involved in applying to and attending dental schools and summarizes general admission requirements; **The Application Process** describes the steps in the application process; and **Special Admissions Topics** addresses the special topics of advanced standing and transferring, combined degree programs, and admissions for international students.

THE DENTAL SCHOOL PROGRAM

A common goal of all dental school programs is to produce graduates who are:

- competently educated in the basic biological and clinical sciences;
- capable of providing quality dental care to all segments of the population; and
- committed to high moral and professional standards in their service to the public.

The traditional dental school program requires four academic years of study, often organized as follows. However, since there is wide variation in the focus and organization of the curricula of dental schools, the schools' descriptions in Part II of this guide show the specifics of courses of study that won't be covered here.

■ Years One and Two

Students generally spend the major part of the first two years studying the biological sciences to learn about the structure and function of the human body and its diseases. Students also receive instruction about dentally oriented biological sciences such as oral anatomy, oral pathology, and oral histology and learn about providing health care to diverse populations. At this time, students learn the basic principles of oral diagnosis and treatment and begin mastery of dental treatment procedures through practice on models of the mouth and teeth. In many programs, students begin interacting with patients and provide basic oral heath care.

■ Years Three and Four

The focus of the final two years of dental school generally concentrates on clinical study. Clinical training, which is broad in scope, is designed to provide competence in the prevention, diagnosis, and treatment of oral diseases and disorders. Students apply basic principles and techniques involved in oral diagnosis, treatment planning, restorative dentistry, periodontics, oral surgery, orthodontics, pediatric dentistry, prosthodontics, endodontics, and other types of treatment through direct patient care. They learn to attend to chronically ill, disabled, special care, and geriatric patients and children. In addition, dental schools provide instruction in practice management and in working effectively with allied dental personnel to provide dental care.

During these two years, students may rotate through various clinics of the dental school to treat patients under the supervision of clinical instructors. They often have an opportunity to acquire additional clinical experience in hospitals and other off-campus, community settings. These experiences give students an appreciation for the team approach to health care delivery through their association with other health professionals and health professions students.

As dental school curricula are designed to meet the anticipated needs of the public, every school continues to modify its curriculum to achieve a better correlation between the basic and clinical sciences. There is, in clinical training, increased emphasis on providing comprehensive patient care—a method of training that permits a student to meet all the patient's needs within the student's existing levels of competence. Widespread efforts also are being made to integrate new subject matter into the curriculum and to allow students free time for elective study, participation in research, and community service.

The D.M.D. and the D.D.S. are equivalent degrees that are awarded to dental students upon completion of the same types of programs.

QUALIFYING FOR DENTAL SCHOOL

At least 56 U.S. and ten Canadian dental schools will be accepting applications to the first year of their Doctor of Dental Medicine (D.M.D.) or Doctor of Dental Surgery (D.D.S.) programs in 2008-09. The D.M.D. and the D.D.S. are equivalent degrees that are awarded to dental students upon completion of the same types of programs.

■ Numbers of Applicants and Enrollees

More than 18,300 students participated in D.M.D. and D.D.S. programs in the United States in 2004-05; of those, 4,612 were enrolled as first-year students. About 47 percent of the 9,433 individuals who applied for admission were enrolled. Women comprised 44 percent of the applicants and 42 percent of the enrollees in 2004. Black/African Americans, Hispanic/Latinos, and Native Americans comprised 12.4 percent of the applicants and 11.6 percent of the enrollees in 2004. These underrepresented minority figures are expected to increase in the future. In Canada, in 2003-04, 1,802 students were enrolled in predoctoral dental school programs. Of these 444 were first-year students.

See Table 2-1 for a comparison of the number of dental school applicants to the number accepted and enrolled for the 2004-05 academic year.

■ General Admission Requirements

Dental schools consider many factors when deciding which applicants to accept into their programs. Utilizing "whole" application review, admissions committees assess biographical and academic information provided by the applicant and by the undergraduate and graduate schools the applicant attended. These committees generally also assess the applicant's results from the Dental Admission Test (DAT), grade point average (GPA), letters of recommendation, and interviews.

All U.S. dental schools require students to take the DAT (all Canadian dental schools require students to take the Canadian Dental Aptitude Test), but other admission requirements vary from school to school. Differences may exist, for example, in the areas of undergraduate courses required, interview policies, and state residency requirements. Each school's individual requirements are specified in Part II of this guide.

Most schools require a minimum of two years of undergraduate education (also called "predental education"). However,

TABLE 2-1. TOTAL U.S. DENTAL SCHOOL APPLICANTS AND FIRST-YEAR ENROLLEES, 2005-06

	Total*	Male/Female	White	African American	Hispanic/ Latino	Native American/ Alaska Native	Asian/Pacific Islander	Other	Not Reported
Applicants	10,731	5,977/4,744	6,111	666	629	76	2,377	529	343
Enrollees	4,558	2,544/1,997	2,768	286	259	28	910	153	254

*Sum of applicants and enrollees by gender and by race/ethnicity do not add to total number of applicants and enrollees because a small number did not provide this information.

Source: American Dental Education Association, Applicant Analysis for the 2005 Entering Class.

dental schools generally accept students who have three or four years of predental education, and most dental schools give preference in the admissions process to individuals who will have earned a bachelor's degree prior to the start of dental school. Of all U.S. students entering dental schools, more than 90 percent have completed four or more years of college, less than 1 percent have just the minimum two-year requirement, and about 8 percent have graduate training.

Individuals pursuing dental careers should take certain science courses. However, you do not have to be a science major to gain admission to a dental school and successfully complete the program. As shown in Table 2-2, most dental students are science majors as undergraduates, but many major in fields not related to science.

■ ADEA Admissions Guidelines

As the primary dental education association in North America, the American Dental Education Association (ADEA) has developed guidelines addressing dental school admission. Although adhering to the guidelines is voluntary, member institutions (which include all U.S. and Canadian dental schools) are encouraged to follow these guidelines as they consider and accept applicants to their schools. The guidelines are as follows:

ADEA encourages dental schools to accept students from all walks of life who, on the basis of past and predicted performance, appear qualified to become competent dental professionals.

ADEA further encourages dental schools to use, whenever possible as part of the admission process, a consistently applied assessment of an applicant's nonacademic attributes.

ADEA urges dental schools to grant final acceptance only to students who have completed at least two years of postsecondary education and the Dental Admission Test. ADEA further suggests that dental schools encourage applicants to earn their baccalaureate degrees before entering dental school.

The recommendation for at least two years of postsecondary education may be waived for students accepted at a dental school under an early selection program. Such a program is one where a formal and published agreement exists between a dental school and an undergraduate institution that a student, at some time before the completion of the student's first academic year at the undergraduate institution, is guaranteed admission to the dental school, provided that the student successfully completes the dental school's entrance requirements and normal application procedures.

ADEA recommends that dental schools notify applicants, either orally or in writing, of provisional or final acceptance on or after December 1 of the academic year prior to the academic year of matriculation.

ADEA further recommends that applicants accepted on or after December 1 be given at least 45 days to reply to the offer; for applicants who have been accepted on or after January 1, the minimum response period should be 30 days; for applicants accepted on or after February 1, the minimum waiting period can be reduced to 15 days. ADEA believes that dental schools are justified in asking for an immediate response from applicants accepted after July 15, or two weeks before the beginning of the academic year, whichever comes first.

TABLE 2-2. UNDERGRADUATE MAJORS OF DENTAL SCHOOL APPLICANTS AND ENROLLEES, 2004-05

Predental Major	Percent of Applicants	Percent of Enrollees	Percent Rate of Enrollment
Biological Sciences	50.4%	54.1%	49.9%
Chemistry/Physics	14.0%	14.1%	49.4%
Engineering	1.7%	2.3%	66.3%
Math/Computer Science	0.8%	0.8%	52.5%
Social Science	0.7%	0.8%	54.1%
Business	3.7%	4.2%	55.6%
Education	0.7%	0.7%	51.4%
Language/Humanities/Arts	2.7%	3.0%	54.1%
Predental/Premedical/Health-Related	14.8%	13.2%	43.7%
Other Major	6.5%	6.3%	47.6%
No Major/Major Not Reported	4.1%	3.3%	39.4%

Source: American Dental Education Association, Applicant Analysis Report for the 2004 Entering Class.

Finally, ADEA recommends that dental schools encourage a close working relationship between their admissions and financial aid staff in order to counsel dental students early and effectively on their financial obligations.

THE APPLICATION PROCESS

The dental school application process involves a number of procedures, but is easily followed once you learn what is needed. This section explains how the application process works in general, recognizing that specific details may vary somewhat from school to school. Once you have a basic framework, however, you will find it easier to adapt to these variations.

There are three main steps in the application process:

- take the Dental Admission Test (or, for Canadian schools, the Canadian Dental Aptitude Test);
- in the vast majority of cases, submit a centralized application form to ADEA's Associated American Dental Schools Application Service (AADSAS) (as of January 1, 2007, four of the 56 U.S. dental schools do not participate in AADSAS); and
- acquire and submit supplemental materials such as letters of evaluation, academic transcripts, and any required institution-specific applications.

Following is a brief description of each step and whom you should contact for more information. This section concludes with advice on how to effectively manage the timing of the application process. Always remember that the application process for an individual school may vary from this general information; see Part II of this guide for specific application requirements by school.

Not sure what to write about in your essay? Consider these ideas.

The AADSAS application requires a personal essay on why you wish to pursue a dental education. Where do you start?

Put yourself in the shoes of the admissions committees that read application essays. They are looking for individuals who are motivated, academically prepared, articulate, socially conscious, and knowledgeable about the profession. What can you tell admissions committees about yourself that will make you stand out?

Here are some possible topics for your essay:

- How did you become interested in studying dentistry? Be honest! If you knew you wanted to be a dentist from the age of six, that's fine, but if you didn't, that's all right too. Explain how you discovered dentistry as a career possibility and what you have done to research the career. Admissions committees are looking for how well thought-out your career plans are.
- What have you done to demonstrate your interest in dentistry? Have you observed or worked in dental offices? Have you talked to practicing dentists? How good of an understanding do you have of general dental practice? How do you envision yourself utilizing your dental degree?
- What have you done to demonstrate your commitment to helping others?
- Do you have any special talents or leadership skills that could be transferable to the practice of dentistry?
- Have you benefited from any special experiences such as participating in research, internships, etc.?
- Did you have to work to pay for your education? How has that made you a stronger applicant?
- Have you had to overcome hardships or obstacles to get where you are today? How has this influenced your motivation for advanced education?

These tips are provided by Dr. Anne Wells, ADEA Associate Executive Director for Application Services and former Associate Dean for Admissions, University of Louisville School of Dentistry.

■ Take the DAT

All U.S. dental schools require applicants to take the Dental Admission Test (DAT). The DAT is designed to measure general academic ability, comprehension of scientific information, and perceptual ability. This half-day, multiple-choice exam is conducted by the American Dental Association (ADA) and is administered on computer at Prometric Testing Centers in various sites around the country on almost any day of the year.

Successful participation in the Dental Admission Testing Program requires completion of at least one year of collegiate education, which should include courses in biology and general and organic chemistry. Advanced level biology and physics are not required. Most applicants complete two or more years of college before taking the exam. ADEA further suggests that, although there is no formal preparation for the test, students who have not taken a basic science course in over two years should review for the DAT.

The ADA suggests that applicants take the DAT well in advance of their intended dental school enrollment and at least one

Submitting your ADEA AADSAS application: words of advice

Before you begin the application process:

- Meet with your health professions advisor to discuss the application process including the timing of application submission and the DAT, services that may be provided by your advisor such as a Pre-Dental Committee Report or other application assistance, and potential dental schools to which you plan to apply.

- Consider the timing of the Dental Admissions Test (DAT). You may submit an AADSAS application before taking the DAT, but you should know that many schools consider you for admission only after they have received your DAT scores. However, you should also be aware that delaying the submission of an AADSAS application prior to taking the DAT can result in a late application and can reduce your chances of being accepted for admission.

- Collect copies of all transcripts and have them at hand for your reference.

- Begin to line up your evaluations/recommendations early. Be sure to plan around school vacations, when faculty advisors may not be available.

- AADSAS staff strongly recommends that you submit your AADSAS application well in advance of the application deadlines of the schools to which you are applying. AADSAS processing, including transcript verification, can take four to eight weeks.

- Remember that the AADSAS application becomes available in mid May.

While completing the application:

- When you set up your account for processing, you will identify a user name and password. Keep these in a safe yet accessible place.

- Be sure to read all application instructions before starting to fill out the application.

- Any time after you set up your account, you can go back into the application (using your user name and password) to add or change information up until the time you submit it for processing.

- Print the Transcript Matching Form from your application. Request that an official transcript from **each** college/university you have attended (even if coursework transferred and is posted to another later transcript) be sent to AADSAS. The Transcript Matching Form must be attached by each college's registrar to the official transcript and mailed by the registrar to AADSAS. AADSAS applications are not processed until all official transcripts are received.

- Remember that AADSAS accepts only official transcripts sent directly from the registrar. AADSAS does not accept student-issued transcripts.

After submitting the application:

- Be sure to check with the schools to which you are applying (and their individual entries in this guide) to find out what supplemental materials or fees are required. These must be submitted directly to the school, not to AADSAS.

- Log on to your AADSAS application to monitor the status of your application while it is being processed at AADSAS and after it has been sent to the dental schools.

- Update any changes of address or other contact information in your application at any time in the application process, even after your application has been sent to your designated schools.

- Remember that AADSAS does not retain application information from year to year. Individuals re-applying for admission to dental school must complete a new application each year, including providing new transcripts and letters of evaluation.

For further information, visit the ADEA website at www.adea.org, and select the AADSAS link.

These recommendations were provided by Dr. Anne Wells, Ms. Cynthia Gunn, and Ms. Chonté James of ADEA AADSAS.

---

year prior to when they hope to enter dental school. See Tables 3.2 and 3.3 in this guide for an overview of individual schools' requirements regarding the DAT and the mean score of their first-time enrollees. The individual school listings in this guide also address their requirements regarding timing and scores on the DAT. You should also note that, effective January 2007, examinees who have attended three or more DAT exams must apply for special permission to take the test again. For details, see the DAT section of the ADA website.

The exam consists of multiple-choice test items presented in the English language and requires four hours and 15 minutes for administration. The four separate parts of the exam cover:

- the natural sciences (biology, general chemistry, and organic chemistry);
- perceptual ability (two- and three-dimensional problem-solving);
- reading comprehension (dental and basic sciences); and
- quantitative reasoning (mathematical problems in algebra, numerical calculations, conversions, etc.).

Most dental schools view the DAT as one of many factors in evaluating candidates for admission. As a result, schools vary in their emphasis on the different parts of the test.

A number of procedures are used to ensure that the DAT is fair to all candidates, regardless of racial, ethnic, gender, or regional background. Further, as part of the scoring process, test question data are analyzed for fairness, and any questions that may appear differentially familiar are evaluated and, if appropriate, modified.

The DAT Candidate's Guide, the DAT Online Tutorial, and the DAT Application and Preparation Materials are available in the DAT section of the ADA website. An online tutorial is also available, as well as a link to the DAT Online Application.

The DAT program has no data on the content or efficacy of test preparation courses designed to prepare candidates to take the DAT. The Department of Testing Services urges individuals considering participating in test preparation courses to review carefully the course materials to ensure that they reflect the current content of the DAT.

Candidates applying to take the DAT must submit to the DAT testing program application information from the DAT section of the ADA website. The fee is $170. After the application and fee payment are processed, the ADA notifies the Prometric Candidate Contact Center that the candidate is eligible for DAT testing. At the same time, the candidate will receive a letter from the ADA including instructions on how to register with the Prometric Candidate Contact Center to arrange the day, time, and place to take the DAT at a Prometric Testing Center. A current listing of testing centers is at www.2test.com. The candidate is eligible to take the test for a 12-month period. If the candidate does not call, register, and take the exam during this period, he or she will have to submit another application and fee in order to take the exam later. Candidates may apply and

TABLE 2-3. DENTAL SCHOOLS PARTICIPATING IN ADEA AADSAS (as of January 1, 2007)

State	Schools
Alabama	University of Alabama
Arizona	Arizona School of Dentistry & Oral Health
California	Loma Linda University University of California, Los Angeles University of California, San Francisco University of the Pacific University of Southern California
Colorado	University of Colorado
Connecticut	University of Connecticut
District of Columbia	Howard University
Florida	University of Florida Nova Southeastern University
Illinois	University of Illinois at Chicago Southern Illinois University
Indiana	Indiana University
Iowa	University of Iowa
Kentucky	University of Kentucky University of Louisville
Maryland	University of Maryland, Baltimore
Massachusetts	Boston University Harvard School of Dental Medicine Tufts University
Michigan	University of Detroit Mercy University of Michigan
Minnesota	University of Minnesota
Missouri	University of Missouri-Kansas City
Nebraska	Creighton University University of Nebraska
Nevada	University of Nevada, Las Vegas
New Jersey	University of Medicine and Dentistry of New Jersey
New York	Columbia University New York University State University of New York at Buffalo State University of New York at Stony Brook
North Carolina	University of North Carolina
Ohio	Case School of Dental Medicine The Ohio State University
Oklahoma	University of Oklahoma
Oregon	Oregon Health & Science University
Pennsylvania	University of Pennsylvania University of Pittsburgh Temple University
South Carolina	Medical University of South Carolina
Tennessee	Meharry Medical College
Texas	Baylor College of Dentistry University of Texas Health Science Center-Houston University of Texas Health Science Center at San Antonio
Virginia	Virginia Commonwealth University
Washington	University of Washington
West Virginia	West Virginia University
Wisconsin	Marquette University
Puerto Rico	University of Puerto Rico
Nova Scotia	Dalhousie University

STUDENT PROFILE

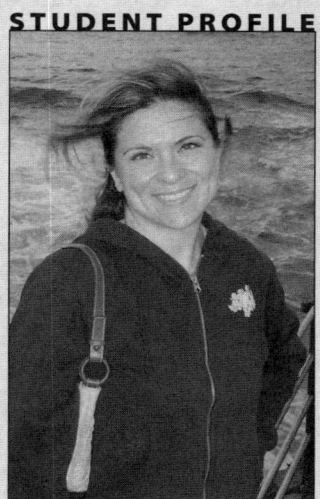

GINA BETITA
UNIVERSITY OF CALIFORNIA, SAN FRANCISCO

Why dentistry?

I've wanted to become a health professional as long as I could remember. The turning point toward dentistry came when a dentist spoke to my class in high school. He told an inspirational story about a woman who never smiled before he worked on her teeth. When he finished her treatment, she looked in the mirror and was so overcome with emotion that she cried because she was finally happy with her physical appearance. That really motivated me for a career in dentistry, in which I could improve people's lives by improving their smile. Additionally, I like the fact that dentistry is such a multi-disciplinary health profession in which you can own your own business, be a doctor, a psychologist, a teacher, a problem-solver, a researcher for new products and techniques, an artist, and do all of this between 9 and 5, four days a week if you wish!

Now that I'm in dental school, I've been involved in a number of dental community outreach projects. UCSF has a high school outreach program that I helped establish whereby dental students visit high schools in underserved counties as far as seven hours away. We teach the students about proper oral hygiene and promote opportunities that exist within the dental field. We also bring these students back to UCSF at the end of the year for an all day hands-on conference with workshops and motivational speakers. Some of the teenagers that we teach have never been to a dentist, so it's very impactful to see the difference we can make in their lives as dental health professionals. I think that dental students have a unique opportunity to reach out and I'm active in ADEA and other organizations so I can help spread this message nationwide.

What are you doing now?

I'm a fourth-year student, and I love being fully involved in clinic. Everything we learned in the first three years is coming together, and we're finally using it all. In your third year, clinic can make you nervous, but by the fourth year you feel comfortable there. My classmates and I really have fun in clinic and enjoy seeing patients.

Where do you see yourself in five years?

In fourth year, everything is dynamic! You don't know exactly where you're going to end up. I'm in the U.S. Air Force Reserves, and I have a Health Professions Scholarship. I'd like to do an AEGD residency in the Air Force after graduation, and then I will have four years to serve back. After that I'd like to go back to school to earn an M.P.H. in oral epidemiology. Dental public health is gaining momentum; so many students are becoming interested in the field and I'm really excited about this change.

I'm hoping that my M.P.H. degree will help me establish a career in dental public policy. Eventually, I see myself working both in private practice and public health. That's more like a 10-year plan. I'd like to work on a large scale — improving dental health care benefits and reaching the underserved — but also working on an individual basis with patients. I don't think I can get away from either one.

Advice to applicants and first-year students

My biology curriculum at UC Irvine required anatomy and histology, and they were incredibly helpful. Pathology and pharmacology classes would also be useful.

You should also get exposure in dentistry. I had a part-time job working for an orthodontist, but volunteer experience is important too. I was involved in Flying Samaritans in Baja California, Mexico. We spent one weekend a month helping to provide dental and medical services at a free clinic. I taught kids about oral health and assisted a dentist, mostly with extractions to take patients out of pain.

Research experience is important, too. Schools like to see that you have the skills to comprehend the present literature that exists within the health fields. It broadens your educational experience and exposes you to investigative techniques that you should become familiar with as a health professional.

Be sure to visit the dental school campuses and feel them out, to find out where you feel comfortable. Explore the summer programs they offer and talk to the faculty and students. If you get an opportunity to work with a faculty researcher, he or she can help you form a network of connections to other faculty and could write you a supportive letter of recommendation to apply.

The first set of finals in dental school was the most difficult academic experience I'd ever had. It was really the support from my classmates that got me through it. As undergrads, you don't have all the same classes together, but in dental school you see all of your classmates every day. It helps to know you're all in the same boat. Dental school is challenging at first, but enjoyable after that.

What do you do for balance in your life?

I live in a beautiful city! It's not difficult to take a break here. The 1000+ acre Golden Gate Park is right next door, and on the weekends my friends and I go out and enjoy the culture, museums, restaurants, and clubs of the city. I am definitely taking advantage of living in San Francisco.

What is the last book you read?

I know you're thinking "Get away from dentistry!" but my mom gave me *Chicken Soup for the Dental Soul*. It's full of heartwarming stories.

Are you married/partnered/single? Any children?

I'm single right now. I'd like to have a family by that 10-year mark, and that seems realistic because dentistry is a lot more flexible than many health professions. I don't have to work long shifts or overnight, and when I'm in practice I can choose my own hours or work part time. I like the fact that you can have a family and enjoy such a great career.

---

retake the test up to three times, but they must submit a new application and fee for each re-examination, and the re-examination must be at least 90 days after the previous exam. Individuals with disabilities or special needs may request special arrangements for taking the DAT. For details, visit the Special Testing Arrangements section of the Dental Admissions Testing page of the ADA website.

The Canadian Dental Association and the Association of Canadian Faculties of Dentistry have developed the Dental Aptitude Test for applicants to Canadian dental schools. All Canadian dental schools require the test. For more information, contact the Canadian Dental Association (L'Association Dentaire Canadienne), 100 Bronson Avenue, Suite 204, Ottawa, Ontario, Canada K1R 6G8; 613-237-6505; www.acfd.ca.

■ Submitting an AADSAS Application

ADEA's AADSAS (pronounced "add-sass," the acronym for the Associated American Dental Schools Application Service) is a centralized application service sponsored and administered by the American Dental Education Association (ADEA). At least 52 of the 56 U.S. dental schools including Puerto Rico participate in AADSAS. One Canadian school also participates in AADSAS.

The Application

The ADEA AADSAS application is available online at www.adea.org/aadsas, May 15 – February 1 each year.

The online AADSAS application requires you to submit information, including:

- Biographical information
- Colleges/universities attended
- Coursework completed and planned prior to enrollment in dental school
- DAT scores, if available
- Personal statement (essay)—a one-page essay in which you present yourself and your reasons for wanting to attend dental school.
- Background information—information about your personal background, including experiences related to the dental profession; extracurricular, volunteer, and community service experiences; honors, awards, and scholarships; and work and research experiences.
- Dental school designations—where you select the dental schools that you want to receive your application.

You will also be required to submit an official transcript from each college/university you have attended to the AADSAS Verification Department.

Letters of evaluation/recommendation may also be submitted with your AADSAS application.

Submission Deadlines

Applications may be submitted beginning mid May. Each school has a specific application deadline date, which is noted in the online AADSAS Application and in the individual school entries in Part II of this guide. Your completed application, transcripts, payment, and other required documents must be received by AADSAS no later than the stated deadline of the schools to which you are applying. Since many schools have a rolling admissions process and begin to admit highly qualified applicants as early as December 1, applicants are encouraged to submit their applications early.

Application Fees

Check the AADSAS website for complete information about application fees. Payment may be by check, money order, or credit card (VISA, MasterCard, Discover, or American Express). All fees must be paid in U.S. currency drawn on a U.S. bank or the U.S. Postal Service.

AADSAS has a fee reduction program for applicants with demonstrated financial hardship. Details may be obtained on the AADSAS website.

AADSAS Schools

The schools that use AADSAS are listed by state in Table 2-3. If you are applying only to the schools that do not participate in AADSAS, you should apply directly to those schools. Individuals applying for advanced standing (i.e., graduates of non-ADA accredited dental schools) or seeking to transfer dental schools should contact the schools directly.

Please note that AADSAS serves as an information clearinghouse only. It does not influence any school's evaluation or selection of applicants, nor does ADEA recommend applicants to dental schools or vice versa.

■ Submit Any Required Supplemental Application Materials

Each school has its own policy regarding the payment of a separate application fee and the submission of additional application materials. These materials may include an institution-specific application form, documentation of dentistry job shadowing, and official academic transcripts. Part II of this guide briefly reviews each dental school's application requirements. In addition, the ADEA AADSAS application instructions include a chart that identifies the supplemental requirements for at least 52 U.S. dental schools and one Canadian dental school that are AADSAS participants.

After you have submitted all of your materials, the dental schools that wish to consider you for a place in the entering class will contact you for a visit to the campus. This visit will likely include an interview with the admissions committee, a tour of the campus and facilities, meetings with faculty and students, and other meetings and activities. When you visit a dental school, at the same time the admissions committee is evaluating you as a prospective student, you will have the opportunity to evaluate the dental school program and environment to determine if you think it would be a good fit for you and your goals.

■ Manage the Timing of the Application Process

The trick to managing the timing of the application process is summed up in two words: DON'T PROCRASTINATE! Most dental schools will fill a large percentage of their 2008 entering classes by December 2007. This means that even though schools have deadlines for completing all the application requirements that range from October 2007 to February 2008, it is not a good idea to wait until the last minute to take the DAT, submit the AADSAS application, or complete any supplemental materials requested by the schools to which you are applying.

The individual dental school information in Part II of this guide includes a timetable for each school's entering class. It is essential that you become familiar with the timetables for the schools to which you are applying and that you make plans to complete the admission application requirements on time.

SPECIAL ADMISSIONS TOPICS

For those of you interested in advanced standing and transferring, combined degree programs, and admission for international students, this section briefly addresses those areas. Part II of this guide provides some additional information on these topics for each dental school, but you should contact the dental schools you are considering for more details.

■ Advanced Standing and Transferring

Advanced standing means that a student is exempted from certain courses or is accepted as a second- or third-year student. Advanced standing is offered at the time of admission to students who have mastered some aspects of the dental school curriculum because of previous training. An individual who has a Ph.D. in one of the basic sciences, such as physiology, for example, may be exempted from taking the physiology course in dental school. Some schools may also grant advanced standing to students who have transferred from other U.S. or Canadian dental schools or who have graduated from international dental schools. In these cases, applicants may be allowed to enter as second- or third-year students.

Each dental school has its own policy on advanced standing and transferring students; see the individual school entries in Part II of this guide. But it is important to be aware that most students do not obtain advanced standing and that very few students transfer from one school to another.

■ Combined Degree Programs

Many dental schools in the United States and Canada offer combined degree programs that give students the opportunity to obtain other degrees along with their D.D.S. or

D.M.D. Degrees that may be combined with the dental degree include:

- a baccalaureate degree (B.A. or B.S.);
- a master's degree (M.A. or M.S.); or
- a doctorate (Ph.D. or M.D.).

Numerous dental schools have formal combined baccalaureate and dental degree programs. Combined degree programs expand career options especially for those interested in careers in dental education, administration, and research. They may also shorten the length of training where specific agreements have been made between the dental school and its parent institution. The undergraduate and dental school portions of some combined degree programs take place at the same university, while other combined programs are the result of arrangements made between a dental school and other undergraduate colleges. Sometimes colleges independently will grant baccalaureate degrees to students who attended as undergraduates and did not finish their undergraduate education but did successfully complete some portion of their dental training.

Many dental schools also sponsor combined graduate and dental degree programs. These programs, which usually take six to seven years to complete, are offered at the masters or doctoral level in subjects that include the basic sciences (biology, physiology, chemistry), public policy, medicine, and other areas. See Table 3-5 in chapter 3 of this guide for a list of dental schools with combined degree programs. If you are interested in more information about combined degree programs, you should contact the schools directly.

■ Admissions for International Students

The term "international student" refers to an individual who is a native of a foreign country and who plans to study in the United States or Canada on a student visa. Students who have permanent residency status in the United States are not considered international students; they have the same rights, responsibilities, and options as U.S. citizens applying for admission to dental school. Generally, international applicants are considered for admission only to the first-year class regardless of previous dental training, although some schools permit international students to apply for advanced standing. (For more information, visit the American Dental Association's website at www.ada.org, and select the links from Dental Professionals, then Licensure, then U.S. Licensure for International Dentists.)

Applicants who have completed coursework outside the United States or Canada (except through study abroad) should supply a copy of their transcripts, translated into English, plus a course-by-course evaluation of all transcripts. Application details for international applicants are contained in the ADEA AADSAS application.

Each dental school has its own policies on admission requirements for international students. However, most dental schools require international students to complete all the application materials mandated for U.S. citizens and permanent residents. In addition, international students may be asked to take the Test of English as a Foreign Language (TOEFL) or demonstrate English language proficiency. They should expect to finance the entire cost of their dental education.

CHAPTER 3
DECIDING WHERE TO APPLY

Selecting the dental schools to which you want to apply is a very personal decision. Every applicant is looking for different characteristics in an educational experience. Your individual decision depends on many factors, such as career goals, personal interests, geographical preference, and family circumstances. For this reason, dental school rankings tend to be misleading, since the education provided by U.S. and Canadian dental schools is of a high quality overall. As a more productive alternative, this chapter offers a framework to help you create your own list of dental schools tailored to your interests and needs. It covers fundamental issues that will help you decide what kind of educational experience you are looking for and begin to identify the schools most likely to offer it.

The general information in chapter 2 provided a broad introduction to the dental school program. However, variations exist across dental schools that will be important when you make your decision about where to apply. If you have a commitment to providing community-based care, for example, you will likely prefer to attend a dental school that offers a public health focus and varied opportunities for gaining experience in community clinics. Similarly, if you are interested in ultimately focusing on oral health research, you will want to look for a dental school with a strong research focus and student research opportunities. Academic dental institutions also offer a range of curriculum options. Some schools offer innovative problem-based curricula and some organize their curricula along more integrative rather than discipline-based lines, while others follow a more traditional discipline-based, classroom instruction-followed-by-clinical training structure. You should therefore consider in what type of educational environment you will feel most comfortable, along with what you think will best prepare you for the kind of career you will choose to follow.

The same approach holds true as you consider dental schools in different areas of the country. You may want to determine whether you are more comfortable in a particular geographical or physical location—a rural versus a big city setting, for example, or if you prefer to attend a school near where you grew up or one in a new area where you may want to remain after graduation. The composition of the study body also varies. Some schools have student bodies made up of individuals from all over the country (and some, even the world); some (primarily those affiliated with state universities) give preference to students from their home state; and some have partnership agreements with states that do not have dental schools, allowing students from those states to attend for the in-state tuition fee.

The key is to define your needs and preferences and then identify dental schools that correspond. To help you do that, here are some questions that can help you think through what you are looking for in a dental school:

What is the focus of the dental school's training, and does it match my interests and needs?

You might say, for example:

- I want to become a general practitioner, either in my own practice or in a group practice environment.
- I have a strong interest in scientific research regarding oral health.
- I am undecided about the type of dentistry I would like to practice, so I want to be in a school where I have a range of options from which to choose.
- My dream is to become a professor, so I'd like opportunities to prepare for an academic career while I'm in dental school.
- I want to prepare myself for eventual specialty training.
- I hope to obtain a combined degree.

What is the structure of the curriculum in terms of what is taught and when?

You might say, for example:

- I would like to start getting hands-on clinical experience as soon as possible.
- I would like the opportunity to take a wide range of electives.
- I am very interested in externships, especially the opportunity to participate in short-term service programs in other countries.
- I am devoted to helping the underserved, so I want to make sure there are plenty of opportunites for community service.
- I plan to return to my home community as a general practitioner, so I want to focus on the training I need for that.

STUDENT PROFILE

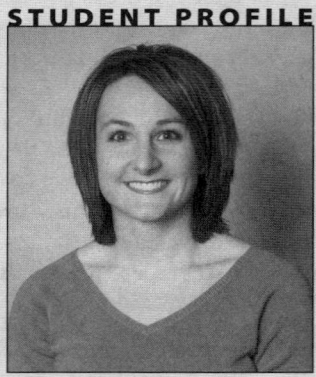

KELLI JOBMAN
UNIVERSITY OF NEBRASKA

Why dentistry?

My dad is a general practice dentist in Huron, South Dakota, and has been for 30 years. My mom is a nurse and his office manager. I wanted to go into a health profession too.

My dad's practice is a great example of how dentistry can be. He's always been there for his patients, and he often sees a toothache over his lunch hour to help a patient get out of pain. I knew I wanted to help people in the same way. When it came time to choose my field, I knew a lot about dentistry, how rewarding it is, and how the hard work can pay off.

As a woman, I also found the flexibility that dentistry offers really appealing. I liked the idea of being a good role model as a female dentist, and I thought as a woman I would bring a lot of positive energy and some fun to the dental field. It has been exciting to see the increase in females in the dental field (I don't think there were any women at all in my dad's dental school class and our class is almost 50:50!).

What are you doing now?

I'm a third year student at the University of Nebraska. Our time is split half and half between clinic and classes. I've really enjoyed the transition into taking care of patients and developing relationships with them. The best feeling is when you meet a new patient and send them off after a positive experience at the dental school.

Of course, some of the days are really long. Sometimes I don't leave until 10 p.m. Dental school may seem harder than undergrad, but it's really not—the classes just cover more information at a quicker rate and in more detail. Also, the lab work definitely shows you how to be a better clinician. I know that if I put in the time now, it'll be worth it in the end.

Where do you see yourself in five years?

It's funny, when you get to your junior year, everyone asks you, "What's the plan?" I see a lot of options, and that's part of what I like about dentistry. I could see myself in a general dentistry private practice somewhere near a good-sized city in the Midwest. I could also see myself in a pediatric residency. I have done some teaching and mentoring (together my dad and I speak to preprofessional students at South Dakota State about dentistry every year), and I would also love to balance a part-time practice with part-time teaching in a dental school. I'd like to start a family in the next five years, and I definitely want to enjoy what I'm doing and the relationships I have with my patients.

Advice to applicants and first-year students

In terms of classes to take, biochemistry, immunology, microbiology, and anatomy and physiology are all musts. It also helps to do something to work on your eye-hand coordination, like playing piano, knitting, or sewing. Also, the more time you spend shadowing or working in a dental office, the more you will learn. I recommend getting a feel for what every specialty is like, in case you might be interested in one of them. You will also find out a lot about how different practices are run from both dental and business viewpoints, and a lot about the teamwork that goes into a practice.

One of the things everybody worries about is, if I get accepted to more than one dental school, how will I decide? If you look carefully at the different programs, you will find the one that seems like the best fit for you. When I got accepted to Nebraska, they said "Welcome to our family." I knew it was the perfect match for me.

What do you do for balance in your life?

My husband and I love to travel! I also enjoy movies and spending time outdoors. I've been playing the piano since I was 5, and have always enjoyed playing whenever I have time. Also, by being involed with ADEA and ASDA events, I've been able to attend some great dental conventions. These have been a great opportunity to meet people from other dental schools. Finally, I take half an hour out of my day to get some exercise and burn some energy.

What is the last book you read?

I have a fun, girlie book in my bag: Mine Are Spectacular! by Janice Kaplan and Lynn Schnurnberger.

Are you married/partnered/single? Any children?

My husband's name is Mark and we've been married for a year. He's a landscape architect and a great dental spouse! We also have a puppy, Gus, who's an 8-pound shipoo, half shih tzu and half poodle.

- I have learned that I learn best in active learning situations, so I want to find a curriculum that focuses on that style of education.

What academic resources are available?

You might say, for example:
- I want to gain experience working with the most state-of-the-art technologies in dentistry.
- I am very interested in having easy access to modern clinical facilities and a large number of patients.
- I would like to get as much experience as possible working in a community setting.
- I would like to get as much experience as possible in a hospital setting.
- I want to have the opportunity to earn a Ph.D. as well as a dental degree.

What services are available to students?

You might say, for example:
- I need to feel comfortable about seeking academic help if I need it.
- I would like to be active in student government.
- I want to attend a school that provides a supportive atmosphere for women and minorities.
- I want to attend a school in which the faculty and administration are sensitive to the stresses dental students experience.
- I want to be able to live on campus or to obtain inexpensive housing near campus.

Where is the school located?

You might say, for example:
- My family situation requires me to attend dental school close to home.
- I prefer attending dental school in an urban setting.
- I need to attend a school where I can benefit from in-state tuition.
- I would like to attend a dental school in an area where hiking and outdoor recreation are easily available.

Your answers to all these questions—and others that you will think of as well—should help you conduct an initial analysis of the information on individual schools in Part II of this book. You can then expand your research by asking for more information directly from each school that you consider a prospect.

To get you started, the tables in this chapter provide an at-a-glance, cumulative comparison of a number of aspects of the individual dental schools:

Table 3-1 presents the number of applicants and enrollees at each school, broken down by gender and racial/ethnic background.

Table 3-2 shows the number of applicants interviewed or accepted and enrollees at each school, broken down by geographical origin (in state or province or out of state or province).

Table 3-3 summarizes specific admissions requirements for each school.

Table 3-4 provides characteristics of the entering class of each school.

Table 3-5 shows where students at each school come from.

Table 3-6 tells which schools offer combined degree programs.

The information in the tables is presented alphabetically by state, territory, and province.

For more information and detailed admission requirements for each school, consult the individual school entries in Part II of this book. As you determine where you plan to send applications, you should contact those dental schools directly for the most complete information about admission requirements. Their telephone numbers, addresses, and websites are included with their entries.

Dental School Rankings

Dental school applicants should be aware that there are proprietary publications available that purport to rank dental schools according to the quality of their programs. The American Dental Education Association and the American Dental Association advise applicants to view these rankings with caution. The bases for these rankings are questionable, and even those individuals most knowledgeable about dental education would admit to the difficulty of establishing criteria for, and achieving consensus on, such rankings.

The accrediting organization for all U.S. dental schools is the Commission on Dental Accreditation. Applicants interested in the current accreditation status of any U.S. dental school should contact the commission at 800-621-8099, ext. 2713.

All schools have their relative strengths. A dental school ideally suited for one applicant might not be appropriate for another. The American Dental Education Association and the American Dental Association recommend that applicants investigate on their own the relative merits of the dental schools they wish to attend.

TABLE 3-1. DENTAL SCHOOLS' APPLICANTS AND ENROLLEES BY GENDER, RACE, AND ETHNICITY—CLASS ENTERING FALL 2006

STATE, TERRITORY, OR PROVINCE	DENTAL SCHOOL	APPLICANTS TOTAL	M	F	AF AMER	HISP	NAT AMER	ASIAN AMER	ENROLLEES TOTAL	M	F	AF AMER	HISP	NAT AMER	ASIAN AMER
ALABAMA	University of Alabama at Birmingham	714	404	310	50	36	3	130	54	31	23	3	1	0	4
ARIZONA	Arizona School of Dentistry & Oral Health	2,915	1,805	1,110	73	136	26	718	54	27	27	0	3	7	8
ARIZONA	Midwestern University	NA	NA	NA	NA	NA	NA	NA	NA	NA	NA	NA	NA	NA	NA
CALIFORNIA	Loma Linda University	2,007	1,203	801	47	110	8	729	95	68	27	1	4	0	40
CALIFORNIA	University of California, Los Angeles	1,743	955	788	44	108	7	655	88	47	41	2	6	1	33
CALIFORNIA	University of California, San Francisco	1,943	1,035	908	48	113	10	745	80	46	34	0	2	0	39
CALIFORNIA	University of Southern California	2,680	1,519	1,161	86	134	10	1,055	144	66	78	5	7	0	49
CALIFORNIA	University of the Pacific	2,944	1,782	1,162	46	125	15	1,045	140	89	51	2	13	1	38
COLORADO	University of Colorado	1,322	804	518	23	73	14	235	50	30	20	0	1	0	2
CONNECTICUT	University of Connecticut	1,363	733	625	52	56	1	422	39	22	17	6	1	0	2
DISTRICT OF COLUMBIA	Howard University	2,159	1,109	1,050	427	109	7	787	90	37	53	54	4	1	21
FLORIDA	Nova Southeastern University	2,285	1,395	890	49	140	13	593	105	64	41	4	15	0	16
FLORIDA	University of Florida	1,319	691	628	46	148	5	302	82	47	35	4	14	0	13
GEORGIA	Medical College of Georgia	267	160	107	27	12	2	39	63	41	22	4	4	1	9
ILLINOIS	Southern Illinois University	681	357	324	41	19	3	170	51	28	23	4	1	0	5
ILLINOIS	University of Illinois at Chicago	1,064	526	538	56	48	3	297	64	31	33	5	7	1	15
INDIANA	Indiana University	1,845	1,145	695	51	60	7	482	100	61	39	2	3	1	10
IOWA	University of Iowa	989	615	374	36	55	4	148	78	44	34	4	5	0	6
KENTUCKY	University of Kentucky	1,454	931	523	41	56	6	245	56	31	25	1	2	0	7
KENTUCKY	University of Louisville	2,428*	1,645	777	58	84	8	452	82	40	42	7	2	0	3
LOUISIANA	Louisiana State University	230	110	120	12	4	0	36	60	38	22	0	0	0	13
MARYLAND	University of Maryland	2,376	1,321	1,053	130	91	6	741	130	70	60	9	4	0	31
MASSACHUSETTS	Boston University	3,913	2,090	1,818	89	179	9	1,505	115	61	54	2	6	1	47
MASSACHUSETTS	Harvard School of Dental Medicine	989*	546	440	32	42	1	346	35	12	23	1	2	0	13
MASSACHUSETTS	Tufts University	3,744	2,073	1,665	110	162	13	1,366	161	85	76	7	11	0	48
MICHIGAN	University of Detroit Mercy	1,516	863	653	73	59	4	503	78	39	39	5	6	1	12
MICHIGAN	University of Michigan	2,169	1,208	961	135	63	5	708	105	68	37	10	4	1	12
MINNESOTA	University of Minnesota	855	486	369	17	17	6	177	96	54	42	2	2	2	7
MISSISSIPPI	University of Mississippi	134	62	72	21	1	100	12	35	17	18	5	1	29	0
MISSOURI	University of Missouri-Kansas City	1,058	639	419	26	42	10	244	102	58	44	4	2	1	3
NEBRASKA	Creighton University	2,845	1,920	925	60	119	20	657	85	50	35	3	3	0	10
NEBRASKA	University of Nebraska	881	546	335	19	34	4	182	47	22	25	2	2	0	1
NEVADA	University of Nevada, Las Vegas	2,635	1,691	944	59	123	16	766	77	52	25	1	3	0	10

Source: Individual schools

Note: The numbers presented above may not match those listed by the individual schools in Part II because of differing reporting procedures. Neither set of numbers is intended to be an exact statistic but is presented to give a sense of the applicant and enrollee profiles of each school.

*Remaining applicants did not wish to report for gender   NR = not reported   NA = not available

CHAPTER 3 DECIDING WHERE TO APPLY

TABLE 3-1. DENTAL SCHOOLS' APPLICANTS AND ENROLLEES BY GENDER, RACE, AND ETHNICITY—CLASS ENTERING FALL 2006 (CONTINUED)

STATE, TERRITORY, OR PROVINCE	DENTAL SCHOOL	APPLICANTS TOTAL	M	F	AF AMER	HISP	NAT AMER	ASIAN AMER	ENROLLEES TOTAL	M	F	AF AMER	HISP	NAT AMER	ASIAN AMER
NEW JERSEY	University of Medicine and Dentistry of New Jersey	1,548	732	816	83	88	2	542	1,548	732	816	83	88	2	542
NEW YORK	Columbia University	2,050	1,014	1,036	59	89	6	867	76	43	33	4	12	1	32
NEW YORK	New York University	3,907	2,069	1,833	110	169	11	1,542	232	134	98	3	4	0	114
NEW YORK	Stony Brook University	1,091*	545	543	36	100	2	384	39	22	17	1	1	0	8
NEW YORK	University at Buffalo	1,708	961	747	42	49	4	629	86	60	26	0	1	0	16
NORTH CAROLINA	University of North Carolina at Chapel Hill	903	490	413	65	43	4	146	81	42	39	13	2	1	8
OHIO	Case School of Dental Medicine	2,940	1,930	1,010	62	81	12	792	70	46	24	3	0	0	17
OHIO	The Ohio State University	1,110	740	370	40	32	6	217	102	72	30	1	1	0	9
OKLAHOMA	University of Oklahoma	598	414	184	2	14	23	53	58	45	13	1	3	6	2
OREGON	Oregon Health & Science University	1,000	654	346	9	31	6	204	75	50	25	0	2	0	10
PENNSYLVANIA	Temple University	3,566	2,072	1,494	173	149	14	1,231	125	83	42	3	10	0	23
PENNSYLVANIA	University of Pennsylvania	2,205	1,159	1,046	68	84	4	845	117	47	70	3	3	1	51
PENNSYLVANIA	University of Pittsburgh	1,844	1,066	777	43	62	6	596	80	52	28	0	8	2	9
PUERTO RICO	University of Puerto Rico	302	162	140	NA	NA	NA	NA	42	15	27	0	40	2	0
SOUTH CAROLINA	Medical University of South Carolina	728	431	297	30	30	4	113	56	33	23	0	1	0	1
TENNESSEE	Meharry Medical College	1,705	809	896	356	79	9	539	62	23	39	48	5	1	5
TENNESSEE	University of Tennessee	466	249	217	64	14	6	72	80	43	37	10	1	0	7
TEXAS	Baylor College of Dentistry	1,457	818	639	60	144	9	383	95	45	50	10	12	3	26
TEXAS	University of Texas Health Science Center at Houston	787	400	387	42	102	5	198	84	47	37	4	14	0	21
TEXAS	University of Texas Health Science Center at San Antonio	1,051	568	483	40	125	7	223	96	55	41	3	12	0	14
VIRGINIA	Virginia Commonwealth University	1,899	1,185	714	69	63	9	460	90	57	33	5	2	0	19
WASHINGTON	University of Washington	1,012*	593	383	14	44	8	252	55	33	22	1	1	1	12
WEST VIRGINIA	West Virginia University	1,236	753	483	34	40	4	326	50	26	24	0	5	0	1
WISCONSIN	Marquette University	2,955	1,850	1,105	99	134	11	714	80	40	40	4	4	0	4
ALBERTA	University of Alberta	322	170	152	NA	NA	NA	NA	34	17	17	NA	NA	NA	NA
BRITISH COLUMBIA	University of British Columbia	290	142	148	NR	NR	NR	NR	40	20	20	NR	NR	NR	NR
MANITOBA	University of Manitoba	285	147	138	NR	NR	NR	NR	29	15	14	NR	NR	NR	NR
NOVA SCOTIA	Dalhousie University	274	131	143	NR	NR	NR	NR	36	17	19	NR	NR	NR	NR
ONTARIO	University of Toronto	530	242	288	NR	NR	NR	NR	68	31	37	NR	NR	NR	NR
ONTARIO	University of Western Ontario	580	NR	NR	NR	NR	NR	NR	55	28	27	NR	NR	NR	NR
QUÉBEC	McGill University	268	114	154	NR	NR	NR	NR	20	NA	NA	NA	NA	NA	NA
QUÉBEC	Université de Montréal	NR	NR	NR	NR	NR	NR	NR	NR	NR	NR	NR	NR	NR	NR
QUÉBEC	Université Laval	423	170	253	NR	NR	NR	NR	48	15	33	NR	NR	NR	NR
SASKATCHEWAN	University of Saskatchewan	347	NA	NA	NR	NR	NR	NR	28	18	10	NR	NR	NR	NR

Source: Individual schools

Note: The numbers presented above may not match those listed by the individual schools in Part II because of differing reporting procedures. Neither set of numbers is intended to be an exact statistic but is presented to give a sense of the applicant and enrollee profiles of each school.

*Remaining applicants did not wish to report for gender   NR = not reported   NA = not available

ADEA OFFICIAL GUIDE TO DENTAL SCHOOLS

TABLE 3-2. DENTAL SCHOOLS' APPLICANTS AND ENROLLEES, IN STATE VERSUS OUT OF STATE—CLASS ENTERING FALL 2006

STATE, TERRITORY, OR PROVINCE	DENTAL SCHOOL	IN STATE OR PROVINCE APPLICANTS TOTAL	NUMBER INTERVIEWED	NUMBER ACCEPTED	OUT OF STATE OR PROVINCE APPLICANTS TOTAL	NUMBER INTERVIEWED	NUMBER ACCEPTED	ENROLLEES IN STATE OR PROVINCE	PERCENTAGE	OUT OF STATE OR PROVINCE	PERCENTAGE
ALABAMA	University of Alabama at Birmingham	125	81	49	589	42	18	45	83	9	17
ARIZONA	Arizona School of Dentistry & Oral Health	NA	70	21	NA	290	33	21	39	33	61
ARIZONA	Midwestern University	NA	NA	NA	NA	NA	NA	NA	NA	NA	NA
CALIFORNIA	Loma Linda University	93	NR	NR	NR	NR	NR	NR	NR	NR	NR
CALIFORNIA	University of California, Los Angeles	1,053	120	105	671	25	23	73	83	15	17
CALIFORNIA	University of California, San Francisco	1,705	213	106	238	86	34	66	83	14	18
CALIFORNIA	University of Southern California	1,248	320	100	1,432	271	44	100	69	44	31
CALIFORNIA	University of the Pacific	1,271	122	93	1,673	67	47	93	66	47	34
COLORADO	University of Colorado	145	70	34	1,177	73	16	34	68	16	32
CONNECTICUT	University of Connecticut	60	23	20	1,302	152	52	19	49	20	51
DISTRICT OF COLUMBIA	Howard University	40	40	24	2,119	231	143	17	19	73	81
FLORIDA	Nova Southeastern University	434	350	105	1,851	NR	NR	62	59	43	41
FLORIDA	University of Florida	463	297	72	836	45	10	72	88	10	12
GEORGIA	Medical College of Georgia	267	139	63	0	0	0	63	100	0	0
ILLINOIS	Southern Illinois University	339	NR	73	342	NR	4	50	98	1	2
ILLINOIS	University of Illinois at Chicago	399	126	81	665	22	14	58	91	6	9
INDIANA	Indiana University	254	161	69	1,591	276	31	69	69	31	31
IOWA	University of Iowa	130	111	63	869	82	15	63	81	15	19
KENTUCKY	University of Kentucky	161	76	59	1,293	58	15	41	73	15	27
KENTUCKY	University of Louisville	177	124	70	2,251	251	90	47	57	35	43
LOUISIANA	Louisiana State University	164	77	58	66	11	2	58	97	2	3
MARYLAND	University of Maryland	178	NR	NR	2,178	NR	NR	70	54	60	46
MASSACHUSETTS	Boston University	120	NR	NR	3,493	NR	NR	9	8	106	92
MASSACHUSETTS	Harvard School of Dental Medicine	49	4	1	840	116	52	1	3	34	97
MASSACHUSETTS	Tufts University	127	53	44	3,617	415	288	29	18	132	82
MICHIGAN	University of Detroit Mercy	365	91	83	1,151	58	45	52	67	26	33
MICHIGAN	University of Michigan	277	NR	74	1,892	NR	121	63	60	42	40
MINNESOTA	University of Minnesota	173	NR	65	682	NR	31	65	68	31	32
MISSISSIPPI	University of Mississippi	124	71	35	10	0	0	35	100	0	0
MISSOURI	University of Missouri-Kansas City	169	85	67	889	129	35	68	67	34	33
NEBRASKA	Creighton University	98	NA	NA	2,747	NA	NA	15	18	70	82
NEBRASKA	University of Nebraska	105	55	37	776	109	20	34	72	13	28
NEVADA	University of Nevada, Las Vegas	147	95	60	2,488	338	65	52	68	25	32
NEW JERSEY	University of Medicine and Dentistry of New Jersey	300	NR	NR	1,248	NR	NR	300	19	1,248	81

Source: Individual schools

Note: The numbers presented above may not match those listed by the individual schools in Part II because of differing reporting procedures. Neither set of numbers is intended to be an exact statistic but is presented to give a sense of the applicant and enrollee profiles of each school.

NR = not reported   NA = not available

TABLE 3-2. DENTAL SCHOOLS' APPLICANTS AND ENROLLEES, IN STATE VERSUS OUT OF STATE—CLASS ENTERING FALL 2006 (CONTINUED)

STATE, TERRITORY, OR PROVINCE	DENTAL SCHOOL	IN STATE OR PROVINCE APPLICANTS TOTAL	NUMBER INTERVIEWED	NUMBER ACCEPTED	OUT OF STATE OR PROVINCE APPLICANTS TOTAL	NUMBER INTERVIEWED	NUMBER ACCEPTED	ENROLLEES IN STATE OR PROVINCE	PERCENTAGE	OUT OF STATE OR PROVINCE	PERCENTAGE
NEW YORK	Columbia University	NA	NA	NA	NA	NA	NA	23	30	53	70
NEW YORK	New York University	NA	NA	NA	NA	NA	NA	23	30	53	70
NEW YORK	Stony Brook University	413	165	35	678	50	4	35	90	4	10
NEW YORK	University at Buffalo	422	134	86	1,286	177	86	47	55	39	45
NORTH CAROLINA	University of North Carolina at Chapel Hill	248	166	65	655	59	16	68	84	13	16
OHIO	Case School of Dental Medicine	204	35	23	2,736	297	225	15	20	61	80
OHIO	The Ohio State University	235	112	88	875	63	48	76	75	26	25
OKLAHOMA	University of Oklahoma	158	114	48	440	49	10	48	83	10	17
OREGON	Oregon Health & Science University	143	70	58	857	76	52	52	69	23	31
PENNSYLVANIA	Temple University	272	120	77	3,294	636	233	40	32	85	68
PENNSYLVANIA	University of Pennsylvania	154	NA	NA	2,051	NA	NA	16	14	101	86
PENNSYLVANIA	University of Pittsburgh	201	57	32	1,445	173	48	32	40	48	60
PUERTO RICO	University of Puerto Rico	80	61	40	222	2	2	40	95	2	5
SOUTH CAROLINA	Medical University of South Carolina	156	113	51	452	7	5	51	91	5	9
TENNESSEE	Meharry Medical College	NA	NA	NA	NA	NA	NA	9	15	53	85
TENNESSEE	University of Tennessee	181	127	58	285	62	44	51	64	29	36
TEXAS	Baylor College of Dentistry	747	299	127	710	22	11	88	93	7	7
TEXAS	University of Texas Health Science Center at Houston	754	241	82	33	2	1	83	99	1	1
TEXAS	University of Texas Health Science Center at San Antonio	785	262	147	266	15	12	89	93	7	7
VIRGINIA	Virginia Commonwealth University	236	81	59	1,663	186	88	55	61	35	39
WASHINGTON	University of Washington	235	128	47	777	31	13	45	82	10	18
WEST VIRGINIA	West Virginia University	75	72	32	1,161	73	31	31	62	19	38
WISCONSIN	Marquette University	177	80	42	2,778	180	66	40	50	40	50
ALBERTA	University of Alberta	198	69	36	124	10	4	31	91	3	9
BRITISH COLUMBIA	University of British Columbia	NR	NR	NR	NR	NR	NR	NR	NR	NR	NR
MANITOBA	University of Manitoba	NR	55	24	NR	28	5	24	83	5	17
NOVA SCOTIA	Dalhousie University	NR	NR	NR	NR	NR	NR	NR	NR	NR	NR
ONTARIO	University of Toronto	NR	NR	NR	NR	NR	NR	NR	NR	NR	NR
ONTARIO	University of Western Ontario	NR	NR	NR	NR	NR	NR	52	95	3	5
QUÉBEC	McGill University	NA	NA	NA	NA	NA	NA	NA	NA	NA	NA
QUÉBEC	Université de Montréal	NR	NR	NR	NR	NR	NR	NR	NR	NR	NR
QUÉBEC	Université Laval	NR	135	48	NR	NR	NR	NR	NR	NR	NR
SASKATCHEWAN	University of Saskatchewan	84	53	22	263	45	6*	22	79	6	21

Source: Individual schools

Note: The numbers presented above may not match those listed by the individual schools in Part II because of differing reporting procedures. Neither set of numbers is intended to be an exact statistic but is presented to give a sense of the applicant and enrollee profiles of each school.

NR = not reported   NA = not available

TABLE 3-3. ADMISSION REQUIREMENTS BY DENTAL SCHOOL

STATE, TERRITORY, OR PROVINCE	DENTAL SCHOOL	NUMBER YRS. REQUIRED PREDENTAL EDUCATION	UNDERGRADUATE COURSES REQUIRED	DAT*	GPA*	INTERVIEW[§]	STATE RESIDENCY REQUIREMENT
ALABAMA	University of Alabama at Birmingham	Formal minimum 3 yrs.	Inorg. & org. chem., bio., physics, math, Eng.	Mandatory	3.3 or above recommended	Yes	Preference to residents of AL and neighboring states
ARIZONA	Arizona School of Dentistry & Oral Health	Minimum 3 yrs.	General bio., general & org. chem., physics, Eng., biochem., physio.	No minimum	2.5	Yes	None
ARIZONA	Midwestern University	Minimum 3 yrs., bachelor's degree recommended	Bio., general &org. chem., physics, Eng., biochem.	Mandatory	Minimum of 2.50, 3.2 or above recommended	Yes, an on-campus interview is mandatory	NR
CALIFORNIA	Loma Linda University	NR	General bio. or zoo., general or inorg. chem. & org. chem, physics, Eng.	NR	NR	NR	NR
CALIFORNIA	University of California, Los Angeles	Minimum 3 yrs.	inorg. & org. chem., physics, bio., Eng., psych., biochem.	NA	NA	NA	NA
CALIFORNIA	University of California, San Francisco	Minimum 3 yrs.	Inorg. & org. chem., bio., biochem., physics, psych., Eng.	Mandatory	Residents with bachelor's degree, 2.4; nonresidents, 3.0	Yes	No specific requirements
CALIFORNIA	University of Southern California	Minimum 2 yrs.;	Bio., inorg. & org. chem., physics, Eng.	15 required	NA	Yes	None
CALIFORNIA	University of the Pacific	Minimum 3 yrs.	Bio., physics, inorg. & org. chem., Eng.	Mandatory	Assessed	Yes	No specific requirements
COLORADO	University of Colorado at Denver	Minimum 3 yrs. plus	General & org. chem., bio., physics, Eng. comp., hum.	Mandatory	No specific requirements	Upon invitation	No specific requirements
CONNECTICUT	University of Connecticut	Minimum 3 yrs.; usual 4 yrs.	Inorg. & org. chem., physics, bio., Eng.	Mandatory	3.0 or above recommended	Yes	No specific requirements
DISTRICT OF COLUMBIA	Howard University	Minimum 4 yrs.	Bio., inorg. & org. chem., Eng.	17 required	2.7	Yes	NA
FLORIDA	Nova Southeastern University	Minimum 90 semester hours	Bio., inorg, & org. chem., physics, Eng. comp & lit.	18 required	3.3	Yes	None
FLORIDA	University of Florida	Bachelor's degree strongly recommended	Inorg. & org. chem., bio., physics, biochem., micro., mole. bio./genetics, Eng., general psych.	Mandatory, minimum15	3.2 or above recommended	Yes	Preference to FL residents
GEORGIA	Medical College of Georgia	Minimum 90 semester hours	Eng., adv. chem., general bio., general or inorg. chem., physics	Academic, at least 14 required; perceptual, at least 14 required	OGPA minimum 2.8, SGPA minimum 2.8	Required	Must be GA residents
ILLINOIS	Southern Illinois University	Formal minimum of 2 yrs.; usual minimum of 3 yrs.	Inorg. & org. chem., bio., physics, Eng.	Mandatory	3.0 or above recommended	By invitation only and required for acceptance consideration	Preference given to IL residents
ILLINOIS	University of Illinois at Chicago	Minimum 3 yrs., degree preferred	Chem., bio., physics, Eng.	Minimum of 15 aca. ave. & 14 PAT	Minimum 2.5/4.0 cumul. & 2.5/4.0 sci.	Mandatory	Preference to IL residents; 10% nonresident

Source: Individual schools

*DAT—Dental Admission Test; GPA—Grade Point Average
[§]Because interview policies vary considerably from school to school, readers are encouraged to review the individual school listings in Part II.

CHAPTER 3 **DECIDING WHERE TO APPLY**

TABLE 3-3. ADMISSION REQUIREMENTS BY DENTAL SCHOOL (CONTINUED)

STATE, TERRITORY, OR PROVINCE	DENTAL SCHOOL	NUMBER YRS. REQUIRED PREDENTAL EDUCATION	UNDERGRADUATE COURSES REQUIRED	DAT*	GPA*	INTERVIEW§	STATE RESIDENCY REQUIREMENT
INDIANA	Indiana University	Minimum 3 yrs.	Bio., general & org. chem., physics, anatomy, physio., biochem., general psych., Eng.	Minimum of 16, 18 in Reading Comprehension	3.0	Yes	No specific requirements
IOWA	University of Iowa	Minimum 3 yrs., 4 yrs. recommended	Bio., chem., physics,	Prefer minimum national average on each section	Prefer above a 3.0 on a 4.0 scale	Required	Preference to IA residents
KENTUCKY	University of Kentucky	Minimum 4 yrs.	Bio., general & org. chem., physics, Eng.	Mandatory	Minimum 3.0	Yes	No
KENTUCKY	University of Louisville	Mimimum 90 credit hours, including 32 science hours	Gen. & org. chem. or org. chem. & biochem., physics, bio	Mandatory	No minimum but 3.0 or above in sciences recommended	Required	No
LOUISIANA	Louisiana State University	Minimum 3 yrs.	Org. chem., physics, Eng.	NR	NR	NR	NR
MARYLAND	University of Maryland	Bachelor's degree strongly recommended	Inorg. & org. chem., bio., physics, Eng. comp., biochem.	NR	NR	NR	NR
MASSACHUSETTS	Boston University	Formal mimimum 3 yrs., usual and recommended 4 yrs.	Inorg. & org. chem., physics, bio., Eng., math w/calculus	Mandatory	3.2 or above recommended	Yes	No specific requirements
MASSACHUSETTS	Harvard School of Dental Medicine	Formal minimum 3 yrs., usual minimum 4 yrs.	Bio., gen. & org. chem., physics, calculus, Eng. (preferably comp.)	Mandatory	3.0 or above	Yes	No specific requirements
MASSACHUSETTS	Tufts University	Bachelor's degree required	General bio., general & org. chem., physics, biochem., writing-intensive humanities course	16 Academic Average, 15 Perceptual Ability, 16 Total Science	Preference given to those above 3.3	Required for acceptance	No specific requirements
MICHIGAN	University of Detroit Mercy	Formal minimum 2 yrs., generally accepted 3+ yrs.	Eng. (comp. & lit.), bio., org. & inorg. chem., physics	Mandatory (recommended 17 or higher in science sections)	No cutoff, but 3.0 or above recommended. 2.95 or above science recommended	Yes, at the discretion of the Admissions Committee	No specific requirements
MICHIGAN	University of Michigan	Formal minimum of 2 yrs., generally acceptable minimum of 2 yrs., usual and recommended 4 yrs.	Inorg. & org. chem., physics, bio., biochem., micro., Eng. comp., psych., sociology	NR	NR	NR	NR
MINNESOTA	University of Minnesota	Formal minimum 3 yrs.; preferred minimum 4 yrs.	General & org. chem., biochem., physics, bio., Eng., psych., math	Mandatory	Minimum 2.5	Yes	Preference to MN residents
MISSISSIPPI	University of Mississippi	Minimum 4 yrs.	Org. & inorg. chem., physics, bio., adv. bio. or chem., statistics, Eng., math	NR	NR	Yes	Preference to MS residents
MISSOURI	University of Missouri-Kansas City	Minimum 90 hrs. at the time of application, degree preferred	Bio., anatomy, physio., cell bio., org. & inorg. chem., physics, Eng. comp.	17 preferred	Science 3.4 preferred	Yes	Preference to residents of MO, KS, AR, NM, HI
NEBRASKA	Creighton University	Formal minimum 2 yrs., generally accepted minimum 4 yrs.	Inorg. & org. chem., bio. or zoo., Eng., physics	Mandatory	Above 3.0 recommended	Not req. for all students	No specific requirements

Source: Individual schools
*DAT—Dental Admission Test; GPA—Grade Point Average
§Because interview policies vary considerably from school to school, readers are encouraged to review the individual school listings in Part II.

TABLE 3-3. ADMISSION REQUIREMENTS BY DENTAL SCHOOL (CONTINUED)

STATE, TERRITORY, OR PROVINCE	DENTAL SCHOOL	NUMBER YRS. REQUIRED PREDENTAL EDUCATION	UNDERGRADUATE COURSES REQUIRED	DAT*	GPA*	INTERVIEW[§]	STATE RESIDENCY REQUIREMENT
NEBRASKA	University of Nebraska	Minimum 3 yrs.	Eng., bio., general & org. chem., physics	NR	NR	Yes	NR
NEVADA	University of Nevada, Las Vegas	Formal minimum 3 yrs., bachelor's degree preferred	Bio., general & org. chem., physics, Eng., biochem.	Mandatory	NA	NR	NA
NEW JERSEY	University of Medicine and Dentistry of New Jersey	Minimum 3 yrs., normal 4 yrs.	Inorg. & org. chem., bio., physics, Eng.	Minimum 18	3.25	Yes	NA
NEW YORK	Columbia University	Preferred minimum 4 yrs., formal minimum 90 credits	Inorg. & org. chem., bio., physics, Eng.	No minimum	No minimum	Yes	NA
NEW YORK	New York University	B.A./B.S. from United States required	Eng., bio., org. chem., physics	18 required	3.2	Yes	No specific requirements
NEW YORK	Stony Brook University	Minimum of 3 yrs., bachelor's degree preferred	Bio., inorg. & org. chem., physics, calc. or stat.	Mandatory; preferably taken within 3 years of application	3.0 or above recommended	Mandatory; scheduled at discretion of Admissions Committee	No specific requirements
NEW YORK	University at Buffalo	Minimum 3 yrs.	Gen. bio., gen. & org. chem., physics, all w/lab; Eng. w/comp.	14 minimum AA, PAT	3.0 min.	Required for all receiving serious consideration	No specific requirements
NORTH CAROLINA	University of North Carolina at Chapel Hill	Minimum 3 yrs.	Inorg. & org. chem., bio., physics, Eng.	17 required	3.0	Yes	No specific requirements
OHIO	Case School of Dental Medicine	Minimum 2 yrs., 4 yrs. suggested	Inorg. & org. chem., physics, bio., Eng.	Mandatory	3.2 or above recommended	Yes	No specific requirements
OHIO	The Ohio State University	Formal minimum 3 yrs., usual acceptable minimum 4 yrs.	Bio., general & org. chem., physics, anatomy, biochem., micro., Eng., adv. writing.	Mandatory, 13 minimum PAT	3.4 or above recommended	Yes	Priority to OH residents
OKLAHOMA	University of Oklahoma	Minimum of 90 semester hours	Bio., physics, psych., general & org. chem., Eng., biochem.	17 minimum	2.5 minimum, 3.0 to be competitive	Yes	Preference to OK residents
OREGON	Oregon Health & Science University	Formal minimum 3 yrs.; usual 4 yrs.; bachelor's degree strongly preferred	Gen. bio., inorg. & org. chem., physics, anat., physiology, biochem., Eng. comp.	Mandatory	3.0 or above recommended	Yes	Priority order: OR residents, WICHE residents, nonresidents, Canadian; int'l. students
PENNSYLVANIA	Temple University	Minimum 3 yrs.	Bio., gen. & org. chem., physics, Eng.	18 required	3.0	Required	No specific requirements
PENNSYLVANIA	University of Pennsylvania	Formal minimum 3 yrs., usual minimum 4 yrs.	Inorg. & org. chem., bio., biochem., physics, math, Eng.	Mandatory	3.2 or above recommended	Yes	No specific requirements
PENNSYLVANIA	University of Pittsburgh	Prefer 4 yrs.	Inorg. & org. chem., bio. w/lab, physics, Eng.	Min of 16 on each section	Min of 3.0	Required	No specific requirements
PUERTO RICO	University of Puerto Rico	Minimum 90 semester credits	Bio., gen. & inorg. chem., physics, Eng., Spanish,	Mandatory	Minimum general and science GPA of 2.5	Yes	NR

Source: Individual schools
*DAT—Dental Admission Test; GPA—Grade Point Average
[§]Because interview policies vary considerably from school to school, readers are encouraged to review the individual school listings in Part II.

TABLE 3-3. ADMISSION REQUIREMENTS BY DENTAL SCHOOL (CONTINUED)

STATE, TERRITORY, OR PROVINCE	DENTAL SCHOOL	NUMBER YRS. REQUIRED PREDENTAL EDUCATION	UNDERGRADUATE COURSES REQUIRED	DAT*	GPA*	INTERVIEW[§]	STATE RESIDENCY REQUIREMENT
SOUTH CAROLINA	Medical University of South Carolina	Minimum 4 yrs., but strongly recommend applicant earn bachelor's degree	Bio., gen. & org. chem., physics, math, Eng.	Mandatory, U.S. version only	No specific requirement	If eligible, applicant would be invited for interview on campus	Strong preference to SC residents
TENNESSEE	Meharry Medical College	Minimum 2 yrs.	Gen. & org. chem., physics, general bio. or botany or zoo.	Mandatory	Minimum 2.0	Yes	NR
TENNESSEE	University of Tennessee	Minimum 4 yrs.	Eng. comp., general bio., general & org. chem., biochem., physics, and hist., micro. or comp. anatomy	17 required	Minimum 3.0	Required	54 TN, 18 AR, 8 other states
TEXAS	Baylor College of Dentistry	Formal minimum 3 yrs., usual minimum 4 yrs.	Bio., inorg. & org. chem., gen physics, biochem., Eng.	Mandatory	3.0 or above recommended	Yes	Preference to TX residents and surrounding states
TEXAS	University of Texas Health Science Center at Houston	Formal minimum 3 yrs., usual minimum 4 yrs.	General & org. chem., physics, bio., Eng., biochem.	Mandatory	3.0 or above strongly recommended	Yes	Preference to TX residents
TEXAS	University of Texas Health Science Center at San Antonio	Minimum 3 yrs.	Inorg. & org. chem., bio., physics	Competitive	Competitive	Yes	No specific requirements
VIRGINIA	Virginia Commonwealth University	Formal minimum of 3 yrs.; generally acceptable minimum of 4 yrs.	General bio., general & org. chem., biochem., physics	Mandatory; should be taken no later than December of the year prior to desired matriculation	No specific requirements	Yes	No specific requirements
WASHINGTON	University of Washington	Minimum 3 yrs., most entering students have 4 yrs.	General & org. chem., biochem., physics, general bio. or zoo., micro.	Mandatory; must be taken no later than Oct. 31 of year prior to admission	GPA needs to be competitive within applicant pool	Applicants are selected after being screened. Approximately 15% of the pool is interviewed.	Preference as follows: Washington residents, residents of WICHE states, residents of other states
WEST VIRGINIA	West Virginia University	Minimum 3 yrs.	Bio., inorg. & org. chem., physics, Eng. comp.	Mandatory	3.0 or above strongly recommended	Yes	Preference to WV residents
WISCONSIN	Marquette University	Formal minimum 3 yrs., usual minimum 4 yrs.	Inorg. & org. chem., bio., physics, Eng.	Mandatory; Canadian DAT accepted	No specific reqt., 3.3+ recommended	Mandatory for acceptance	50% in state 50% out of state
ALBERTA	University of Alberta	Minimum 2 yrs. (10 full course requirements)	General & org. chem., bio., physics, Eng., stat., biochem.	Canadian DAT mandatory; minimum score is 5/30 for Reading Comprehension, PAT, MAN	Minimum 3.0 out of 4	A personal interview is required of all competitive applicants annually	A maximum of three out-of-province Canadian residents and one foreign applicant may be accepted
BRITISH COLUMBIA	University of British Columbia	Minimum 3 yrs.	General & org. chem., physics, bio., biochem., Eng., math	Mandatory; Canadian DAT only	Minimum 70%	100 candidates invited for an interview	NA

Source: Individual schools
*DAT—Dental Admission Test; GPA—Grade Point Average
[§]Because interview policies vary considerably from school to school, readers are encouraged to review the individual school listings in Part II.

TABLE 3-3. ADMISSION REQUIREMENTS BY DENTAL SCHOOL (CONTINUED)

STATE, TERRITORY, OR PROVINCE	DENTAL SCHOOL	NUMBER YRS. REQUIRED PREDENTAL EDUCATION	UNDERGRADUATE COURSES REQUIRED	DAT*	GPA*	INTERVIEW[§]	STATE RESIDENCY REQUIREMENT
MANITOBA	University of Manitoba	Minimum 2 yrs.	General & org. chem., biochem., physics, bio, Eng.	Mandatory	Minimum 2.5 in core science courses	Yes	NA
NOVA SCOTIA	Dalhousie University	Minimum 2 yrs.	General & org. chem., physics, bio., physiology, microbio., biochem.	Mandatory	Minimum 3.5 to be competitive	Yes	Preference to Atlantic Province residents
ONTARIO	University of Toronto	Minimum 3 yrs.	Biochem., physiology	Mandatory	Minimum 2.7	Yes	NR
ONTARIO	University of Western Ontario	Minimum 2 yrs.	Bio., physics, general & org. chem., physio., biochem.	Mandatory	3.0	Yes	NR
QUÉBEC	McGill University	Minimum 4 yrs.	Bio., general & org. chem., physics	Mandatory	3.5 minimum	Yes	NA
QUÉBEC	Université de Montréal	NR	NR	NR	NR	NR	NR
QUÉBEC	Université Laval	Minimum 2 yrs.	Chem., physics, bio., math,	17,2/30	31,735	Yes	Yes
SASKATCHEWAN	University of Saskatchewan	Minimum 2 yrs. predentistry courses	General bio., general & org. chem., physics, biochem.	Mandatory; 25% weight on CDA DAT scores on Reading Comprehension, Perceptual Ability, Carving, Academic Average. Academic Average a reqt. effective 2007.	3.0. 65% weight on 2 best years	Yes, 10% weight	NR

Source: Individual schools
*DAT—Dental Admission Test; GPA—Grade Point Average
[§]Because interview policies vary considerably from school to school, readers are encouraged to review the individual school listings in Part II.

TABLE 3-4. CHARACTERISTICS OF THE CLASS ENTERING FALL 2006 BY DENTAL SCHOOL

STATE, TERRITORY, OR PROVINCE	DENTAL SCHOOL	AGE OF STUDENTS (FIRST-TIME ENROLLEES) MEAN	RANGE	# OVER 30	PREDENTAL EDUCATION OF ALL FIRST-YEAR STUDENTS 2 YRS.	3 YRS.	4 YRS.	BACC.	MAST.	PH.D.	MEAN DAT (FIRST-TIME ENROLLEES) ACAD.	PAT	MEAN GPA (FIRST-TIME ENROLLEES) OVERALL	SCI.
ALABAMA	University of Alabama at Birmingham	NA	NA	NA	NA	NA	NA	NA	NA	NA	19.2	18.3	3.58	3.5
ARIZONA	Arizona School of Dentistry & Oral Health	25	20-36	12	0	3	2	47	2	0	18.59	18.13	3.46	3.21
ARIZONA	Midwestern University	NA	NA	NA	NA	NA	NA	NA	NA	NA	NA	NA	NA	NA
CALIFORNIA	Loma Linda University	NA	NA	NA	NA	NA	NA	NA	NA	NA	20	19.7	3.27	3.24
CALIFORNIA	University of California, Los Angeles	NA	NA	NA	NA	NA	NA	NA	NA	NA	22	20	3.65	3.6
CALIFORNIA	University of California, San Francisco	NR	NR	NR	0	0	1	75	4	0	20.6	19.2	3.61	3.57
CALIFORNIA	University of Southern California	NA	NA	NA	NA	NA	NA	NA	NA	NA	20	19	3.47	3.37
CALIFORNIA	University of the Pacific	25	19-34	NR	7	6	4	108	11	0	20.5	19.7	3.37	3.29
COLORADO	University of Colorado	NA	NA	NA	NA	NA	NA	NA	NA	NA	19.6	19.6	3.71	3.66
CONNECTICUT	University of Connecticut	24	22-28	NR	0	0	0	39	0	0	20	18.3	3.57	3.5
DISTRICT OF COLUMBIA	Howard University	NA	NA	NA	NA	NA	NA	NA	NA	NA	17	16	3.09	3.0
FLORIDA	Nova Southeastern University	NA	NA	NA	NA	NA	NA	NA	NA	NA	19	18	3.6	3.58
FLORIDA	University of Florida	23	21-34	1	0	4	1	75	1	1	19	18	3.6	3.5
GEORGIA	Medical College of Georgia	NA	NA	NA	NA	NA	NA	NA	NA	NA	19	19	3.5	3.5
ILLINOIS	Southern Illinois University	NA	NA	NA	NA	NA	NA	NA	NA	NA	19	18.1	3.64	3.6
ILLINOIS	University of Illinois at Chicago	NA	NA	NA	NA	NA	NA	NA	NA	NA	19.3	18.74	3.45	3.35
INDIANA	Indiana University	25	22-42	14	0	2	16	73	9	0	18.72	18.46	3.52	3.44
IOWA	University of Iowa	23	21-37	3	0	28	0	47	3	0	19	18	3.7	3.63
KENTUCKY	University of Kentucky	25	21-40	5	0	0	0	54	2	0	18.44	17.64	3.52	3.37
KENTUCKY	University of Louisville	24	21-38	5	0	2	5	70	5	0	18	17	3.57	3.46
LOUISIANA	Louisiana State University	NR	NR	NR	NR	2	3	55	NR	NR	19.1	19.2	3.56	3.48
MARYLAND	University of Maryland	24	22-37	5	0	0	1	122	6	1	20	18.7	3.5	3.4
MASSACHUSETTS	Boston University	24	19-46	4	0	3	1	103	8	0	20	20	3.23	3.11
MASSACHUSETTS	Harvard School of Dental Medicine	NA	NA	NA	NA	NA	NA	NA	NA	NA	24.4	21.6	3.77	3.77
MASSACHUSETTS	Tufts University	24	20-41	8	0	1	0	153	6	1	19	18.1	3.41	3.33
MICHIGAN	University of Detroit Mercy	NA	NA	NA	NA	NA	NA	NA	NA	NA	19	18	3.54	3.51
MICHIGAN	University of Michigan	NA	NA	NA	NA	NA	NA	NA	NA	NA	19.58	19.25	3.51	3.41
MINNESOTA	University of Minnesota	NA	NA	NA	NA	NA	NA	NA	NA	NA	19.4	19.1	3.63	3.57
MISSISSIPPI	University of Mississippi	NA	NA	NA	NA	NA	NA	NA	NA	NA	17.4	16.9	3.63	3.55
MISSOURI	University of Missouri-Kansas City	27	21-37	5	0	1	11	87	1	0	18.3	NR	3.64	3.6
NEBRASKA	Creighton University	24	21-36	3	0	9	4	72	3	0	18.92	19.07	3.53	3.42
NEBRASKA	University of Nebraska	24	21-36	3	0	7	5	32	3	0	18.6	18.1	3.78	3.7
NEVADA	University of Nevada, Las Vegas	NA	NA	NA	NA	NA	NA	NA	NA	NA	19.27	18.78	3.51	3.26
NEW JERSEY	University of Medicine and Dentistry of New Jersey	NA	NA	NA	NA	NA	NA	NA	NA	NA	19.28	17.58	3.47	3.4
NEW YORK	Columbia University	NR	NR	NR	0	0	0	69	6	0	22.16	19.06	3.49	3.44

Source: Individual schools

NR = not reported   NA = not available or not applicable

ADEA OFFICIAL GUIDE TO DENTAL SCHOOLS

TABLE 3-4. CHARACTERISTICS OF THE CLASS ENTERING FALL 2006 BY DENTAL SCHOOL (CONTINUED)

STATE, TERRITORY, OR PROVINCE	DENTAL SCHOOL	AGE OF STUDENTS (FIRST-TIME ENROLLEES) MEAN	RANGE	# OVER 30	PREDENTAL EDUCATION OF ALL FIRST-YEAR STUDENTS 2 YRS.	3 YRS.	4 YRS.	BACC.	MAST.	PH.D.	MEAN DAT (FIRST-TIME ENROLLEES) ACAD.	PAT	MEAN GPA (FIRST-TIME ENROLLEES) OVERALL	SCI.
NEW YORK	New York University	NA	NA	NA	NA	NA	NA	NA	NA	NA	19.06	17.8	3.29	3.16
NEW YORK	Stony Brook University	NR	NR	NR	NR	NR	NR	NR	NR	NR	21	19	3.71	3.72
NEW YORK	University at Buffalo	NR	NR	NR	NR	NR	NR	NR	NR	NR	19.35	19.11	3.57	3.56
NORTH CAROLINA	University of North Carolina at Chapel Hill	24.7	21-41	8	1	1	0	79	0	0	19.7	18.1	3.6	3.53
OHIO	Case School of Dental Medicine	NR	NR	NR	NR	NR	NR	NR	NR	NR	19.36	18.5	3.5	3.45
OHIO	The Ohio State University	NR	NR	NR	NR	NR	NR	NR	NR	NR	18.98	18.98	3.52	3.39
OKLAHOMA	University of Oklahoma	NR	NR	NR	NR	NR	NR	NR	NR	NR	19.51	18.33	3.63	3.54
OREGON	Oregon Health & Science University	26	21-37	12	0	0	0	75	2	NR	19.55	18.87	3.58	3.57
PENNSYLVANIA	Temple University	24	21-36	4	0	3	6	112	4	0	18.8	18.7	3.33	3.19
PENNSYLVANIA	University of Pennsylvania	23	20-29	0	0	3	0	113	1	0	21	19	3.68	3.63
PENNSYLVANIA	University of Pittsburgh	NR	NR	NR	NR	NR	NR	NR	NR	NR	19.83	18.64	3.54	3.43
PUERTO RICO	University of Puerto Rico	25	20-49	3	0	8	0	33	1	0	15	16	3.45	3.33
SOUTH CAROLINA	Medical University of South Carolina	NR	NR	NR	NR	NR	NR	NR	NR	NR	19.3	19.89	3.59	3.58
TENNESSEE	Meharry Medical College	NR	NR	NR	NR	NR	NR	NR	NR	NR	16	15	3.1	2.9
TENNESSEE	University of Tennessee	23	21-29	NR	NR	NR	NR	NR	NR	NR	18	18	3.45	3.36
TEXAS	Baylor College of Dentistry	24	20-36	NR	0	1	0	90	3	0	19.5	17.8	3.51	3.44
TEXAS	University of Texas Health Science Center at Houston	24.5	19-43	10	0	2	0	82	0	0	19.19	17.8	3.59	3.52
TEXAS	University of Texas Health Science Center at San Antonio	NA	NA	NA	NA	NA	NA	NA	NA	NA	19	18	3.74	3.6
VIRGINIA	Virginia Commonwealth University	25	19-38	NR	0	0	0	89	1	0	19	18	3.36	3.25
WASHINGTON	University of Washington	25	21-31	6	0	0	2	53	2	0	21.22	20.33	3.45	3.46
WEST VIRGINIA	West Virginia University	24	21-35	2	0	11	12	26	1	0	18	17	3.54	3.4
WISCONSIN	Marquette University	23.5	20-37	4	0	16	64	NR	0	0	18.44	18.08	3.5	3.43
ALBERTA	University of Alberta	NR	NR	NR	NR	NR	NR	NR	NR	NR	24.1	20.1	3.8	3.84
BRITISH COLUMBIA	University of British Columbia	24	20-29	0	0	3	36	NA	1	0	20.9	21.7	3.65	NR
MANITOBA	University of Manitoba	23.5	20-46	1	2	5	0	20	2	0	20.08	19.35	4.01	3.92
NOVA SCOTIA	Dalhousie University	NR	NR	NR	NR	NR	NR	NR	NR	NR	20	17	3.7	3.7
ONTARIO	University of Toronto	NA	NA	NA	0	21	41	NA	3	0	21	19	3.83	NA
ONTARIO	University of Western Ontario	NR	NR	NR	NR	NR	NR	NR	NR	NR	NR	NR	3.9	NR
QUEBEC	McGill University	NR	NR	NR	NR	NR	NR	NR	NR	NR	NA	NA	NA	NA
QUEBEC	Université de Montréal	NR	NR	NR	NR	NR	NR	NR	NR	NR	NR	NR	NR	NR
QUEBEC	Université Laval	NR	NR	NR	NR	NR	NR	NR	NR	NR	17.2	15	NA	NA
SASKATCHEWAN	University of Saskatchewan	NR	NR	NR	NR	NR	NR	NR	NR	NR	NR	19.79	NR	NR

Source: Individual schools

NR = not reported   NA = not available or not applicable

TABLE 3-5. THE CLASS ENTERING FALL 2006 AT DENTAL SCHOOLS BY STATE OF RESIDENCE

DENTAL SCHOOL		TOTAL 1ST YEAR ENROLLEES	IN-STATE	OUT-OF-STATE+	
ALABAMA	University of Alabama at Birmingham	54	45	9	GA-3, NC-2, MS-2, FL-1, TN-1
ARIZONA	Arizona School of Dentistry & Oral Health	54	21	33	CA-7, ID-1, IL-1, IN-3, LA-1, MD-1, ME-1, MT-2, ND-2, NM-1, OH-2, OK-1, OR-2, TX-2, UT-1, VA-3, WA-2
ARIZONA	Midwestern University	NA	NA	NA	NA
CALIFORNIA	Loma Linda University	95	NR	NR	NR
CALIFORNIA	University of California, Los Angeles	88	73	15	AZ-2, CO-1, FL-2, GA-1, IL-2, PA-1, TX-1, UT-4, VA-1, WA-1
CALIFORNIA	University of California, San Francisco	80	66	14	AZ-2, HI-1, ID-1, IL-1, NJ-1, OR-1, TX-1, UT-3, WA-1, other-2
CALIFORNIA	University of Southern California	144	NR	NR	Numbers not specified: AZ, FL, HI, WA, MI, UT, GA, MN, WI, IL
CALIFORNIA	University of the Pacific	140	93	47	AZ-8, Canada-3, CO-1, GA-2, HI-4, ID-1, MN-1, NC-2, NM-2, NV-6, OR-2, PA-2, UT-9, WA-4
COLORADO	University of Colorado	50	34	16	AZ-8, NM-3, ND-2, AK-1, HI-1, MT-1
CONNECTICUT	University of Connecticut	39	19	20	DE-2, GA-1, MA-5, ME-5, NJ-1, RI-4, VA-1, Trinidad and Tobago-1
DISTRICT OF COLUMBIA	Howard University	90	17	73	AZ-1, CA-4, CO-1, FL-4, GA-4, IL-2, LA-2, MD-14, MI-2, MN-1, NY-9, NJ-2, NC-2, OH-1, OR-1, PA-2, SC-1, TN-2, TX-3, UT-1, VA-6, WA-2, Canada-3, Grand Bahama-1, St. Lucia-1
FLORIDA	Nova Southeastern University	105	62	43	AZ-4, CA-9, GA-1, ID-2, international-1, KS-1, LA-1, MI-1, NC-2, NE-1, NJ-1, NV-1, PA-2, SC-1, UT-9, VA-1, WA-1, WY-2, Canada-2
FLORIDA	University of Florida	82	72	10	AZ-1, GA-2, ID-1, IN-1, MI-1, NC-1, TN-1, UT-1, WI-1
GEORGIA	Medical College of Georgia	63	63	0	NA
ILLINOIS	Southern Illinois University	51	50	1	MO-1
ILLINOIS	University of Illinois at Chicago	64	58	6	CA-2, IN-1, NM-1, MI-1, WI-1
INDIANA	Indiana University	100	69	31	AZ-3, AR-1, BC-1, CA-2, ID-3, MA-1, MI-2, NV-2, NC-1, OH-1, OR-2, PR-1, TX-5, UT-2, WA-3, WI-1
IOWA	University of Iowa	78	63	15	CO-1, FL-1, GA-1, HI-1, ID-2, MD-1, MT-1, ND-1, NV-1, UT-1, WI-2, WY-1, international-1
KENTUCKY	University of Kentucky	56	41	14	IL-2, VA-2, 1 each NC, OH, UT, CA, GA, MO, TN, IN, Canada, China
KENTUCKY	University of Louisville	82	47	34	AL-1, AZ-1, AR-2, CA-1, FL-1, GA-7, ID-1, IL-2, IN-4, MI-1, MO-1, NV-1, PA-1, SC-1, TN-1, UT-7, WA-2
LOUISIANA	Louisiana State University	60	58	2	AR-2
MARYLAND	University of Maryland	130	NR	NR	NR
MASSACHUSETTS	Boston University	115	9	106	AZ-3, CA-16, CO-1, DE-1, FL-13, GA-4, HI-1, ID-1, IL-1, LA-1, MD-2, MI-1, MT-1, NC-2, NH-1, NJ-2, NY-13, OH-1, OR-1, PA-4, RI-1, SC-2, TX-2, UT-2, VA-2, WA-3, WI-1, plus Canadian and international
MASSACHUSETTS	Harvard School of Dental Medicine	35	1	35	CA-8, CO-2, CT-1, FL-3, GA-1, IL-1, MD-1, MI-2, NC-2, NJ-1, NY-3, OH-1, PA-1, UT-1, Canada-4, Korea-1, Taiwan-1
MASSACHUSETTS	Tufts University	161	29	132	AK-1, AZ-3, CA-17, CO-1, CT-6, DE-1, FL-13, GA-4, ID-2, IL-3, IN-2, KS-1, ME-5, MI-1, MN-2, MS-1, MT-1, NC-3, NE-1, NH-3, NJ-7, NY-9, OR-3, PA-2, RI-3, TN-2, TX-6, UT-4, VA-1, Bulgaria-1, Ethiopia-1, Korea-10, Monaco-1, Nigeria-1
MICHIGAN	University of Detroit Mercy	78	52	25	AB-2, BC-1, ONT-11, FL-1, IL-1, Iran-1, NC-1, OH-2, OR-1, TX-3, WI-1
MICHIGAN	University of Michigan	105	63	42	AZ-2, CA-10, DC-1, GA-2, ID-1, IL-1, MO-1, MT-1, NV-1, NJ-2, NM-1, OH-5, UT-6, WA-4, WI-3, nonresident-1
MINNESOTA	University of Minnesota	96	NR	NR	NR
MISSISSIPPI	University of Mississippi	35	35	0	NA
MISSOURI	University of Missouri-Kansas City	102	68	34	KS-27, HI-1, NM-3, AR-2
NEBRASKA	Creighton University	85	15	70	AL-1, AZ-1, CA-5, CO-4, HI-1, ID-8, IL-2, IN-1, IA-2, KS-1, MN-3, MO-2, MT-1, NV-1, NM-5, NY-1, ND-6, PA-1, RI-1, SD-5, TX-1, UT-11, WA-4, WI-1, WY-1
NEBRASKA	University of Nebraska	47	NR	NR	NR
NEVADA	University of Nevada, Las Vegas	77	NR	NR	NR
NEW JERSEY	University of Medicine and Dentistry of New Jersey	1,548	58	38	AZ-1, CA-4, GA-1, MI-1, NY-29, OH-1, PA-1

Source: Individual schools   NR = not reported   NA = not available or not applicable

TABLE 3-5. THE CLASS ENTERING FALL 2006 AT DENTAL SCHOOLS BY STATE OF RESIDENCE (CONTINUED)

	DENTAL SCHOOL	TOTAL 1ST YEAR ENROLLEES	IN-STATE	OUT-OF-STATE+	
NEW YORK	Columbia University	76	NA	NA	NA
NEW YORK	New York University	232	NR	NR	NR
NEW YORK	Stony Brook University	39	35	4	IN-1, KY-1, RI-1, UT-1
NEW YORK	University at Buffalo	86	47	39	AZ-4, CA-4, WA-4, CO-3, MA-3, MI-3, TX-3, UT-3, NH-2, NJ-2, PA-2, ID-1, MD-1, MN-1, ONT-1, VA-1, WI-1
NORTH CAROLINA	University of North Carolina at Chapel Hill	81	69	13	CA-1, FL-1, GA-1, ID-1, LA-1, NV-1, SC-1, TN-1, UT-3, VA-2
OHIO	Case School of Dental Medicine	70	15	54	AZ-1, CA-2, CO-1, ID-5, IN-3, MA-1, MD-1, MI-4, MN-1, NV-1, PA-1, TN-1, TX-1, UT-12, VA-2, WA-7, WY-1, Canada-6, Korea-3
OHIO	The Ohio State University	102	76	26	UT-13, ID-4, CA-2, IN-2, AZ-1, DE-1, NV-1, WA-1, WV-1
OKLAHOMA	University of Oklahoma	58	48	10	CA-2, MN-1, UT-7
OREGON	Oregon Health & Science University	75	52	23	AZ-9, ID-3, AK-2, MT-2, NM-2, CA-1, HI-1, NV-1, WA-1, WY-1
PENNSYLVANIA	Temple University	125	40	85	AZ-3, CA-7, CO-2, CT-1, DE-3, FL-10, GA-2, ID-3, IL-2, IN-1, MD-1, NC-3, NH-1, NJ-9, NM-1, NY-5, OH-2, OR-2, TX-1, UT-17, VA-6, WA-2, WI-1
PENNSYLVANIA	University of Pennsylvania	117	16	101	AK-1, AZ-3, CA-9, CT-1, FL-8, GA-2, IL-7, KY-1, MA-1, MD-2, MI-4, MN-1, MT-1, NC-1, NJ-12, NY-11, OH-4, OR-1, TN-1, TX-4, UT-2, VA-6, WA-3, WI-1, WV-1, Canada-3, Ecuador-1, Indonesia-1, Korea-5, Singapore-1, Syria-1, Trinidad-1
PENNSYLVANIA	University of Pittsburgh	80	35	43	AK-1, AZ-4, CA-10, FL-3, ID-3, IN 1, MA-1, MD-2, MI-4, NJ-1, NY-4, OH-1, OK-1, TX-1, UT-4, VA-1, WA-3
PUERTO RICO	University of Puerto Rico	42	40	2	AZ-1, UT-1
SOUTH CAROLINA	Medical University of South Carolina	55	51	4	PA, NC, TN, GA, ID
TENNESSEE	Meharry Medical College	62	9	53	AL-1, AZ-1, CA-4, CO-1, FL-1, GA-8, IL-1, IN-1, LA-3, MD-1, MI-2, MS-2, NC-6, NJ-1, NV-2, OK-1, PR-2, SC-1, TX-9, VA-1, International-4
TENNESSEE	University of Tennessee	80	51	29	AL-2, AR-19, GA-2, KS-1, MS-3, TX-2
TEXAS	Baylor College of Dentistry	95	88	7	AZ-1, CA-1, IL-1, NM-2, OK-1, UT-1
TEXAS	University of Texas Health Science Center at Houston	84	83	1	NM-1
TEXAS	University of Texas Health Science Center at San Antonio	96	89	7	ID-2, UT-4, WA-1
VIRGINIA	Virginia Commonwealth University	90	NR	NR	Numbers not specified: CA, FL, ID, IN, MA, NC, NH, NJ, NV, NY, PA, UT
WASHINGTON	University of Washington	55	45	10	AK-1, CA-3, HI-1, ID-1, MT-2, LA-1, KY-1
WEST VIRGINIA	West Virginia University	50	31	19	FL-1, GA-1, LA-1, MD-1, NM-2, NY-3, OR-1, PA-3, PR-1, UT-2, VA-1, Korea-1, Kuwait-1
WISCONSIN	Marquette University	80	40	40	AK-4, CA-3, CO-1, FL-1, IL-10, LA-1, MI-5, MN-1, MO-1, NM-2, NY-1, NC-1, ND-1, OH-1, OR-2, PA-1, TN-1, TX-1, UT-3
ALBERTA	University of Alberta	34	31	3	NR
BRITISH COLUMBIA	University of British Columbia	40	NR	NR	NR
MANITOBA	University of Manitoba	29	24	5	AB-3, BC-2
NOVA SCOTIA	Dalhousie University	36	NR	NR	NR
ONTARIO	University of Toronto	68	NR	NR	4 int'l. (all from U.S.)
ONTARIO	University of Western Ontario	55	NR	NR	NR
QUEBEC	McGill University	20	NR	NR	NR
QUEBEC	Université de Montréal	NR	NR	NR	NR
QUEBEC	Université Laval	48	NR	NR	NR
SASKATCHEWAN	University of Saskatchewan	28	22	6	AB–1, BC-2, MB-1, ONT-2

Source: Individual schools   NR = not reported   NA = not available or not applicable

TABLE 3-6. COMBINED AND OTHER DEGREE PROGRAMS BY DENTAL SCHOOL

STATE, TERRITORY, OR PROVINCE	DENTAL SCHOOL	Ph.D.	M.S.	M.P.H.	M.D.	Other	B.A./B.S.	Additional Information
ALABAMA	University of Alabama at Birmingham	Yes*	Yes	Yes	No	Yes	No	*An integrated clinician scientist training program where students earn both a D.M.D. and a Ph.D. degree in a biomedical science.
ARIZONA	Arizona School of Dentistry & Oral Health	No	No	No	No	No	No	Certificate in Public Health required during D.M.D. program.
ARIZONA	Midwestern University	No	No	No	No	No	No	
CALIFORNIA	Loma Linda University	Yes	Yes	No	No	No	Yes	
CALIFORNIA	University of California, Los Angeles	Yes	Yes	No	No	Yes	No	
CALIFORNIA	University of California, San Francisco	Yes	Yes	No	Yes	Yes	Yes	
CALIFORNIA	University of Southern California	Yes	Yes	No	No	Yes	Yes	
CALIFORNIA	University of the Pacific	No	No	No	No	No	No	
COLORADO	University of Colorado	No	No	No	No	No	Yes	
CONNECTICUT	University of Connecticut	Yes	Yes	Yes	Yes	No	Yes	
DISTRICT OF COLUMBIA	Howard University	No	No	No	No	No	Yes*	*Combination six-year program for Howard University students admitted into the Dental School after the second year of undergraduate studies.
FLORIDA	Nova Southeastern University	No	No	Yes	No	No	No	
FLORIDA	University of Florida	No	Yes	Yes	No	No	Yes	
GEORGIA	Medical College of Georgia	Yes	Yes	No	No	No	No	
ILLINOIS	Southern Illinois University	Yes	Yes	Yes	No	No	Yes	
ILLINOIS	University of Illinois at Chicago	Yes*	Yes*	No	No	No	Yes	*Seven-year program. **Four- to five-year program.
INDIANA	Indiana University	Yes	No	Yes	No	No	No	
IOWA	University of Iowa	Yes	Yes	Yes	No	No	Yes	
KENTUCKY	University of Kentucky	Yes	Yes	No	No	No	No	
KENTUCKY	University of Louisville	Yes	Yes	No	Yes	No	No	M.P.H. may be pursued through U of L Graduate School.
LOUISIANA	Louisiana State University	Yes	No	No	No	No	No	
MARYLAND	University of Maryland	Yes	No	No	No	No	Yes*	*B.S./D.D.S. with schools within the University of Maryland system.
MASSACHUSETTS	Boston University	Yes	Yes	No	No	Yes	Yes	
MASSACHUSETTS	Harvard School of Dental Medicine	Yes	Yes	Yes	Yes	Yes	No	Additional degrees may be pursued through other Harvard University schools, including the Harvard School of Public Health, the Kennedy School of Government, and Harvard Medical School. A new Ph.D. program, Biological Sciences in Dental Medicine, was introduced in 2001 in conjunction with Harvard's Graduate School of Arts and Sciences. In addition, HSDM students have pursued the Ph.D. degree at the Massachusetts Institute of Technology.
MASSACHUSETTS	Tufts University	No	Yes	Yes	No	Yes	Yes	
MICHIGAN	University of Detroit Mercy	No	No	No	No	Yes	Yes	Six-year B.S./D.D.S. program for eligible high school students seeking matriculation to the undergraduate university (College of Engineering and Science)
MICHIGAN	University of Michigan	Yes	No	No	No	No	Yes	
MINNESOTA	University of Minnesota	Yes	No	No	No	Yes	No	
MISSISSIPPI	University of Mississippi	No	No	No	No	No	No	
MISSOURI	University of Missouri-Kansas City	Yes	Yes	No	No	No	Yes	
NEBRASKA	Creighton University	No	No	No	No	No	No	
NEBRASKA	University of Nebraska	Yes	Yes	No	No	No	No	
NEVADA	University of Nevada, Las Vegas	No	No	No	No	Yes*	No	*M.B.A.

Source: Individual schools

TABLE 3-6. COMBINED AND OTHER DEGREE PROGRAMS BY DENTAL SCHOOL (CONTINUED)

STATE, TERRITORY, OR PROVINCE	DENTAL SCHOOL	Ph.D.	M.S.	M.P.H.	M.D.	Other	B.A./B.S.	Additional Information
NEW JERSEY	University of Medicine and Dentistry of New Jersey	Yes	Yes	Yes	No	Yes	Yes	
NEW YORK	Columbia University	Yes	Yes	Yes	Yes	Yes	No	
NEW YORK	New York University	Yes*	Yes	Yes**	No	Yes	Yes	* Ph.D. in Epidemiology. **M.P.H. in Global Public Health and D.D.S./M.P.H. program.
NEW YORK	Stony Brook University	Yes	Yes	Yes	Yes*	No	No	*M.D. awarded as part of OMFS.
NEW YORK	University at Buffalo	Yes	Yes	Yes	No	No	Yes	
NORTH CAROLINA	University of North Carolina at Chapel Hill	Yes	No	Yes	No	No	No	
OHIO	Case School of Dental Medicine	No	No	Yes	Yes*	No	Yes	*D.M.D./M.D. in conjunction with the Case School of Dental Medicine; five-year program followed by a one-year residency in medicine required prior to licensure.
OHIO	The Ohio State University	Yes	Yes	No	No	No	No	
OKLAHOMA	University of Oklahoma	No	Yes	No	No	Yes	Yes	
OREGON	Oregon Health & Science University	No	Yes	No	No	No	No	
PENNSYLVANIA	Temple University	No	Yes	No	No	Yes*	Yes	*M.S. in Oral Biology, D.M.D./M.B.A.
PENNSYLVANIA	University of Pennsylvania	Yes	Yes	Yes	Yes*	Yes*	Yes	*Oral surgery is a six-year M.D.-certificate program
PENNSYLVANIA	University of Pittsburgh	No	No	No	No	Yes*	Yes	*M.B.A.
PUERTO RICO	University of Puerto Rico	Yes	No	No	No	No	No	
SOUTH CAROLINA	Medical University of South Carolina	Yes	No	No	No	No	No	
TENNESSEE	Meharry Medical College	Yes	No	No	No	No	No	
TENNESSEE	University of Tennessee	Yes	Yes	Yes	Yes*	No	Yes	*In combination with Oral & Maxillofacial Surgery program.
TEXAS	Baylor College of Dentistry	Yes	Yes	No	No	No	Yes	
TEXAS	University of Texas Health Science Center at Houston	Yes	Yes	No	No	No	Yes	
TEXAS	University of Texas Health Science Center at San Antonio	Yes	Yes	Yes	Yes	No	Yes	
VIRGINIA	Virginia Commonwealth University	Yes	Yes	No	No	No	No	
WASHINGTON	University of Washington	Yes*	Yes	Yes	No	No	No	*Seven-year D.D.S./Ph.D. program for students committed to an academic or research career in dentistry and dental research.
WEST VIRGINIA	West Virginia University	Yes	Yes	No	No	No	Yes	
WISCONSIN	Marquette University	Yes	Yes	No	No	No	Yes	
ALBERTA	University of Alberta	No	No	No	No	Yes*	No	*B.Med.Sc.
BRITISH COLUMBIA	University of British Columbia	No	No	No	No	No	No	
MANITOBA	University of Manitoba	No	No	No	No	Yes*	No	*B.Sc.Dent.
NOVA SCOTIA	Dalhousie University	No	Yes	No	Yes	Yes*	No	*D.D.S. qualifying program.
ONTARIO	University of Toronto	Yes	Yes	No	No	No	No	
ONTARIO	University of Western Ontario	Yes	Yes	No	No	No	No	
QUEBEC	McGill University	No	Yes	No	No	No	No	
QUEBEC	Université de Montréal	Yes	Yes	No	No	Yes	No	
QUEBEC	Université Laval	Yes	Yes	Yes	No	No	No	
SASKATCHEWAN	University of Saskatchewan	No	No	No	No	Yes	Yes	

Source: Individual schools

CHAPTER 4
FINANCING YOUR DENTAL EDUCATION

As we explained in chapter 1, one of the benefits of becoming a dentist is the high level of professional income you can expect to earn over the course of your career. But if you're a prospective student without significant personal or family resources and are already, perhaps, carrying student loans from your undergraduate studies, you may think, "How can I possibly get there from here?" There is no denying that dental school is expensive, and it's easy for prospective students to see this cost as an insurmountable obstacle and to wonder how in the world they can afford such an expense. The basic message is, "you can!"

Regardless of your socioeconomic background you can afford a dental education through a combination of financial aid and wise management of your money. It is important for you to keep four things in mind regarding the cost of dental school.

- First, as a dentist, your anticipated income will enable you to repay educational loans in a timely fashion. The most recent American Dental Association survey of dentists who graduated in the last ten years found that only 17 percent needed to extend their repayment periods beyond the standard ten years, while 27 percent had been able to accelerate their payments to pay off their loans early.

- Second, a dental education is a sound investment that will pay off in both significant lifetime income and other professional benefits. Dentists are in the top five percent of the nation's wage earners. Though incomes vary across the country and depend on type of practice, in 2002 the average net income for new dentists graduating from U.S. dental schools between 1999 and 2001 was $142,461; for graduates between 1996 and 1998 it was $153,174; and for graduates between 1992 and 1995 it was $174,565.

- Third, you are not alone in needing help in financing your dental education. Most dental students rely on financial assistance to help pay for dental school.

- And, fourth, funds to help you pay for dental school are readily available. While grants, scholarships, and loan assistance are certainly not inexhaustible, their availability means that a shortage of money should not be an insurmountable obstacle to your attending dental school.

As you will see in the individual dental school entries in Part II of this book, tuition and fees vary widely from school to school. One of the biggest factors is the cost of tuition, which depends on whether the school is a private or state-supported institution. Living expenses will also vary as they reflect the cost of living in the area where the school is located.

Your particular needs will depend on your family's financial circumstances and where you pursue your dental education. This chapter will introduce you to the financing basics: how to apply for student aid; what loan, scholarship, and grant options are available; how to plan to repay your student debt; and how to build and keep good credit. The chapter ends with a glossary of terms related to student aid. It can help you communicate effectively with the experts who will assist you with this important process.

TYPES OF FINANCIAL AID

Financial aid programs are available to cover the education costs you or your family cannot pay for. Two major types are available to dental students: 1) scholarships and grants, both of which are gift aid and can be based on merit, special interests, or financial need; and 2) loans, which are funds that must be repaid. Later in this chapter we will explain different types of scholarships and grants. This section focuses on applying for federal aid, open to U.S. citizens and eligible permanent residents, which constitutes the majority of all available financial aid.

Need-based programs can include subsidized, low-interest loans, grants, scholarships, and work-study programs (which allow you to work, usually on campus around your class schedule). The amount of total need-based aid you can receive is determined by the following formula: Cost of Attendance – Expected Family Contribution = Financial Need.

The cost of attendance is determined by the dental school where you enroll. The calculated family contribution is based on the financial information that you (and perhaps your family) provide on the school's financial aid application forms.

Most need-based aid is sponsored by the federal government and is administered by the U.S. Department of Education (ED) in the case of Title IV aid and the U.S. Department of Health and Human Services (HHS) in the case of Title VII aid. Many dental schools offer institutional need-based assistance, as do a number of states. Loans are usually either low interest or interest-free while you are enrolled in school. To receive need-based funds from federally sponsored programs, you must meet other eligibility criteria including being a U.S. citizen or permanent resident and maintaining satisfactory academic progress.

Cost-based aid (also referred to as non-need based aid) is different from need-based aid because it does not require you or your family to demonstrate financial need. Instead, cost-based aid is determined as follows: Cost of Attendance – Estimated Financial Aid = Cost-Based Eligibility

As a result, cost-based financial aid can serve as a useful financing mechanism for students who may not qualify for adequate need-based assistance and have minimal financial resources of their own to pay for the full cost of their dental education. The federal government, private organizations, and some dental schools offer cost-based loan assistance programs. Note that cost-based aid consists **primarily** of loans, and creditworthiness is usually a criterion for eligibility. A student's total education loan debt may also be a factor in determining eligibility for cost-based aid.

Merit-based and other non-need-based grants and scholarships are given to students who meet certain criteria. These funds may be awarded by the dental school itself, private organizations, and individual states.

APPLYING FOR FINANCIAL AID

To begin the process, you will need to complete and submit a Free Application for Federal Student Aid (FAFSA). This U.S. Department of Education form is designed to determine your eligibility for federal and state financial aid and should be completed as soon as possible after January 1 of the year you plan to begin dental school. There is no charge for acquiring or submitting the form. You can obtain a copy of the FAFSA on the web at www.fafsa.ed.gov or from your college or university. **It is best to submit the FAFSA electronically.** This website provides a worksheet and also answers a range of questions.

At about the same time, using the information in Part II of this guide, you should contact the dental schools where you plan to apply to ask if you need to fill out additional financial aid forms or submit other materials. Application requirements vary from school to school. You may be required to submit the FAFSA application, an institutional application, and tax returns. Some schools may require parental financial information for you to be considered for institutional or need-based financial aid. Parental information is required if you want to be considered for federal Title VII financial aid programs (see glossary).

You must meet schools' application deadlines to be considered for the most favorable types of financial aid. Be aware that meeting deadlines could make the difference in the type of financial aid you receive, *so find out what they are and don't procrastinate!*

The financial aid application process may seem complicated. Remember that most dental students receive financial aid, and that financial aid officers at dental schools are prepared to serve as resources.

■ Basis for Awarding Financial Aid

Financial aid funds are awarded to students on the basis of financial need, cost, merit, group association, or on a combination of factors. Dental students are generally considered independent students (that is, not dependent on their parents) and are expected to contribute their own income and assets toward educational costs. Financial aid officers will conduct a need analysis of your and, if applicable, your spouse's information. In some cases, your parents' financial information will also be used to determine whether you are eligible for financial aid.

You may be required to submit copies of your (and your spouse's) tax returns to substantiate the information you provided on your FAFSA. Depending on the type of financial aid programs for which you are applying, you may be required to provide your parents' financial information on the FAFSA as well as copies of their tax returns. Schools may also have additional forms, such as an institutional financial aid application and may request other documentation from both you, your spouse, and, possibly, your parents.

Income tax returns reveal certain kinds of untaxed income, such as interest from tax-exempt bonds, untaxed portions of pensions and social security benefits, and earned income credits. Tax returns can also be useful in interpreting more complex situations, especially when income is derived from sources other than wages or salaries from employment. Wage statements (W-2 forms) are also useful in documenting income, especially for earnings of non-tax filers and tax-deferred income. Descriptions of situations affecting your ability to pay, such as unusual medical and dental expenses, child care costs, and unreimbursed employee business expenses may also be requested.

■ Use of Professional Judgment

The financial aid officer (FAO) at the dental school you attend may make adjustments to your need analysis in a process called "professional judgment." If your FAO believes it is appropriate, for instance, he or she may adjust your cost of attendance or the information used to calculate your Expected Family Contribution to take into account circumstances that might affect the amount you're expected to contribute toward your education. These circumstances could include unusual medical or dental expenses. Also an adjustment may be made if you plan to apply for Title VII aid and a parent has been recently unemployed. If conditions such as these apply to you or your family, contact your FAO. There must be very good reasons for

TABLE 4-1. FORMS OF FINANCIAL AID

Loan
The primary source of financial aid for dental students. Must be repaid by the recipient.

Gift aid (scholarships/grants)
Merit-based or need-based aid. Does not have to be repaid by the recipient.

Research fellowships or traineeships
These offer stipends to students who conduct scientific research.

Commitment service scholarships
Commitment service scholarships provide support for educational and living expenses while a student is in school. In exchange, recipients are required to serve in the military or in health care shortage areas after graduation. Limited availability.

Loan repayment programs
After education is completed, a borrower who works in a health care shortage area providing care to underserved populations may be eligible for a federal or state loan repayment program. Examples include the Indian Health Service, National Health Service Corps, Faculty Loan Repayment program, National Institutes of Health, or state loan repayment program. The Armed Forces offers a loan repayment to eligible military personnel.

Education tax breaks
Student Loan Interest Deduction, Lifetime Learning Tax Credits, Tuition and Fees Deduction, and Education IRAs.

Work-study
Provides students an opportunity to work part time. (Because the dental school curriculum is demanding, dental students are often not able to take advantage of work-study support.)

the FAO to make any adjustments, and you will be required to provide adequate proof to support adjustments.

You can calculate your estimated financial need by visiting www.finaid.org/calculators and clicking on financial need estimation. The need analysis formula used by this estimation program is a slight simplification and has no official standing, so do not expect that the results represent the exact financial aid you will receive. It is possible that you will receive less aid than the figures reported by this form because of the aid granting institution's limited funds. However, this website is useful in giving you an estimate to work with, and it can also help you figure out how much attending dental school will cost and how much you need to save.

■ Determining What You Need

The purpose of federally authorized student financial aid is to assist a student in meeting costs associated with obtaining his or her education. It is not intended to support a spouse or dependents. Students need to understand that a financial aid award package anticipates that a student's spouse will contribute financially to support the household.

Obtaining a dental education represents a substantial financial commitment. It's important for you to plan a budget and stick to it for a number of years. While you should view all your student loans to pay for dental school as an investment in your future that will pay handsome returns, you will nevertheless want to be as prudent as possible to minimize what you have to pay back.

First, understand your current financial status by taking stock of all your financial commitments prior to entering dental school. The easiest way to do this is by making a log of all outstanding debt, including undergraduate student loan and consumer debt (such as car loans and credit cards). Write down the total dollar amount owed for each loan along with the amount of any interest that has accrued, the current interest rate, and the amount you must pay monthly. (See an example in Table 4-2.) Once this is done, you will be better able to determine your ability to handle additional debt.

Second, you should evaluate your financial resources. Write down anticipated annual income during school that you will receive from employment (if any) along with any other income to which you will have access (like spouse's income). Next, determine what other resources are available to help pay for school such as savings, parent contributions, gifts, scholarships and grants that you've been awarded, and tuition waivers.

Third, you should determine what your expenses will be during dental school. The financial aid office at your dental school will already have developed an estimate of what you will need. While you can use this estimate as a guide, you should go through the exercise yourself to ensure you come up with the same or a similar figure. Cost of attendance typically includes tuition, books, fees, room and board, transportation, miscellaneous personal expenses, and child care (if applicable). Credit card debt cannot be included in the cost of attendance. After you have made an accurate estimate of your first year's expenses, you can probably estimate the cost for four years by adding five percent per year. Your FAO can assist you if you need help. Table 4-3 is an example of a budget work sheet that may help you determine your needs.

Finally, the Financial Aid Office, after careful review of your application materials, will notify you about your financial aid award package. This notice usually pro-

TABLE 4-2. EXAMPLE OF A STUDENT'S LOG OF OUTSTANDING DEBT ON ENTERING DENTAL SCHOOL

Loan/debt	Current Balance	Interest Rate	Monthly Payment	Repayment Period
Stafford Loans	$16,000	6.8%	$185	10 years
Perkins Loans	$4,000	5%	$42	10 years
Credit card**	$8,000	18%	$173	Monthly

While attending dental school full time, you are eligible to apply for an in-school deferment on federal student loans (Stafford and Perkins Loans).

**Credit card payments cannot be included in a dental student budget.

Source: Columbia University

vides details on financial aid programs for which you qualified and the dollar amount awarded or the recommended amount to borrow in federal loans (Perkins, Stafford, Graduate PLUS, etc.) and private/alternative loans. You should review the financial aid award package and follow instructions to secure the recommended funds to meet your budget. Once you've estimated your current financial obligations, what resources may be available, and what you will need, you will be better able to determine how much you will need to borrow. Most educational loan programs limit borrowing to cover the cost of attendance as determined by the institution's financial aid office.

Everyone is concerned about borrowing. You can look for places to reduce personal expenses while you are in dental school. Some strategies are to find a roommate to share housing; reduce entertainment and dining out expenses; use public transportation instead of a car; and avoid using credit cards if you cannot pay the bill in full at the end of each month.

■ Know the Players Involved in Your Student Loans

When you borrow for school, several parties are involved in the transaction with you. They typically are the lender, the federal government, the guaranty agency, the financial aid office, the holder of the loan or the secondary market, and the servicer. It is understandable to wonder how all these entities are involved with your student loan.

The U.S. Department of Education (ED) plays a major role in student lending through the Federal Family Education Loan Program (FFEL) and the Federal Direct Student Loan Program (FDSL). Both programs include federal subsidized and unsubsidized Stafford Loans and Graduate PLUS. FFEL loans are made by banks and other lenders. FDSL loans are made by ED through colleges and universities. The dental school will inform you if they participate in either the FDSL or FFEL loan programs. If they participate in the FFEL programs, they will normally provide students with a list of recommended lenders. Both programs are guaranteed by the federal government in case a borrower defaults on a loan.

A guaranty agency verifies that you are qualified for a particular federal loan program and insures loans for the lender. The guaranty agency is an organization that agrees to reimburse a lender for any portion of a student loan that is not repaid by a borrower. If a borrower defaults, the guaranty agency pays the lender the remaining amount owed and collects the balance directly from the borrower. Like lenders, many guaranty agencies offer debt counseling services and money management programs that can help you avoid default.

The lender is the provider of student loans. The lender mails a check or transfers funds to your school electronically. Check with the financial aid officer at the school you will attend for direction in choosing a lender, as most will have a list of recommended lenders.

The holder of a student loan is the owner of the promissory note (prom note) that you sign to receive a loan. The holder may be the original lender or another company that has purchased the loan. The purchasers are known collectively as the secondary market.

A servicer is a company contracted by a lender to handle all the administrative aspects of the loan. This means collecting loan payments, taking inquiries about loans, corresponding with borrowers, coordinating address changes, providing loan status updates, etc.

The Financial Aid Officer (FAO) at your school plays a major role in helping you obtain information on financing your dental education. The FAO will determine your eligibility for many different types of financial aid: grant aid, scholarships, and loans. The FAO also certifies your eligibility for student loans. An FAO provides information on your student loan portfolio including your lenders and billing servicers. The FAO's guidance on the repayment process can be helpful even after you graduate by providing information about postponing payments through deferment or forbearance arrangements. The FAO will work with you because he/she doesn't want your loan to go into default! If you encounter problems down the road and need guidance, your FAO is a great place to start.

TABLE 4-3. EXAMPLE OF A STUDENT'S BUDGET WORKSHEET

	Expense/ Month	Year 1 Total*
Mortgage or rent	$550	$6,600
Utilities: electric, gas, sewer, phone	$75	$900
Food: groceries, dining out	$350	$4,200
Personal (laundry, clothing, etc.)	$75	$900
Car payment, maintenance, gas, repair, parking, insurance	$300	$3,600
Home/apartment insurance	$25	$300
Life insurance	$50	$600

Examples of expenses that are not allowable in a student budget include: credit card payments; alimony; household goods and furnishings; interview expenses (suits, travel, etc.); student loan repayment; savings/emergency fund.

After you have made an accurate estimate of your first year's expenses, calculate the cost for four years of dental education by adding 5% to each subsequent year to account for inflation.

*Assumes a 12-month budget. Check with your school for the length of the academic year.

AN OVERVIEW OF STUDENT LOAN PROGRAMS

It's important to realize that, although student loans must be repaid by the borrower, they are considered financial aid. Financial aid cannot exceed a student's cost of education as determined by the school. Student loans differ from other types of consumer loans because most defer repayment of both the loan's principal and interest while you are enrolled. Also, most have grace periods so that you will have a period of time after graduation (or withdrawal) to prepare financially for repayment. Interest rates on student loans are usually lower than most other types of consumer credit and come with additional benefits such as deferment of repayment of the loan if you continue your education after graduation. Table 4-4 is a quick reference guide to some of the programs available to dental students.

The government pays the interest on the Subsidized Stafford loan while you're in school and during grace or other deferment periods. Since the Perkins, Health Professions Student Loan (HPSL), Loans for Disadvantaged Students (LDS), and most institutional loans do not assess interest while you are in school or during grace or deferment periods, they are sometimes also called "subsidized loans."

Unsubsidized loans, on the other hand, accrue interest during school, grace, and deferment periods. Although you can usually postpone payment during these periods, it is ultimately your responsibility to repay both the principal and accrued interest. You should keep in mind that all accrued unpaid interest will eventually be capitalized. You can contact your lender to find out when the first capitalization will occur and how frequently thereafter. Examples of unsubsidized loans are unsubsidized Stafford or Grad PLUS loans.

TABLE 4-4: QUICK REFERENCE GUIDE TO LOAN PROGRAMS

	Annual Limit	Aggregate Limit	Interest rate while enrolled in school	Interest rate while in repayment (July 1, 2006-June 30, 2007)	Grace Period (months)	Repayment Term
Federal Stafford Loan (Subsidized)+	$8,500	$65,500	6.8% (interest is paid by the federal government)	6.8%	6 months	10 years
Federal Stafford Loan (Unsubsidized)+	$40,500 (minus Subsidized Stafford Loan Amount)	$189,125 (includes subsidized Stafford borrowing)	6.8% (interest payments can be postponed until start of repayment)	6.8%	6 months	10 years
Federal Perkins Loan	$6,000	$40,000	No interest is assessed while in school	5% Fixed Rate	9 months	10 years
Health Professions Student Loan (HPSL)	Can't exceed student's annual COA - EFC	None	No interest is assessed while in school	5% Fixed Rate	12 months	10 years
Loans for Disadvantaged Students (LDS)	Can't exceed student's annual COA - EFC	None	No interest is assessed while in school	5% Fixed Rate	12 months	10 years
Institutional Loans	Varies by School	Varies by School	Usually interest free or low interest rate	Usually interest free or low interest rate	Varies by School	Varies by School
Private/Alternative Loan Programs	Up to cost of attendance minus other financial aid	Varies by Lender	Varies by Lender	Some lenders increase interest rates when loans go into repayment	Varies by Lender	Varies by Lender
Graduate PLUS	Can't exceed student's annual COA-OFA	None	8.5%	8.5%	None	10 years

NOTES:

See glossary for definitions of terms you do not understand.

+ Terms apply to FFEL Staffords and William Ford Direct Staffords.

* Repayment periods on Stafford Loans can extend up to 25 years.

U.S. citizens and permanent residents studying at dental schools in Canada are eligible to apply for Stafford Loans as well as other federal student aid programs. If you need additional monies you may have to rely on private/alternative loans. International students generally have fewer options available for financing.

■ Federal Stafford Loan Program

The interest rate for Stafford Loans (whether subsidized or unsubsidized) first disbursed on or after July 1, 2006, is fixed for the life of the loan at 6.8%. You may have a fee of up to 2.5 percent (assumes 1.5% origination fee and up to 1% guarantee fee) deducted proportionately from each disbursement of your loan. A portion of this fee goes to the federal government to help reduce the cost of the loans. Many lenders and guaranty agencies waive all or part of this fee.

Generally, repayment begins after a six-month grace period that starts at graduation. Repayment can be postponed during some postgraduate programs and in certain other situations. When you start repaying, the monthly amount due will depend on the principal you owe at that time and the length of your repayment period. You have the option of repaying your loan using a fixed, graduated, or income-sensitive repayment plan. The standard repayment term is ten years, but if your Stafford Loan is greater than $30,000, you may have up to 30 years to repay based on educational debt.

Stafford Loans are either subsidized or unsubsidized. The subsidized Stafford Loan is awarded on the basis of financial need, which is determined by the information you provide on the FAFSA and other supporting financial aid application materials your school may require. If you qualify for a subsidized loan, the federal government pays interest on the loan (subsidizes the loan) while you are in school at least half time and during grace and deferment periods. Dental students may qualify to borrow up to $8,500 in subsidized Stafford Loans annually. The aggregate amount of subsidized Stafford Loans a dental student can owe throughout his or her education (from undergraduate freshman through postgraduate training) is $65,500.

Although the Financial Aid Office is required to first determine a student's eligibility for a Subsidized Stafford Loan, the Unsubsidized Stafford Loan is not awarded on the basis of financial need. If you qualify for an unsubsidized loan, you will be charged interest from the time the loan is disbursed until it is paid in full. You may choose to pay the interest while you are in school or allow it to accumulate ("accrue"). If you allow the interest to accrue, it will be added to the principal amount of your loan ("capitalized") and will increase the amount you have to repay. If you pay the interest before it capitalizes, you'll repay less in the long run. You're obligated to pay the interest on an unsubsidized loan—even the amount that accrues while you are in school and during times of grace and deferment. The annual outstanding maximum Unsubsidized Stafford Loan a dental student can borrow is $40,500 minus the amount of a Subsidized Stafford Loan a student is eligible to borrow.

■ Federal Perkins Loan Program

The Federal Perkins Loan Program provides long-term, low-interest loans to students with exceptional financial need. The annual maximum loan amount is $6,000 and the cumulative amount a borrower can owe is $40,000. Loans are made through a school's financial aid office. The school is the lender. This loan has an interest rate of five percent. The borrower is not charged interest during in-school, grace, or deferment periods and has a fixed ten-year repayment term. There is a nine-month grace period. Repayment can be postponed during some post graduate programs and in certain other situations. Check with the financial aid office at the school you plan to attend to determine application and repayment procedures.

■ Health Professions Student Loan Program (HPSL)

HPSL offers loans made from revolving loan funds administered by participating schools. These loans are federally funded, and parental financial information is required to determine eligibility. Borrowers may qualify for loans up to the cost of attendance. Because of funding limitations, HPSL awards will probably be much smaller than cost of attendance. HPSL has an interest rate of five percent. The borrower is not charged interest during in-school, grace, or deferment periods and has a fixed ten-year repayment term. There is a 12-month grace period, and repayment may be deferred for postgraduate training and up to three years for service in the military. Check with the financial aid office at the school you plan to attend to determine application and repayment procedures.

■ Loans for Disadvantaged Students Program (LDS)

LDS is open to students who demonstrate financial need and who meet the criteria of "disadvantaged student." Terms of the loan are identical to HPSL. This loan program is not available at all institutions. Check with the financial aid office at the school where you are applying to determine application and repayment procedures.

■ Graduate PLUS

Graduate PLUS loans are federal loan funds that a student can borrow as an alternative to private education loans. This is an unsubsidized loan, so interest accrues while the student is enrolled in school and during any eligible deferment period. There is no annual or aggregate loan limit. The loan amount you're eligible to borrow annually is based on your yearly cost of attendance as determined by the school minus other financial aid that you will be receiving. Students must have maximized their Stafford Loan annual borrowing limits before they can access "Grad PLUS." In addition, Grad PLUS borrowers are required to undergo a credit check to ensure no adverse credit history. The credit criteria for Grad PLUS are less stringent than some private education loan programs. However, if a potential borrower is denied Grad PLUS funds, he or she can add a qualified "endorser." This loan has no grace period and a maximum repayment term of 10 years. Borrowers with a cumulative Grad PLUS debt of $30,000 or more can request extended repayment

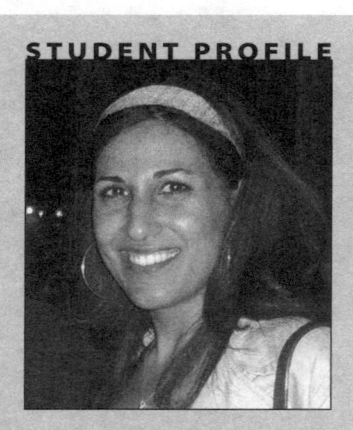

STUDENT PROFILE

SUMMER TOTONCHI
SOUTHERN ILLINOIS UNIVERSITY

Why dentistry?
I knew I wanted to be in a health profession, because I wanted to make people feel better and guide them to better health. Then I found that there are so many options within the field of dentistry. It's both science — ortho is like physics for teeth! — and art. You can be a generalist, or you can specialize.

The first and second years of dental school are not easy. You really have to be determined to stick with it. It can be hard to adjust to the workload and to learn to manage your time. But I don't focus on being first in the class, I focus on doing my best and working up to my abilities. It's rewarding to see how I have improved when I look back over a semester or a year. In clinic, the patients will notice your improvement too. And the teachers definitely notice — then they give you harder things to do!

What are you doing now?
I'm a third-year student at Southern Illinois University, and I love clinic. It can be intimidating to get into, and it takes time. I still haven't done all the procedures yet. But once you get over the hump where you're sitting there looking at the patient, thinking "Oh no, I've forgotten everything I learned in the past two years," it's exciting to apply your knowledge and work to solve the patient's problems.

Where do you see yourself in five years?
Working in a private practice. I don't know if my fiancé and I will work together or not — he would like to pursue a specialty. I know that I want to work at least part time in academia. I have always enjoyed tutoring and helping other students.

Advice to applicants and first-year students
Concentrate on the sciences. Take the prerequisites and any extra courses you might have to take in dental school, like microbiology. It does help to be exposed to the material more than once.

Observe at a dental office. It definitely pushed me more into the field. I shadowed several days a week over several weeks.

Get some research experience. That kind of independent problem solving really teaches you to work through a problem and connect the dots. It's just like dental school in that you get lots of bits and pieces the first two years, then in clinic you put them all together in a treatment plan.

Once you're in dental school, it's good to be involved in dental school activities. In fact, if I didn't attend ADEA meetings, I wouldn't have met my fiancé! But it's also great to interact with people from other dental schools and see their accomplishments and obstacles. It gives you good ideas to bring back to your own school.

And it's never too late to ask for help if you are not doing as well as you wanted to. Over time you will gain self-confidence and be able to say, "Yes, I can do this!" That will help you continue in what can be a stressful field.

What do you do for balance in your life?
That's hard to do when your life partner is also in dental school! Right now I divide my free time between exercise and wedding planning.

What is the last book you read?
Angels and Demons by Dan Brown – I only read half *The DaVinci Code,* but this is a different style of writing.

Are you married/partnered/single? Any children?
My fiancé is in dental school in California, and we're getting married in summer 2007. We have to figure out where we will live after I finish dental school. I was born in Baghdad, Iraq, but I moved to Chicago when I was 14 and have lived in Illinois ever since.

Ed Note: Ms. Totonchi is the student representative on the ADEA Annual Session Planning Committee.

schedules of up to 25 years. The interest rate on Grad PLUS loans is fixed at 8.5% for the life of the loan if taken from a FFELP lender, or 7.9% if borrowed under Direct Loans. Repayment can be deferred if you meet certain criteria such as continued enrollment as at least a half time student or economic hardship.

■ Institutional Loans

Some dental schools have institutional loan programs. Most often school loans have favorable terms and conditions. Check with the financial aid office at the school where you are applying to determine application and repayment procedures.

■ Private/Alternative Loans

Private/alternative loans are used to bridge the gap between the total cost of attendance and available resources. These loans should only be considered after you have exhausted all other possible funding sources. Private loans are available from banks and other lenders. When comparing these programs, we recommend that you compare the different loan terms including interest rates, fees, repayment options, capitalization policies, and deferment and forbearance options. A wide variety of loan features are available from one loan program to another. A standardized method, called Annual Percentage Rate (APR), exists to compare loan programs. APR is designed to calculate the yearly cost of loans, taking into account fees and other costs associated with securing a loan. APRs give you a way to assess the true cost of each loan program.

Private lenders usually require a credit check, and a cosigner may be an option. The interest rate on private loans is always variable, usually without a cap. Borrowers usually have up to 20 to 25 years to repay. Private loans are unsubsidized, so they should be repaid as quickly as possible. The loan servicer may allow principal payments to be made during the in-school and grace periods.

■ Master Promissory Note

A Master Promissory Note (MPN) opens a line of credit for an educational loan. Currently the most common use of a MPN is for Stafford Loans and Graduate PLUS. Schools may also use a MPN for Perkins, HPSL, and LDS loans. Using a MPN simplifies the loan application and promissory note process by reducing paper requirements and providing faster turnaround time when the multiyear feature is used. You will not be required to sign a new promissory note each time you request an additional loan where you have already completed a MPN as long as you remain with the same lender. If you change schools, you may be asked to sign a new MPN if the school has a different "preferred" lender; however, you may tell the new school that you wish to stay with your old lender.

OTHER AID

■ Federal Work-Study Program

This program provides jobs for students who are enrolled at least half time and have financial need. A participating educational institution arranges jobs on or off campus. Federal Work-Study earnings go toward meeting the financial need of a student. Because of the rigorous academic demands on dental students, many schools do not participate in this program, and those that do only make awards to students who request them. For more information, contact the financial aid offices at the dental schools to which you plan to apply.

■ "Outside" Scholarships (Those Not Awarded by a Dental School)

There are a variety of scholarship search databases available on the Internet. These websites allow an individual to enter demographic, academic, and personal data into a search engine that will identify scholarships for which that individual might meet eligibility criteria. Information on how to apply for the scholarships is then provided. A central site with links to several of these search locations is www.finaid.org/scholarships. It provides a free, comprehensive, independent, and objective guide to student financial aid. You should never pay for any scholarship search.

SOURCES OF AID FOR CANADIAN AND INTERNATIONAL STUDENTS

The availability of financial assistance for international students coming to the United States for academic study is limited. Federal student aid is restricted to U.S. citizens or permanent residents. Individual dental schools may have scholarships or grants for international students, but these are not common. Students should contact the school they are interested in applying to for specific information on any available institutional assistance.

International students can access private loan programs offered by banking institutions, but almost all programs require a credit-worthy U.S. citizen or permanent resident co-signer. There may also be restrictions on the type of visa (F1 or J1). In addition to the loans listed below, certain international students (e.g., permanent U.S. residents with a green card) may be eligible for Federal Stafford and PLUS loans. A resource currently available to international students exploring financing options is the Internet. An extensive compilation of financial aid for international students can be found at www.edupass.org/finaid/loans/phtml. International students may be eligible for private scholarships based on academic interest or merit. International students are also encouraged to contact the cultural section of their embassy or ministry of education to find out about funding available from their country's government.

The following are some private loan programs available to Canadian and other international students studying dentistry in the United States.

- Canadian Higher Education Loan Program (CanHELP), 888-296-4332; www.internationalstudentloan.com/canadian_student/
- GATE Student Loan Program (Guaranteed Access To Education), 800-895-4283; www.gateloan.com/
- Global Student Loan Corporation (GSLC), 212-736-9666; www.globalslc.com/
- International Student Loan Program (ISLP), 888-296-4332; www.internationalstudentloan.com/intl_student/
- Massachusetts Educational Financing Authority Loan program (MEFA), 800-449-6332; www.mefa.org/index.php
- TERI Education Loans, 800-255-TERI; www.teri.org/lp_health.html

FEDERALLY FUNDED SCHOLARSHIPS

■ Scholarships for Disadvantaged Students Program (SDS)

The SDS program provides funds to U.S. citizen and permanent residents who are full-time, financially needy students from disadvantaged backgrounds enrolled in health professions programs. Funds are awarded to eligible schools by HHS. The schools are responsible for selecting recipients, making reasonable determinations of need and disadvantaged student status, and making awards. The maximum award cannot exceed a student's financial need. Students interested in applying for this scholarship must provide parental income information, regardless of age or marital status, and should contact a student financial aid office at schools they are interested in for any special application procedures. Please note that not all schools qualify for SDS funding.

■ National Health Service Corps (NHSC) Scholarship Program

The NHSC mission is to help meet the health care needs of underserved communities. Only applicants who share the NHSC's commitment and who agree to provide oral health services for a minimum of two years in any underserved community identified by the NHSC will be competitive for a scholarship award. The NHSC scholarship pays tuition and fees, books, supplies, and equipment and includes a monthly stipend. For more information, visit http://nhsc.bhpr.hrsa.gov/.

■ Armed Forces Health Professions Scholarships

The U.S. Armed Services offer scholarships to dental students that pay tuition fees, books, instruments, and a stipend. To qualify, applicants must be U.S. citizens between the ages of 21 and 40 (although age limits can be waived in certain cases) and be a graduate of a dental school accredited by the American Dental Association. The service obligation is at least three years of active duty depending on the program under which the applicant receives his or her commission.

- The Armed Forces Health Professionals Scholarship Program provides full tuition for up to four years of dental training, including all school-required fees and expenses, books, and equipment (excludes food, housing, and computers). It also includes a monthly stipend.

- The Financial Assistance Program provides extra payment and a monthly stipend for dentists in residency. Residents also receive their current residency pay. After residency, dentists in this program agree to serve for a certain time. Once in the military, the pay is competitive and includes a signing bonus and fringe benefits.

For further information, contact a local recruiter for the military service in which you're interested.

■ National Institute of Dental and Craniofacial Research (NIDCR) Short-Term Training Awards

NIDCR offers numerous training programs for dental students who have an interest in dental research. For general information about training programs offered by the National Institutes of Health (NIH) and the NIDCR, contact Dr. Deborah Philp, 301-594-6578, dphilp@dir.nidcrnih.gov, or visit www.nidcr.nih.gov/Funding/Training/.

Dual Degree Programs (D.D.S. or D.M.D./Ph.D.). This program provides support to institutions to train dental students who want to pursue careers in biomedical research and academic dentistry. Students participate in an integrated program of graduate training in the biomedical sciences and clinical training offered through participating dental schools. Graduates receive a combined D.D.S. or D.M.D./Ph.D. degree. Funding is awarded directly to participating institutions, which then select the trainees. Trainees must be U.S. citizens, noncitizen nationals, or permanent residents. For more information, visit www.nidcr.nih.gov/Funding/Training/t32Contacts_Dual_Degree.htm.

NIDCR Summer Dental Student Award. To expose future dentists to research careers, NIDCR offers an outstanding research training opportunity for dental students. The Summer Dental Student Award is designed to promote the professional careers of talented dental students through exposure to the latest advances in oral health research. Selected candidates will be assigned to mentors who conduct research in the students' areas of interest. Students will gain hands-on experience in basic or clinical research. Participation in the program may result in presentation of research findings at a scientific meeting or co-authorship of scientific publications. The NIDCR provides a competitive stipend for a minimum of eight weeks during the summer. Student nomination and application begins in mid November each year. The application deadline is mid January each year. For more information on how to apply, interested candidates may visit: http://www.nidcr.nih.gov/Funding/Training/SummerDentalStudentAward.htm or contact Dr. Deborah Philp, Program Director, dphilp@dir.nidcr.nih.gov, 301-594-6578.

NIH Clinical Research Training Program. This program is designed to attract research-oriented dental and medical students to the campus of the National Institutes of Health in Bethesda, Maryland. Fellows spend a year engaged in a mentored clinical research project in an area that matches their personal interests and goals. An annual stipend is provided, and moving expenses are reimbursed. Candidates must have completed a year of clinical rotations prior to starting the program. U.S. citizenship or permanent residence is required. For more information, visit www.training.nih.gov/crtp/.

> *Interest rates on student loans are usually lower than most other types of consumer credit and come with additional benefits such as deferment of payment while the student is enrolled and for a grace period after graduation.*

Howard Hughes Medical Institutes Research Scholars Program. Participants of the NIH Howard Hughes Medical Institutes joint program work in NIH laboratories as part of a research team and are given the opportunity to attend conferences and meetings. Most students participate in the year-long program after their second or third year of dental or medical school. Candidates must be in good standing at a U.S. dental or medical school and must receive permission from their school to participate. An annual salary is provided. Joint Ph.D. candidates are not eligible. For more information, visit www.hhmi.org/science/cloister/.

Individual Predoctoral Dental Scientist Fellowship (F30). This fellowship provides a maximum of five years' support to students pursuing both D.D.S. or D.M.D. and Ph.D. degrees. An annual stipend and partial tuition are provided. Additional funds are available for other training-related expenses. Applicants must be enrolled in a D.D.S. or D.M.D. program at an accredited U.S. dental school and accepted in a related scientific Ph.D. (or equivalent degree) program. Students attending any accredited U.S. dental school may apply. Applicants must be U.S. citizens, noncitizen nationals, or permanent residents at the time of award. For more information, visit www.grants.nih.gov/grants/guide/pa-files/PA-02-004.html.

Individual Predoctoral Fellowship for Minority Students and Students with Disabilities (F31). This program provides a maximum of five years' support to students pursuing a Ph.D. degree. An annual stipend and partial tuition are provided. Additional funds are available for other training-related expenses. Applicants must be enrolled in a graduate school at an accredited U.S. university and be from an underrepresented minority group or have a disability. Applicants must also be U.S. citizens, noncitizen nationals, or permanent residents at the time of award. For more information, contact Lorrayne W. Jackson, 301-594-2616, jacksonl@mail.nih.gov or visit www.grants1.nih.gov/grants/guide/pa-files/PA-00-069.html.

Institutional NRSA Research Training Grant (T32). This grant provides support to institutions for several types of research training: 1) up to five years of support to individuals pursuing only a Ph.D.; 2) up to five years of support (with possibility of extension) to individuals pursuing a combined D.D.S. or D.M.D./Ph.D. degree; 3) up to one year of support for dental students wishing to interrupt their studies to engage in full-time research; and 4) up to three months per year to dental students or faculty wishing to gain research experience. Funding is awarded directly to participating institutions, which then select the trainees. Trainees must be U.S. citizens, noncitizen nationals, or permanent residents. For more information, visit www.grants.nih.gov/grants/guide/pa-files/PAR-00-116.html.

Graduate Partnerships Program. Prospective Ph.D. students wishing to pursue a doctoral degree in the biomedical sciences can apply to university programs that have a formal partnership with NIH. A stipend is provided. U.S. citizenship or permanent residence is required. For more information, visit www.gpp.nih.gov/.

PRIVATELY FUNDED SCHOLARSHIPS AND OTHER HELPFUL RESOURCES

There are a variety of scholarship search databases available on the Internet. To use them you must enter demographic, academic, and personal data into a search engine. A central site with links to several of these search locations is www.finaid.org/scholarships. It provides a free, comprehensive, independent, and objective guide to student financial aid. You should never pay for any scholarship search. Two other free scholarship search engines are www.FastWeb.com and www.wiredscholar.com.

■ Repaying Student Loans

Repayment of student loans is your responsibility, even if the lender is unable to locate you. Prevent loan default, a bad credit history, and other negative actions by being proactive about loan repayment. Depending on the loan program repayment begins either after graduation from dental school, when you leave school, or when you drop below full-time or half-time enrollment. This section will review the borrower's and lender's responsibilities in this process.

■ The Borrower's Responsibilities

There are some steps you can take to help reduce the amount and kinds of debt you take on. Often it isn't until students begin repaying student loans or seek additional funds to set up a dental practice that they review their records and discover how much they have borrowed (or charged on credit cards). It doesn't have to be that way. You can begin taking steps early on in your borrowing to monitor your spending habits and student loan portfolio. Students who keep track of their borrowing from the start are in a better position to manage repayment successfully.

Borrowing means that you have the benefit of someone else's money now, in exchange for paying it back with interest at a later date. Repaying your loans is a legal and professional obligation. Individuals who default on their loans face financial and legal consequences that can have negative effects both personally and professionally. Before applying for a loan, you should be aware of your responsibilities as a borrower. You are the key to making your borrowing experience a positive one. If you keep good records, open your mail, make sure your lenders and their billing servicers have your current address, and contact your lenders immediately if you have trouble paying, you should have success.

After you sign a promissory note and once funds have been disbursed, you are legally obligated to repay the loan according to the terms of the note. The promissory note is a binding legal document and states that you must repay the loan—even if you do not complete your dental education, are not able to get a job after you complete the program, fail to succeed in practice, are dissatisfied with or feel you did not receive the education you paid for, dislike the dental school you attend, or receive notification that the loan has been sold to another party by your lender. If you do not repay your loan on time or according to the terms in the note, you may go into default. You must make payments on your loan(s) even if you do not receive a bill or repayment notice. If you apply for a deferment or forbearance, you must continue to make payments until you are notified that the request has been granted.

It is your responsibility as a borrower to keep lenders informed about your enrollment status and your current address. You must notify the school, agency, lender, or billing servicer that manages your loan when you graduate, withdraw from school, or drop below half-time status; change your name, address, or Social Security number; or transfer to another school. If you borrow Perkins Loan, HPSL, LDS or institutional loans, these loans will be managed by the school that loaned the money or by an agency that the school assigns to service (billing servicer) the loan.

Repaying your student loans affects your credit rating. Bad credit can adversely affect your ability to borrow money to set up a dental practice in the future and to buy an existing practice, a home, or a car. If you cannot meet your monthly repayment obligations, you have options to defer or postpone payment for postgraduate training. Also, you may request forbearance on your loan, as discussed below.

If your lender does not have your current contact information, you run the risk of becoming delinquent and defaulting on your loan. The consequences of default are serious. If you default on a student loan, there are programs that will allow you to regain your financial aid eligibility or get out of default. You will want to contact the guaranty agency that holds your defaulted loan to inquire about reinstatement and rehabilitation programs. Remember, it takes time and commitment to fix the problem.

Believe it or not, your repayment of student loans also affects other borrowers attending dental school. If you do not repay your student loans and go into default, your dental school's ability to participate in various student loan programs can be limited. Furthermore, it can adversely affect future dental students' ability to borrow for their education.

Regardless of the type of loan, you must receive entrance counseling before you are given the first loan disbursement, and you must receive exit counseling before you leave school. These counseling sessions will either be administered by your school's financial aid office, or you may be asked to complete an online program that will provide you with important information about your loan(s).

The good news is that the vast majority of dental students successfully repay their loan obligations. Table 4-5 is an example of the type of student loan log that you can develop for yourself to help in managing your portfolio. You may also want to add columns for terms and conditions of your student loans such as the number of years you have to repay the loan, deferment and forbearance provisions, how often interest is capitalized, and the length of the grace period.

■ The Lender's Responsibilities

Lenders owe you more than the money they have agreed to lend to you when you sign on the dotted line. They must provide you with a copy of the promissory note. As discussed above, this document explains the conditions of your loan in detail and is the legal document requiring you to repay the loan with interest. KEEP THIS DOCUMENT. The lender should also provide a disclosure statement before or at the time your loan is disbursed. This document states the amount of your loan (principal), fees that may be deducted from the principal amount, fees that may be added at the time of repayment, the interest rate, and an estimate of the total amount you will have to repay, if you follow the standard repayment terms.

It is not uncommon for lenders to sell your loan to another entity after you have taken out the loan. If that happens, your lender will send you a notification of loan transfer with addresses, phone numbers, and other information you need in order to make payments and communicate with the new holder of your loan or their billing servicer. KEEP THIS NOTICE.

Prior to beginning repayment of your student loan, the lender or servicer will send you a detailed repayment schedule. This document will state the principal balance you owe along with the total amount of estimated interest over the period of repayment. In addition, it will tell you the amount and number of your monthly payments and the date your first payment is due. KEEP THIS DOCUMENT.

Because taking out loans means you will have many important papers and documents that you will need after you graduate, it may be helpful to use a loose leaf binder or accordion file to house all of your student loan documents. It is important to keep copies of all documents you receive pertaining to your student loans, including correspondence you send to your lender or servicer regarding your loans. You should also keep a log of student loans you borrow, how much you borrow each year, the interest rate on each loan, and the lender's and servicer's name, telephone number, and address. If you do this, you undoubtedly will save yourself countless hours of painstaking work to reconstruct your borrowing portfolio.

If you need help finding information about your Title IV borrowing (Stafford, Perkins, and Consolidation loans) the National Student Loan Data System stores information on student aid recipients and their current status. The database is maintained by the U.S. Department of Education and can be accessed at www.nslds.ed.gov. Title VII aid, administered by the U.S. Department of Health and Human Services, and private educational loans are not included in the database.

TABLE 4-5. EXAMPLE OF FIRST-YEAR DENTAL STUDENT'S LOAN LOG

Loan	Amount	Interest Rate	Date Repayment Begins	Lender/Website/Servicer/Website
Stafford Subsidized (undergraduate)	$16,000	6.8%	Dec. 2011	Lender X
Perkins (undergraduate)	$4,000	5%	Feb. 2012	My College
Stafford Subsidized (dental school)	$8,500	4.7%	Dec. 2011	Lender Y
Stafford Unsubsidized (dental school)	$18,000	4.7%	Dec. 2011	Lender Y
Perkins (dental school)	$6,000	5%	Feb. 2012	My Dental School
Health Professions Student Loan (dental school)	$6,500	5%	June 2012	My Dental School
Graduate PLUS	$10,000	8.5%	June 2012	Lender Y

Another resource to locate educational loans, although not necessarily complete, can be found at www.loanlocator.org.

THE IMPORTANCE OF BUILDING AND KEEPING GOOD CREDIT

If you are like most students during dental school, you will take out student loans and charge purchases on credit cards. When you apply for a student loan or for other credit, your credit file will be examined, and you will be assigned a credit score based on information provided by credit reporting agencies. There are three kinds of loan approval tests widely used: credit-blind (no checking at all); credit-ready (no credit bureau file exists with any payment history); and credit-worthy (a file exists with one or more good reports and minimal bad reports). The borrower or cosigner, if needed, may have to also meet a debt-to-income ratio and other lender requirements.

A credit score is a number that indicates how likely you are to repay a loan or debt from a credit card purchase. While it is only one piece of information lenders use when evaluating your loan application, it may be the basis for approval or rejection.

Credit bureaus and credit reporting agencies provide credit information to banks and businesses to help them decide whether to issue a loan or extend credit. This information may include your payment habits, number of current and past credit accounts, balance of those accounts, place of employment, length of employment, records of financial transactions, your payment history, and a history of past credit problems. People who make all their payments on time are considered good credit risks. People who are frequently delinquent in making their payments are considered bad credit risks. Defaulting on a loan can negatively affect your credit rating.

With the exception of the Graduate PLUS loan, your credit rating is not checked for eligibility for federal student loan programs; but, eligibility for private loans and some institutional loans may depend on your credit history. Students who have defaulted on previous federal educational loans may be required to agree to repay the loan and begin making payments before they can become eligible for further federal aid.

The Fair Credit Reporting Act and the Equal Credit Opportunity Act help ensure that lenders rely on "likelihood of repayment" as their chief criterion when granting credit. Scoring models do not consider race, gender, nationality, religion, whether you are married, single, or divorced, or other prohibited factors. For more information about credit scores visit, www.myFICO.com.

The majority of credit bureau information is accurate, but you have the right to examine your file and to explain or correct the information it contains.

■ Checking Your Credit Record

All U.S. consumers are eligible to obtain a free copy of their credit report through the only authorized site, AnnualCreditReport.com. You are encouraged to obtain a copy of your credit report annually to make sure there are no errors. It is important that the information on your report be accurate, as errors could possibly affect both your credit rating and your credit score. Annual review of your credit record is also a good way to monitor identity theft.

The Consumer Credit Counseling Service (800-747-4222; debtfreeforme.com) offers free or low-cost debt and credit counseling.

■ Cautions About Credit Cards

If you are like most students, you've received numerous credit card offers promising low interest rates and credit lines of several thousand dollars. If you have accepted these offers and presently carry a balance on one or more such credit cards, you should carefully examine your card use. Although having a credit card is beneficial, problems can arise when you don't pay the bills on time and begin carrying a balance that can balloon into a mountain of debt.

While in school, pay with cash if possible. It may be helpful to ask yourself, "If I can't afford to purchase it with cash now, what is the likelihood that I will be able to pay the credit card bill when it arrives?"

Here are some helpful hints on using credit cards:

- Before you buy an item, evaluate whether you really need it; if not, don't buy it.
- If you make a purchase with a credit card, pay the balance at the end of the month. Don't carry balances. Some cards charge 20 percent or more in interest (usually called finance charges on your statement).
- If you accumulate credit card debt, you may want to transfer debt from high-interest cards to lower-rate cards.
- Read your statements carefully and call the company right away if you have questions about a charge.
- Avoid taking cash advances. The finance charge on a cash advance often starts applying the moment you receive it, not after the next statement closing.
- Be aware of annual fees. Many companies charge $25 and more for the privilege of using their card.
- Be aware of introductory offers. Usually low interest rates are offered in the beginning, only to increase dramatically after the introductory period expires.

OTHER HELPFUL RESOURCES

For further information about financial aid, you may want to consult the following helpful resources.

- *Opportunities for Minority Students in U.S. Dental Schools,* published by ADEA, includes practical information of special interest to minority students considering a career in dentistry. This publication explains the scope of career opportunities available to minorities in dentistry, dental school admissions requirements, financing a dental education, deciding where to apply, and school-specific information directed to minority applicants. Available from ADEA Publications Department, 1400 K Street, NW, Suite 1100, Washington, DC 20005.
- *The Big Book of Minority Opportunities* cites programs including scholarship and other financial aid programs of special interest to Black, Asian, Hispanic, and Native American students. Available from Garrett Park Press, P.O. Box 190, Garrett Park, MD 20896.
- The Student Aid Alliance website provides up-to-date information on federal aid programs and opportunities for students to let their voices be heard on Capitol Hill regarding funding for student aid. Visit www.studentaidalliance.org.
- *The Chronicle Financial Aid Guide* provides information on financial aid programs available to high school, undergraduate, graduate, and adult learners. Available from Chronicle Guidance Publication, www.chronicleguidance.com.
- *The Scholarship Book* lists private sector scholarships, grants, loans, fellowships, internships, and contest prizes covering every major field of study. Visit www.800headstart.com.
- *Foundation Grants to Individuals* finds sources of scholarships, fellowships, grants, awards and other financial support online. Visit http://gtionline.fdncenter.org.

Acknowledgments for Chapter 4

We acknowledge the expertise and contributions of Deborah Philp, National Institute of Dental and Craniofacial Research; Christopher Halliday, Indian Health Service; Paul Koch, Indiana University; Sandra Pearson, Tufts University; Ellen Spilker, Columbia University; the U.S. Department of Education; U.S. Air Force; U.S. Army; and U.S. Navy.

A GLOSSARY OF TERMS
EVERY STUDENT BORROWER SHOULD KNOW

Accrued Interest: Interest assessed on the unpaid balance of the loan principal and payable by the borrower. In the case of subsidized Stafford Loans, paid by the federal government during in-school, grace, and deferment periods.

Aggregate Debt: The total amount a student owes under a particular loan program. This term can also refer to the total amount a student owes under all loan programs.

Aggregate Loan Limits: Refer to the borrower's total borrowed principal still owed. It can refer to the total from only one educational loan type, as in the case of Stafford Loans, William Ford Direct Loans, and Federal Perkins Loans. Alternative loan programs normally consider ALL of a student's education loan when they have an aggregate limit.

Aid Package: Combination of financial aid (scholarships, grants, loans, and/or work study) determined by a school's financial aid office.

Alternative/Private Loans: Educational loan programs established by private lenders. Interest accrues from disbursement, but repayment is usually deferred until some time after graduation. Interest rates are variable, usually without a cap.

Amortization: The process of retiring debt over an extended period of time through periodic installments of principal and interest.

Annual Percentage Rate (APR): A calculation that reflects the total cost of a loan (interest plus all fees) on an annual basis.

Appeal: A formal request to have a financial aid officer review your aid eligibility and possibly use professional judgment to adjust the figures. An example of when an appeal is appropriate is if you believe the information on your financial aid application does not reflect your family's current ability to pay (for example due to the death of a parent, unemployment, or other unusual circumstances). The financial aid officer may require documentation of the special circumstances or other information on your financial aid application.

Asset: An item of value, such as a family's home, business and farm equity, real estate, stocks, bonds, mutual funds, cash, certificates of deposit (CDs), bank accounts, trust funds, and other property and investments.

Award Letter: An official document that lists all of the aid you have been awarded.

Award Year: The academic period for which financial aid is requested and awarded.

Borrower: A student who obtains money from a lending institution by the extension of credit for a period of time. The borrower signs a promissory note as evidence of the debt.

Borrower Benefits/Rewards/Repayment Incentives: Lenders sometimes reduce the cost of loans to borrowers with good repayment behavior. Contact lenders for details.

Budget: Total cost of attending a postsecondary institution for an award year. It usually includes tuition, fees, room, board, books, supplies, equipment, travel, and personal expenses. Each institution develops its own student budget, also known as the "Cost of Attendance".

Campus-Based Aid: Financial aid programs awarded directly by the dental school. This may include both federal programs such as the Perkins Loan, HPSL, LDS, SDS, and Federal Work-Study, and institutional grants and loans. Note that there is no guarantee that every eligible student will receive financial aid through these programs, because the awards are made from a limited pool of money.

Capitalization: The process of adding accrued, unpaid interest to the principal of a loan. Capitalizing the interest increases the monthly payment and the amount of money you will eventually have to repay. Capitalization is sometimes called compounding.

Collateral: Collateral is property used to secure a loan. If the borrower defaults on the loan, the lender can seize the collateral. For example, a mortgage is usually secured by the house purchased with the loan. Education loans are not collateralized unless you are required to have a cosigner.

Compound Interest: The frequency with which accrued unpaid interest is added to the principal balance.

Cosigner: A cosigner on a loan assumes responsibility for the loan if the borrower should fail to repay it. A cosigner may also be referred to as a co-borrower or co-maker.

Cost of Attendance (COA): Total cost of attending a postsecondary institution for an award year. It usually includes tuition, fees, room, board, books, supplies, equipment, travel, and personal expenses. Each institution develops its own student budget, also known as the budget.

Credit Bureau: An agency that compiles, maintains, and distributes credit and personal information to potential creditors/lenders. Lenders check to learn whether a potential borrower is likely to repay based upon the way other credit obligations have been handled in the past.

Credit Rating/Credit Score: An evaluation of the likelihood that a borrower will repay on time.

Default: The failure of a borrower either to make installment payments when due or to comply with other terms of the promissory note. A loan is in default when the borrower fails to pay a number of regular installments on time or otherwise fails to meet the terms and conditions of the loan. Default also may result from failure to submit requests for deferment or cancellation on time. If you default, your school, the lender or agency that holds your loan, the state, and the federal government may all take action to recover the money, including garnishing your wages, withholding income tax refunds, and notifying national credit bureaus of your default. Defaulting on a government loan will make you ineligible for future federal financial aid unless a satisfactory repayment schedule is arranged. It will also affect your credit rating for a long time, making it difficult to borrow funds to buy a car or a house.

Deferment: A period during which the repayment of the principal amount of the loan is suspended as a result of the borrower meeting one of the requirements established by law or regulation and/or contained in the promissory note. During this period, the borrower may or may not have to pay interest on the loan. If you have a subsidized type of loan, either the federal government pays the interest charges during the deferment period or the lender does not charge any to the borrower. If you have an unsubsidized loan, you are responsible for the interest that accrues during the deferment period. You can usually postpone in-school payments by paying the interest charges or by capitalizing the interest, which increases the size of the loan. You can't get a deferment if your loan is in default. If you borrowed during undergraduate school and then worked for a year and entered repayment before beginning dental school, you are eligible to defer payment of student loans as long as you remain a full-time student. Most federal loan programs allow students to defer their loans while they are in school at least half time. There are other activities for which you can obtain deferments. These vary from loan to loan and are itemized on your promissory note. If you don't qualify for a deferment, you may be able to get forbearance.

Delinquent Borrower: If a borrower fails to make a payment on time, the borrower is considered delinquent, and late fees may be charged. Usually delinquencies greater than 30 days are reported to credit bureaus. Once the delinquency exceeds a specific number of days (varies depending on the loan program) the loan goes into default.

Disadvantaged Background (definition from the U.S. Department of Health and Human Services [HHS]): An individual from a disadvantaged background is defined as one who comes from an environment that has inhibited the individual from obtaining the knowledge, skill, and abilities required to enroll in and graduate from a health professions school or a program providing education or training in an allied health profession or who comes from a family with an annual income below a level based on low income thresholds according to family size published by the U.S. Bureau of Census, adjusted annually for changes in the Consumer Price Index, and adjusted by the Secretary of HHS for use in health professions and nursing programs. The school you plan to attend is generally responsible for making a determination of your disadvantaged status.

Disbursement Date: The date on which the lender issues a student the loan proceeds, either by check or by electronic funds transfer to the student's school account.

Disclosure Statement: Lenders are required to provide the borrower with a disclosure statement at the time the loan is made. A statement provides information about the actual loan costs, including the interest rate, origination fees, insurance fees, loan fee, and any other kind of finance charges.

Electronic Funds Transfer (EFT): Electronic funds transfer is used by most schools for Stafford Loans. The money is transferred electronically instead of using paper checks, and hence is available to a student sooner.

Eligible Non-Citizen: Someone who is not a U.S. citizen but is nevertheless eligible for federal student aid. Eligible non-citizens include U.S. permanent residents who are holders of valid green cards, U.S. nationals, holders of form I-94 who have been granted refugee or asylum status, and certain other non-citizens. Non-citizens who hold a student visa or an exchange visitor visa are not eligible for federal student aid.

Endowment: Funds owned by an institution and invested to produce income to support its operations. Many educational institutions use a portion of their endowment income for financial aid. A school with a larger ratio of endowment per student is more likely to give larger financial aid packages.

Enrollment Status: An indication of whether you are a full-time or part-time student. Generally, you must be enrolled at least half time (and in some cases full time) to qualify for financial aid.

Expected Family Contribution (EFC): The amount of money the family is expected to contribute to a student's education, as determined by the Federal Methodology formula approved by Congress. Some schools determine eligibility for non-federal school funds with Institutional Methodology. The EFC is a student/spouse contribution and depends on family size, number of family members in school, taxable and non-taxable income, and assets. Parent information is required for funds authorized by the U.S. Department of Health and Human Services and may also be required by some schools for institutional funds.

FAFSA: See Free Application for Federal Student Aid.

Fees: Origination fees, also referred to as insurance fees, loan fees, points, or guaranty fees, are usually expressed as a percentage of the amount borrowed, and are usually deducted from the loan proceeds at disbursement. Some alternative/private loans add the fees to the principal borrowed. Some loans also include an additional fee (sometimes referred to as a "kicker"), which is charged at the time the loan enters repayment to help offset additional administrative costs relative to billing. Usually these 'back-end' fees are added to the total amount owed.

Financial Aid Officer (FAO): A college or university employee who is involved in the administration of financial aid. Some schools call these individuals financial aid advisors or financial aid counselors.

Financial Aid Package: A collection of grants, scholarships, loans, and work-study employment from all sources (federal, state, institutional, and private) offered to enable a student to attend the college or university.

Financial Need: A student's financial need is the gap between the cost of attending school and a student's resources. A financial aid package is based on the amount of a student's financial need. The process of determining the need is known as need analysis. Cost of Attendance

(COA) - Expected Family Contribution (EFC) = Financial Need.

Fixed Interest Rate: In a fixed interest loan, the interest rate stays the same for the life of the loan. For example, a 5 percent fixed interest rate loan means that the interest rate will be 5 percent from the day the borrower takes out the loan until the day the borrower finishes repaying the loan.

Forbearance: During forbearance the lender allows the borrower to postpone temporarily or reduce the payment on a student loan. Because less is paid during forbearance, it takes longer to repay the loan. Since interest charges continue to accrue, even on subsidized loans, it may increase the total cost of the loan. It may also mean capitalization of accrued and unpaid interest during this time, thus increasing both the balance owed and the monthly repayments required after the forbearance period has ended. Forbearances are granted at the lender's discretion, usually in cases of extreme financial hardship or other unusual circumstances when the borrower does not qualify for a deferment. You can't receive forbearance if your loan is in default.

Free Application for Federal Student Aid (FAFSA): This U.S. Department of Education form is used to apply for all federally sponsored student financial aid and federal need-based aid. The form is available at www.fafsa.ed.gov, and it can be submitted electronically or by mail. When filing a paper FAFSA, be sure to use an original not a photocopy, because photocopying alters the alignment of the forms, interfering with the imaging technology used to process them. As the name suggests, no fee is charged to file a FAFSA. When sending an electronic FAFSA be certain to print a copy for your records.

Gift Aid: Financial aid, such as grants and scholarships, that does not need to be repaid.

Grace Period: A brief period after graduation during which the borrower is not required to begin repaying his or her student loans. The grace period may also kick in if the borrower leaves school for a reason other than graduation or drops below half-time or full-time (depends on the program) enrollment. The length of the grace period depends on the loan program. Not all loans have grace periods; some require repayments to begin directly upon graduation or separation.

Interest Rate Caps: Refers to the maximum interest a borrower may be charged over the life of the loan. For instance, current federal statute specifies that Stafford Loan interest rates cannot exceed 8.25% even though the rate is reset each July 1 based on a formula. A fixed interest rate loan will always have the same rate throughout the life of the loan. Alternative/private loan programs usually do not have an interest rate cap and their interest rates fluctuate periodically, often on a quarterly basis if based on an index such as the 91-day Treasury Bill, or the Loudon InterBank Offering Rate (LIBOR), or the prime rate.

Loan Terms: The specific conditions of a loan, including requirements governing receipt and repayment. It is often used more specifically to refer to the charges for the loan, such as interest, fees, etc.

Minority: According to the U.S. Government, an individual whose race/ethnicity is classified as American Indian or Alaskan Native, Asian or Pacific Islander, Black, or Hispanic. See also *Underrepresented Minority*.

Outside Resource: Funds available to a student because they are in school; examples include outside scholarships, prepaid tuition plans, and Veterans Affairs (VA) educational benefits. This category does not include school-based aid.

Outside Scholarship: A scholarship that comes from a source other than the school.

Out-of-State Student: A student who has not met the legal residency requirements for the state in which the dental school that she/he will attend is located. Out-of-state students are often charged a higher tuition rate at public dental schools.

Overaward: A student who receives federal support may not receive awards totaling more than $400 in excess of his or her financial need.

Prepayment: Paying off all or part of a loan before it is due. Prepayment without penalty is allowed for all federally sponsored loans and other educational loans at any time during the life of the loan.

Principal and Interest: The principal is the total amount of money borrowed or remaining unpaid on a loan. Interest is charged as a percentage of the principal. When a borrower takes out a loan of $10,000, for example, the $10,000 is the principal.

Professional Judgment (PJ): For need-based federal aid programs, the financial aid officer can adjust the Expected Family Contribution (EFC) or Cost of Attendance (COA) when extenuating circumstances exist. For example, if a parent becomes unemployed, disabled, or deceased, the financial aid officer can decide to use estimated income information for the award year instead of the actual income figures from the base year. This delegation of authority from the federal government to the financial aid officer is called professional judgment.

Promissory Note: A binding legal document that must be signed by a student borrower (and a cosigner, if applicable), agreeing to repay the loan according to specified terms. It must be signed before loan funds will be disbursed by the lender. The promissory note states the terms and conditions of the loan, including when repayment will begin, interest rate, deferment and forbearance options, and cancellation provisions. A student should keep this document until the loan has been repaid.

Renewable Scholarships: A scholarship awarded for more than one year. Usually a student must maintain certain academic standards to be eligible for subsequent years. Some renewable scholarships require a student to reapply each year; others will just require a report on a student's progress toward a degree.

Repayment Schedule: This schedule shows the monthly payment, interest rate, total repayment obligation, payment due dates, and term of the loan.

Repayment Term: The period during which the borrower is required to make payments on his or her loans. While payments are made monthly, the term is usually given as the total number of payments or years.

Sallie Mae: Sallie Mae, also known as the Student Loan Marketing Association (SLMA), is the nation's largest secondary loan market for educational loans.

Satisfactory Academic Progress (SAP): A student must be making SAP to continue receiving federal aid. If a student fails to maintain academic standing consistent with the school's SAP policy, he or she is unlikely to meet the school's graduation requirements and may be ineligible to receive federal financial aid.

Secondary Market: An organization that buys loans from lenders, thereby providing the lender with the capital to issue new loans. Selling loans is a common practice among lenders, so the bank to which you make your payments may change during the life of the loan. The terms and conditions of your loan do not change when it is sold to another holder.

Servicer: An organization that acts as an agent for the lender, collecting payments on a loan and performing other administrative tasks associated with maintaining a loan portfolio. Loan servicers disburse funds, monitor loans while the borrowers are in school, collect payments, process deferments and forbearances, respond to borrower inquiries, and ensure that the loans are administered in compliance with federal regulations and guaranty agency requirements.

Simple Interest: Interest paid only on the principal balance of the loan and not on any accrued interest. Most federal student loan programs offer simple interest, but capitalizing the interest on an unsubsidized Stafford Loan is a form of compounded interest.

Statement of Educational Purpose: In this legal document, a student agrees to use the financial aid for educational expenses only. This form is part of the certification a student attests to on the FASFA.

Student Aid Report (SAR): This report summarizes the information included in the FAFSA and must be provided to your school's Financial Aid Officer (FAO). The SAR will also indicate the Expected Family Contribution (EFC). You should receive a copy of your SAR four to six weeks after you file your FAFSA. Review your SAR and correct any errors on part two of the SAR. Keep a photocopy of the SAR for your records. To request a duplicate copy, call 800-4-FED-AID.

Subsidized Loan: With a subsidized loan, such as the Subsidized Stafford Loan, the government pays the interest on the loan while a student is in school, during the grace period, and during any deferment periods. Subsidized loans are awarded based on financial need and may not be used to finance the family contribution. With other subsidized loans types, such as the Perkins and HPSL, interest is not charged while a student is in school, in grace, or in deferment.

Term: The number of years (or months) over which the loan is to be repaid.

Title IV Loans: Education loan programs that are collectively referred to as the William D. Ford Federal Direct Loan Program (FDSL), the Federal Family Education Loan Program (FFELP), the Federal Stafford Loans (subsidized and unsubsidized), and Federal Consolidation Loans.

Title IV School Code: When you fill out the Free Application for Federal Student Aid (FAFSA), you need to supply the Title IV Code for each school to which you are applying.

Title VII Aid: Education loan programs that are collectively referred to as the Loans for Disadvantaged Students (LDS), Health Professions Student Loans (HPSL), Scholarships for Disadvantaged Students (SDS), Primary Care Loans (PCL). Dental students are not eligible for PCL. Title VII aid is administered by the U.S. Department of Health and Human Services.

Underrepresented Minority: According to the U.S. Government, means with respect to a health profession.

Unmet Need: In an ideal world, the financial aid office would be able to award or recommend financial aid to each student for the entire difference between his or her ability to pay and the cost of education. Due to budget constraints, the financial aid office may provide less than a student's need. This gap is known as the unmet need.

Unsecured Loan: A loan not backed by collateral and hence representing greater risk to the lender. Lenders may require a cosigner on the loan to reduce their risk. If you default on the loan, the cosigner will be held responsible for repayment. Most educational loans are unsecured loans. In the case of federal student loans, the federal government guarantees repayment of the loans. Other examples of unsecured loans include credit card charges and personal lines of credit.

Unsubsidized Loan: With an unsubsidized loan, such as the unsubsidized Stafford Loan, the government does not pay the interest that accrues while a borrower is in school, in grace or in deferment. Private/alternative loans are also unsubsidized loans. The borrower is responsible for the interest on an unsubsidized loan from the date the loan is disbursed. Students may have the option while in school of capitalizing the interest. Unsubsidized loans are not based on financial need and may be used to finance the family contribution.

U.S. Department of Education (ED): This department administers several federal student financial aid programs, including the federal Work-Study Program, the federal Perkins Loans, and the federal Stafford Loans.

U.S. Department of Health and Human Services (HHS): This department administers several health education scholarship and loan programs, including the Scholarships for Disadvantaged Students (SDS), Loans for Disadvantaged Students (LDS), and Health Professions Student Loans (HPSL).

Variable Interest: A loan on which the interest rate changes periodically. Fluctuations are usually tied to certain monetary measures such a 91-day Treasury Bill, the London Inter Bank Offering Rate (LIBOR), or the prime rate. Points are then added to the base (1 point equals 1 percent). For example, the interest rate for a Stafford Loan for a student in school is pegged to the cost of a 91-day Treasury Bills + 1.7 percent. Variable rates are updated monthly, quarterly, semi-annually, or annually.

Verification: A review process in which the Financial Aid Officer (FAO) determines the accuracy of the information provided on a student's financial aid application. During the verification process a student and spouse, if applicable, will be required to submit documentation on the application. Such documentation may include signed copies of the most recent federal and state income tax returns for you, your spouse (if any), and your parents, proof of citizenship, proof of registration with Selective Service, and copies of Social Security benefit statements and W-2 and 1099 forms, among other things. Financial aid applications are randomly selected by the federal processor for verification, with most schools verifying at least one-third of all applications. If there is an asterisk next to the Expected Family Contribution (EFC) figure on your Student Aid Report, your SAR has been selected for verification. Schools may select additional students for verification if they suspect fraud. Some schools perform 100 percent verification. If any discrepancies are uncovered, the financial aid office may require additional information. Such discrepancies may cause your final financial aid package to be different from the initial package described on the award letter you received from the school. If you refuse to submit the required documentation, your financial aid package can be cancelled and no aid awarded.

W-2 Form: Employers are required by the IRS to issue a W-2 form for each employee before January 31. The form lists the employee's wages and taxes withheld.

CHAPTER 5
GETTING MORE INFORMATION

This book provides a foundation for anyone who is considering dentistry as a career and wants to know more about obtaining a dental education. Although the information included here is extensive, you probably will want additional details to answer questions that are specific to your situation. This chapter gives you lists of individuals, organizations, and references that will help answer those questions.

INDIVIDUALS WHO CAN HELP

One very effective way of getting more information is to talk to the individuals who are involved in dental education and are interested in encouraging others like you to consider dentistry as a career.

Practicing Dentists

Dentists are knowledgeable about the variety of careers in dentistry and about the education and skills needed. They can tell you what the day-to-day work is like, the kinds of benefits they receive, and how they deal with any shortcomings. In addition, an excellent way of learning more about the profession and whether it feels right for you is to arrange for an internship or a "shadowing" opportunity in a dental office. To pursue such an opportunity, discuss the possibility with your own dentist or other practitioners in your area.

Prehealth Advisors

Prehealth advisors can assist in a broad range of issues about dental education and dental schools. They are especially important in the admission process because they can inform you about the academic preparation necessary to be accepted into a dental school. In addition, these advisors are often involved in providing or coordinating letters of recommendation.

Science Professors

Science professors, especially those in the biological sciences, can be helpful in the same way as prehealth advisors in terms of academic preparation and letters of recommendation. They are particularly important to students at undergraduate schools that do not have an official prehealth advisor.

Dental School Admissions Officers

Admissions officers are especially knowledgeable about their own dental schools and the requirements to gain admission. They can provide you with catalogs and admission information. They can also describe the emphasis of the academic programs, support services to help students succeed, and other features of their schools.

Dental School Minority Affairs Officers

These officers play an important role in collecting and sharing information about what their dental schools are doing to increase minority enrollments and to make minority students who choose their schools feel welcome. They will also have information about the academic program, support services, and other features of their schools.

Financial Aid Administrators

Financial aid administrators are very knowledgeable about how to pay the cost of attending dental school. They will be able to help you understand the financial aid application process and eligibility requirements for government, institutional, and private sources of financial aid. They can assist in securing the funds for which you are eligible.

Dental Students

Dental students are usually forthright in sharing their perceptions of the education they are receiving at their schools. They also will tell you their views of the nonacademic aspects such as student support services and social atmosphere.

Since these individuals' perspectives differ from each other, the information they share can be enormously helpful. You should not hesitate to approach them in order to benefit from their knowledge and points of view.

ORGANIZATIONS THAT CAN HELP

A number of organizations can also offer information about careers in dentistry, preparing for admission, and financial aid for dental students.

American Dental Education Association
1400 K Street, NW, Suite 1100
Washington, DC 20005
Phone: 202-289-7201
Fax: 202-289-7204
www.adea.org

ADEA can provide you with information about the application process for admission to dental school and the application process for postdoctoral programs. ADEA sponsors the ADEA Application Service (AADSAS, see chapter 2) and the Postdoctoral Application Support Service (PASS, see chapter 1). In addition to the *ADEA Official Guide to Dental Schools,* ADEA publishes the *Journal of Dental Education* (a monthly scholarly journal), the *Bulletin of Dental Education Online* (a monthly newsletter), and *Opportunities for Minority Students in Dentistry* (an every-other-year guide). Ordering information is available on the ADEA website. Dental students may belong to ADEA at no charge by going to www.adea.org and selecting "Join ADEA."

Academy of General Dentistry
211 East Chicago Avenue, Suite 900
Chicago, IL 60611-1999
Phone: 888-243-3368
Fax: 312-440-0559
www.agd.org

Founded in 1952, the AGD serves the needs and represents the interests of general dentists, promotes the oral health of the public, and fosters the continued proficiency of general dentists through quality continuing dental education to help them better serve the public. The AGD also sponsors a 24-hour, online message board where consumers can post questions answered by a dentist and a dentist referral service.

American Academy of Oral & Maxillofacial Pathology
214 North Hale Street
Wheaton, IL 60187
Phone: 888-552-2667
Fax: 630-510-4501
www.aaomp.org

The AAOMP promotes all activities involving the practice of oral and maxillofacial pathology, the specialty of dentistry and pathology that deals with the nature, identification, and management of diseases affecting the oral and maxillofacial regions.

American Academy of Oral & Maxillofacial Radiology
P.O. Box 1010
Evans, GA 30809-1010
Phone: 706-721-2607
Fax: 706-721-4937
www.aaomr.org

The AAOMR promotes and advances the art and science of radiology in dentistry and provides a forum for communication among and professional advancement of its members.

American Association of Oral and Maxillofacial Surgeons
9700 West Bryn Mawr Avenue
Rosemont, IL 60018-5701
Phone: 800-822-6637, 847-678-6200
Fax: 847-678-6286
www.aaoms.org

Founded (under a different name) in 1918, AAOMS provides a means of self-government relating to professional standards, ethical behavior, and responsibilities of its fellows and members; contributes to the public welfare; advances the specialty; and supports its fellows and members through education, research, and advocacy.

American Academy of Pediatric Dentistry
211 East Chicago Avenue, Suite 1700
Chicago, IL 60611-2663
Phone: 312-337-2169
Fax: 312-337-6329
www.aapd.org

The AAPD represents the specialty of pediatric dentistry. Its members serve as primary care providers for millions of children from infancy through adolescence and provide advanced, specialty care for patients of all ages with special health care needs.

American Academy of Periodontology
737 North Michigan Avenue, Suite 800
Chicago, IL 60611-6660
Phone: 312-787-5518
Fax: 312-787-3670
www.perio.org

The AAP advocates, educates, and sets standards for advancing the periodontal and general health of the public and promoting excellence in the practice of periodontics, one of the ten dental specialties.

American Dental Association
211 East Chicago Avenue
Chicago, IL 60611-2678
Phone: 312-440-2500
Fax: 312-440-2800
www.ada.org

The ADA is the professional association of dentists committed to the public's oral health, ethics, science, and professional advancement. The ADA has information about dental licensure and postdoctoral study. In addition, the ADA sponsors the Dental Admission Test (DAT), which every applicant to a U.S. dental school must take (see chapter 2).

American Association for Dental Research
1619 Duke Street
Alexandria, VA 22314-3406
Phone: 703-548-0066
Fax: 703-548-1883
www.iadr.com

The AADR advances research and increases knowledge for the improvement of oral health. The AADR also sponsors student research fellowships to encourage dental students to conduct research.

American Association of Endodontists
211 East Chicago Avenue, Suite 1100
Chicago, IL 60611-2691
Phone: 800-872-3636, 312-266-7255
Fax: 866-451-9020, 312-266-9867
www.aae.org

The AAE promotes the exchange of ideas on the scope of the specialty of endodontics, stimulates endodontic research studies among its members, and encourages the highest standard of care in the practice of endodontics.

American Association of Hospital Dentists
211 East Chicago Avenue, Suite 740
Chicago, IL 60611-2616
Phone: 800-852-7921, 312-440-2660
Fax: 312-440-2824
www.scdonline.org/displayconnon.cfm?an=9

The AAHD, founded in 1937, helps hospital dentists develop the skills, knowledge, creativity, and leadership they need to make their practices thrive and advance in their profession. This association also helps shape national health policy on hospital dentistry by providing advocacy at the federal and state levels.

American Association of Orthodontists
401 North Lindbergh Boulevard
St. Louis, MO 63141-7816
Phone: 314-993-1700
Fax: 314-997-1745
www.aaortho.org

The AAO supports research and education leading to quality patient care and promotes increased public awareness of the need for and benefits of orthodontic treatment.

American Association of Public Health Dentistry
National Office
P.O. Box 7536
Springfield, IL 62791-7536
Phone: 217-391-0218
Fax: 217-793-0041
www.aaphd.org

Founded in 1937, the AAPHD provides a focus for meeting the challenge to improve the oral health of the public. Its broad base of membership provides a fertile environment and numerous opportunities for the exchange of ideas and experiences.

American Association of Women Dentists
216 West Jackson Boulevard, Suite 625
Chicago, IL 60606
Phone: 800-920-2293
Fax: 312-750-1203
www.aawd.org

Formed in 1921, the AAWD celebrates the rich history of women dentists and represents women dentists across the United States, internationally, and in the uniformed forces.

American College of Dentists
839J Quince Orchard Boulevard
Gaithersburg, MD 20878-1614
Phone: 301-977-3223
Fax: 301-977-3330
www.acd.org

Founded in 1920, the ACD is the oldest national honorary organization for dentists. The ACD promotes excellence, ethics, professionalism, and leadership in dentistry.

American College of Prosthodontists
211 East Chicago Avenue, Suite 1000
Chicago, IL 60611-2637
Phone: 312-573-1260
Fax: 312-573-1257
www.prosthodontics.org

Founded in 1970, the ACP represents the needs and interests of prosthodontists within organized dentistry and to the public by providing a means for stimulating awareness and interest in the field of prosthodontics.

American Student Dental Association
211 East Chicago Avenue, Suite 1160
Chicago, IL 60611-2687
Phone: 800-621-8099 x 2795, 312-440-2795
Fax: 312-440-2820
www.asdanet.org

The ASDA is a student-run organization that protects and advances the rights, interests and welfare of students pursuing careers in dentistry. It provides services, information, education, representation, and advocacy.

Association of Schools of Public Health
1101 15th Street, NW, Suite 910
Washington, DC 20005
Phone: 202-296-1099
Fax: 202-296-1252
www.asph.org

ASPH represents the deans, faculty, and students of the accredited member schools of public health and other programs seeking accreditation as schools of public health. ASPH collects information on careers in public health, which is useful to individuals interested in pursuing careers in dental public health.

Hispanic Dental Association
1224 Centre West, Suite 400B
Springfield, IL 62704
Toll free: 800-852-7921
Phone: 217-793-0035
Fax: 217-793-0041
www.hdassoc.org

Established in 1990, the HAD provides a voice for the Hispanic oral health professional, promotes the oral health of the Hispanic community, fosters research and knowledge concerning Hispanic oral health problems, and encourages the entry of Hispanics into the oral health profession.

National Dental Association
3517 16th Street, NW
Washington, DC 20010
Phone: 202-588-1697
Fax: 202-588-1244
www.ndaonline.org

The NDA, which is made up of African American dentists, sponsors minority student scholarships for both undergraduate and postgraduate dental students. The NDA also sponsors a student organization, the SNDA, and distributes a career development tape that is available for use by schools, dentists, and other groups.

National Institute of Dental and Craniofacial Research
National Institutes of Health
Bethesda, MD 20892-2190
Phone: 301-496-4261
Fax: 301-496-9988
www.nidcr.nih.gov

The NIDCR provides grants for research training for high school, college, dental, and postgraduate dental students. It is the major source of research funding to dental schools and offers both intramural and extramural research grants and training opportunities.

Oral Health America
410 North Michigan Avenue, Suite 352
Chicago, IL 60611
Phone: 312-836-9900
Fax: 312-836-9986
www.oralhealthamerica.org

Oral Health America develops, implements, and facilitates educational and service programs designed to improve the oral health of all Americans.

Society of American Indian Dentists
P.O. Box 15107
Phoenix, AZ 85060
Phone: 602-954-5160
www.aaip.org/about/said.html

Founded in April 1990 by six American Indian dentists, SAID has grown to approximately 65 members representing 41 different tribes. The society promotes dental health in the American Indian community, encourages American Indian youth to pursue a career in dentistry, promotes American Indian heritage and traditional values, and promotes and supports the unique concerns of American Indian dentists.

Special Care Dentistry Association
401 North Michigan Avenue
Chicago, IL 60611
Phone: 312-527-6764
Fax: 312-673-6663
www.SCDAonline.org

SCDA is the only national organization where oral health and other professionals meet, communicate, exchange ideas, and work together to improve oral health for people with special needs. SCDA had its origin in a federation of three long-standing independent organizations: the American Association of Hospital Dentists, the Academy of Dentistry for Persons with Disabilities, and the American Society for Geriatric Dentistry. These founding organizations remain as components of SCDA, pooling resources to attain overlapping goals.

OTHER RESOURCES

College, university, and public libraries generally have a range of publications about careers, undergraduate and graduate education, and financial aid. As a result, it is worthwhile to visit a library to gather information about careers in dentistry, dental educational programs, and sources of student assistance. Some of the publications you may find there include the following. If you prefer to acquire copies yourself, contact the organizations as noted.

Dental Admission Testing Program Application and Preparation Materials
In addition to the application form that students must complete to take the DAT, this publication contains information that will help students prepare for the test.

Available from: Dental Admission Testing Program, 211 East Chicago Avenue, Suite 1846, Chicago, IL 60611; 312-440-2689; 800-232-2162; or online at www.ada.org/prof/ed/testing/index.asp.

Getting Through Dental School: ASDA's Guide for Dental Students
This biennial reference volume includes information on scholarships and loans, grants, public health and international opportunities, as well as ASDA membership benefits and leadership opportunities.

Getting into Dental School: ASDA's Guide for Predental Students
This resource guide specifically targets the needs of predental students and those considering careers in dentistry. It is a reference volume of facts on applying to dental school, financial aid, ASDA membership benefits, debt management and more. The handbook also includes career options in the dental field and a survival guide for passing the DAT.

ASDA Guides to Postdoctoral Programs Vol. 1-3
This set of publications offers information about general practice residencies, advanced education in general dentistry, and other postdoctoral training programs.

These two publications are available from American Student Dental Association, 211 East Chicago Avenue, Suite 1160, Chicago, IL 60611; 312-440-2795; or online at www.asdanet.org/store.

ON TO PART II

The five chapters in Part I have helped you learn the basics about careers in dentistry; meeting criteria for acceptance into dental school; paying for the costs of a dental education; deciding to which dental schools to apply; and finding additional information to answer the particular questions you have. Part II, Learning about Dental Schools, will give you an opportunity to put this general information to use by introducing you to every dental school in the United States and Canada.

PART II
LEARNING ABOUT DENTAL SCHOOLS

PART TWO **LEARNING ABOUT DENTAL SCHOOLS**

Part II provides an individual introduction to each U.S. and Canadian dental school. We have developed a format for Part II that is relatively consistent from school to school to make it easier for readers to gather information. However, the text is provided by the dental schools themselves so that you can discern the distinctive qualities of each institution.

Every dental school in the United States and Canada is accredited. The Commission on Dental Accreditation accredits U.S. schools, and the Commission on Dental Accreditation of Canada accredits Canadian schools.

HOW TO USE PART II

The school entries are presented alphabetically *by state*.

Information about each school is organized into the areas that tend to be of most interest to dental school applicants:

■ **General Information** describes the type of institution, history of the dental school, location, size, facilities, relationship of the dental school to other health professions schools in the university, and other programs conducted by the school.

■ **Admission Requirements** presents the school's requirements with respect to:
- predental education (number of years, limitations on community college work, required courses, and suggested additional preparation);
- Dental Admission Test (DAT);
- grade point average (GPA);
- residency requirements; and
- advanced standing policies.

■ **Selection Factors** explain how the dental school takes applicant information into consideration, including DAT scores, GPAs, letters of recommendation, and interviews. (Note that in no cases is selection based on an applicant's race, creed, gender, or national origin.) The text may also disclose a school's participation in regional compacts, other interstate agreements, or (for private schools) an in-state agreement.

■ **Timetable** informs readers of the timetable for submitting application materials for admission. The chart also states the fees (if any) applicants must pay to the dental school and when applicants can expect to be notified.

■ **The Dental Program** provides an introduction to the dental school's educational program. Dental schools generally use this section to discuss length of the program, goals, and objectives. The section also informs readers about:
- the degree offered by the school (D.D.S. or D.M.D.);
- alternate degrees that may be available, such as combined degree programs;
- the dental curriculum and its structure; and
- other programs at the school, including fellowships, research, and externship opportunities.

■ **Academic and Other Assistance** describes assistance programs that are available to students of this dental school.

■ **Costs and Financial Aid** allows schools to briefly describe their financial aid policies. The section may also have a chart showing estimated expenses for both residents and nonresidents of the state in which the dental school is located. Schools often include another chart that indicates the number and percent of first-year students receiving financial aid, the average award, and the range of awards. The costs given are for the most recent academic year the school has reported; you should adjust your estimated costs upward for the 2008-09 academic year.

■ **For Further Information** usually lists the names, addresses, and telephone numbers for the dental school's admissions office, financial aid office, minority affairs office, and housing office.

ALABAMA

UNIVERSITY OF ALABAMA AT BIRMINGHAM
SCHOOL OF DENTISTRY

Dr. Huw F. Thomas, Dean

GENERAL INFORMATION

The University of Alabama School of Dentistry (UASD), located on the campus of the University of Alabama at Birmingham, is an integral part of the large complex of medical facilities on this urban campus at the periphery of downtown Birmingham (metropolitan population: approximately one million). The School of Dentistry was created in 1945 by an act of the state legislature, and the first class matriculated in 1948. Students at the UASD pursue their professional education utilizing modern equipment in recently renovated facilities. The renovations include state-of-the-art lecture rooms, new patient receiving and business areas, dental chairs and delivery systems, student lounge, research labs, a new lobby, front entrance, and preclinical laboratory. The clinical facilities of the School of Dentistry Building contain more than 125,000 square feet of clinical teaching space. Teaching of the basic biomedical sciences is accomplished in Volker Hall. This multipurpose complex houses five lecture halls ranging in size from 125 to 700 seats and utilizes innovative audiovisual equipment and teaching aids, as well as wet and dry laboratories.

Joint basic science departments and close working relationships with the School of Medicine and other academic units of the medical center contribute to a curriculum emphasis on comprehensive health care. Research opportunities at both undergraduate and postdoctoral levels are available and encouraged.

In addition to the program leading to the D.M.D. degree, residencies, fellowships, and postgraduate positions are offered in most of the dental specialties as well as in the area of general practice.

ADMISSION REQUIREMENTS

NUMBER OF YEARS OF PREDENTAL EDUCATION: Formal minimum three; usual minimum four.

LIMITATIONS ON COMMUNITY COLLEGE WORK: Maximum of 60 semester hours, all earned before a student enters the third year of study toward a baccalaureate degree.

REQUIRED COURSES:

With lab required	(semester/quarter hrs)
Organic chemistry	8/12
Inorganic chemistry	8/12
Biology	12/18
Physics	8/12

Other courses	
Mathematics	6/9
English	6/9
Nonscience	30/45

All required courses must be acceptable for fulfillment of requirements for a major in these disciplines.

SUGGESTED ADDITIONAL PREPARATION: It is strongly recommended that elective courses be chosen from the following: biochemistry, upper division biology courses (histology, cell biology, embryology, comparative anatomy, and physiology), quantitative analysis, calculus, literature, art, and sculpting. Required nonscience coursework should be selected from courses in the social sciences, philosophy, psychology, history, economics, or foreign languages.

DAT: Mandatory.

GPA: No specific requirements, but 3.3 or above recommended.

RESIDENCY: No specific requirements, but preference is given to Alabama residents.

ADVANCED STANDING: None.

Timetable for the Class Entering Fall 2008

	Earliest Date	Latest Date	School Fee
Application Submission	6/1/07	12/1/07	$50*
Acceptance Notification	12/1/07	8/15/08**	$200***

* Waiver may be granted in special cases, depending on circumstances.
** Late notification given only if there are withdrawals from original roster.
***Applies toward tuition and is nonrefundable.

Required Response:
45 days after notification if received between 12/1 and 12/31
30 days after notification if received between 1/1 and 1/31
15 days after notification if received on or after 2/1 (preferred time, two weeks)

FOR FURTHER INFORMATION
Offices of Admissions, Financial Aid,
Minority Affairs, and Housing
Cindy Edwards
205-934-3387
University of Alabama
School of Dentistry
SDB 125, UAB Station
Birmingham, AL 35294-0007

www.dental.uab.edu

UNIVERSITY OF ALABAMA AT BIRMINGHAM SCHOOL OF DENTISTRY **ALABAMA**

THE DENTAL PROGRAM

The objectives of the dental curriculum are: 1) to produce a health professional whose primary career will be the preservation of oral health; and 2) to provide an academic environment in which the student is educated in the process of inquiry and the scientific method of problem-solving.

YEARS 1 AND 2. The basic sciences are presented in the traditional manner during the first two years. At appropriate times during this first two-year period, interdisciplinary programs are presented that emphasize the application of the basic sciences to various clinical problems. For example, in the last portion of the first quarter of the freshman year, there is a two-week, in-depth discussion of the problem of caries of the enamel and dentin, which is based on the basic science courses already presented. Applications of basic sciences to other clinical problems are presented later in the curriculum, after the students have completed their studies of the basic sciences involved. Among these problems are nutrition, occlusion, and periodontal disease.

The preclinical dental courses are also presented during the first two years. Small groups of students are assigned to a faculty member who is responsible for instruction in preclinical techniques and who serves as a general role model for the group. Initial clinical experience is provided during the first year and at intervals during the second year in a preventive context.

YEAR 3. The major portion of clinical experience is acquired during the third and fourth years.

YEAR 4. During the fourth year, the philosophy of comprehensive patient care is emphasized. Off-campus clinical experiences are included in this year. Students are also permitted to participate in a variety of elective programs throughout the year.

■ Degrees Offered
DENTAL DEGREE: D.M.D.

ALTERNATE DEGREES: D.M.D./M.S., D.M.D./M.P.H., D.M.D./M.B.A., or D.M.D./Ph.D. degree with a major in anatomy, biochemistry, microbiology, pharmacology, or physiology and biophysics; program length is six to nine years.

COSTS AND FINANCIAL AID

A wide range of need-based and merit-based funds is available through the University of Alabama at Birmingham School of Dentistry and federal and state agencies.

Financial Aid Awards to First-Year Students in 2006-07
■ TOTAL NUMBER OF RECIPIENTS: 50   ■ 95% OF CLASS

	Average Award	Range of Awards
Residents	$33,032	$4,703-$56,986
Nonresidents	$8,500	$8,500-$8,500

Estimated School-Related Expenses for Academic Year 2006-07

	YEAR 1	YEAR 2	YEAR 3	YEAR 4	TOTAL
Tuition, resident	$10,308	$10,308	$10,881	$12,027	
Tuition, nonresident	$30,924	$30,924	$32,643	$36,081	
Fees (defined)					
Building Fee	$888	$888	$888	$888	
Student Service Fee	$372	$372	$372	$372	
Recreation Center Fee	$144	$144	$144	$144	
Student Health Service Fee	$225	$225	$225	$225	
Student Dental Fee	$102	$102	$102	$102	
Clinic Fee	$126	$126	$774	$774	
Liability Insurance	n/a	$25	$25	$25	
Anatomy Lab Fee	$387	0	0	0	
Preclinical Lab Fee	$501	$501	0	0	
Prosthodontic Lab Fee	0	0	$300	$300	
Breakage Deposit	0	0	0	$15	
National Board Exam*	0	$220	0	$295	
ASDA Voluntary Dues	$80	$80	$80	$80	
PCD Lab Fee	0	0	$25	$25	
Printed Materials Fee	$126	$126	$126	$126	
Technology Fee	$222	$222	$222	$222	
Hospitalization Insurance	0	0	0	0	
Diploma Fee	0	0	0	$20	
Graduation Fee	0	0	0	$40	
Dental Implant Course Fee	0	0	$442	$492	
Occlusion II Course Fee	0	0	0	$84	
Equipment	0	0	0	0	
Dental Kits	$6,950	$4,718	$3,542	0	
Instrument Case Rental	0	0	$99	$99	
Hospitalization Insurance	$1,220	$1,220	$1,220	$1,220	
TOTAL EXPENSES RESIDENT	**$21,651**	**$19,277**	**$19,467**	**$17,575**	
TOTAL EXPENSES NONRESIDENT	**$42,267**	**$39,893**	**$41,229**	**$41,039**	

*Subject to change based on cost of exam.
**One third of annual amount for dental kits is charged each quarter—fall, winter, and spring.

SELECTION FACTORS

Preference is given to bona fide residents of Alabama and neighboring states. Selection is based on numerous criteria, including academic grades, strength of recommendations from the predental advisory committee and science instructors, DAT scores, and personal characteristics. The best-qualified applicants will have maintained a GPA of B+ or better; have a strong science background; give sound evidence of personal integrity, maturity, and motivation; and show promise of success in dentistry. Applicants whose credentials indicate they may be qualified for the study of dentistry will be invited for a personal interview with the Admissions Committee. This school offers equal educational opportunities to all qualified individuals regardless of gender, race, creed, color, or national origin.

See chapter 3 of this guide for information regarding numbers of applicants and enrollees to each dental school, along with their race, gender, age, type of predental education, mean DAT and GPA, and state of origin.

ACADEMIC AND OTHER ASSISTANCE

Academic and personal counseling is available to all students through assignment to faculty advisors in the School of Dentistry or through the University Counseling Service. It is anticipated that problems the student might experience can be identified and confronted before they become compounded. Tutorial assistance is available if necessary. This institution has the capability to graduate every student accepted into the freshman class and makes every effort to do so. Faculty and students alike are committed to this mutual goal. Students accepted into the School of Dentistry should be prepared to support the entire expense of their dental education. The Student Loan Committee will strive to distribute equitably all available funds, so that those most in need of aid will receive as much help as is practicable.

The UASD conducts a program designed to interest, recruit, and retain disadvantaged minority students and other individuals from groups traditionally underrepresented in the profession. Advice and special counseling are given to these individuals, once identified, in the application procedure. Several faculty members sharing responsibility in this area are also members of the Admissions Committee and are therefore able to contribute to the total evaluation of these applicants.

ARIZONA SCHOOL OF DENTISTRY & ORAL HEALTH

Dr. Jack Dillenberg, Dean

GENERAL INFORMATION

The Arizona School of Dentistry & Oral Health prepares caring, technologically adept dentists to become community and educational leaders. The school offers students an experience-rich learning environment where health professionals approach patient health as part of a team. The Arizona School of Dentistry & Oral Health is part of A.T. Still University, which also includes the Kirksville College of Osteopathic Medicine, Arizona School of Health Sciences, and the School of Health Management.

The 23-acre campus is situated on a 90-acre health and technology park that provides the latest in educational innovations and easy access to Phoenix metropolitan activities. The campus provides a learning environment that is a leader for teaching advanced health professionals. Students, faculty, local dentists, and national oral health leaders have the advantages of broadband wireless and wired digital access, virtual and traditional library services, distance education technologies, and a sophisticated dental simulation lab.

Situated in the East Valley of Arizona's dynamic Phoenix Metropolitan Area, the Arizona School of Dentistry & Oral Health is Arizona's first dental school. The beautiful Sonoran desert, numerous lakes and mountains, urban activities of the nation's sixth largest community, and year round mild climate make Arizona one of the world's most desirable destinations.

ADMISSION REQUIREMENTS

NUMBER OF YEARS OF PREDENTAL EDUCATION: A formal minimum of three years (90 semester hours or 135 quarter hours), but a baccalaureate degree is preferred.

LIMITATION ON COMMUNITY COLLEGE WORK: Courses taken at an accredited community college are applicable if they are equivalent to predental courses at a four-year college.

REQUIRED COURSES:

With lab required	(semester hrs)
General biology	8
(zoology or microbiology are acceptable alternatives)	
General chemistry	8
Organic chemistry	8
Physics (algebra-based)	8
Biochemistry	8
Physiology	8

Other courses
English composition/Technical writing — 3

SUGGESTED ADDITIONAL PREPARATION: Applicants are advised to have a baccalaureate degree, although no specific major is required. Broad preparation with a liberal arts background is recommended. Electives should be chosen from courses that extend the content of biomedical sciences such as anatomy and microbiology. Additional courses that may enhance students' ability to practice dentistry include social sciences, management, business, fine arts, foreign language, and communications. Demonstrated community service through volunteerism or service-oriented employment is preferred. Preference is given to individuals with a demonstrated interest in practicing in underserved areas. Computer literacy is required.

DAT: All applicants are required to take the Dental Admission Test (DAT) and submit their scores. No scores older than three years will be accepted. Canadian DAT scores are not accepted.

GPA: Applicants must have a minimum cumulative and science grade point average of 2.50 on a four-point scale. The overall and science GPA, the school(s) attended, and the rigor of the academic course load are all assessed on an individual basis.

RESIDENCY: Must be a U.S. citizen or permanent resident to apply.

ADVANCED STANDING: The school does not have an established advanced standing program for transfer students or graduates of foreign dental schools.

ARIZONA

Timetable for the Class Entering Fall 2008

	Earliest Date	Latest Date	School Fee
Application Submission	6/1/07	12/1/07	$60
Acceptance Notification	12/1/07		

Required Response:

30 days after notification if received between 12/1 and 1/31
15 days after notification if received between 2/1 and 4/30
7 days after notification if received after 4/30

FOR FURTHER INFORMATION

Office of Admissions
Donna Sparks
Associate Director of Admissions
660-626-2237

Office of Financial Aid
Steve Jorden
Director, Financial Assistance
660-626-2529

Arizona School of Dentistry & Oral Health
5850 E. Still Circle
Mesa, AZ 85206
480-219-6000

Office of Student Services
Beth Poppre
Asst. VP, Student Services
A.T. Still University
480-219-6000
Arizona School of Dentistry & Oral Health
5850 E. Still Circle
Mesa, AZ 85206

www.atsu.edu

THE DENTAL PROGRAM

The curriculum at the Arizona School of Dentistry & Oral Health is designed to produce graduates who are technologically adept, professionally competent, patient-centered, and compassionate.

The curriculum emphasizes patient care experiences through simulation, integration of biomedical and clinical sciences, and problem solving scenarios to achieve clinical excellence. The curriculum includes a strong component of public health, leadership, and practice through weekly learning modules. Students have the opportunity to interact with faculty, practicing dentists, and national leaders to discuss cases in a regularly scheduled "grand rounds" format.

■ Community Service and Patient Care

Students receive fourth-year clinical training offsite alongside dentists practicing in community health centers, American Indian clinics, and other community-based organizations.

■ Clinical Training

YEAR 1. Integrated Human Sciences with preclinical dental simulation.

YEAR 2. Integrated Clinical Sciences with preclinical didactic courses and clinical experiences.

YEAR 3. Mentored on-site clinical experience with clinical didactic courses.

YEAR 4. Continuation of on-site mentored clinical experiences, interspersed with a variety of off-site community-based experiences with community clinical partners providing rich cultural and socio-economic experiences.

■ Degrees Offered

DENTAL DEGREE: Doctor of Dental Medicine (D.M.D.) with a Certificate in Public Health Management

COSTS AND FINANCIAL AID

Estimated Total Expenses for Academic Year 2006-07

Tuition	$39,680
Educational technology fee	$1,050
Computer	$1,900
Educational supplies	$7,725
Room	$11,341
Board	$3,542
Transportation	$3,036
Insurance (health, life, auto)	$3,212
Personal	$4,006
TOTAL	**$75,672**

SELECTION FACTORS

Applicants are evaluated on academic coursework, performance on the DAT, AADSAS essay, letters of evaluation (predental advisory committee when applicable), interviews, leadership, and personal characteristics. Demonstrated community service through volunteerism or service-oriented employment is preferred. The school actively seeks minority applicants who are underrepresented in the dental profession.

See chapter 3 of this guide for information regarding numbers of applicants and enrollees to each dental school, along with their race, gender, age, type of predental education, mean DAT and GPA, and state of origin.

ARIZONA

MIDWESTERN UNIVERSITY
COLLEGE OF DENTAL MEDICINE

Dr. Richard J. Simonsen, Dean

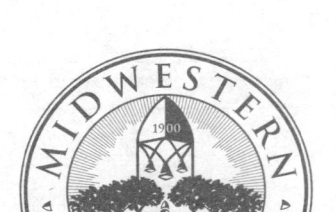

GENERAL INFORMATION

The College of Dental Medicine is part of the campus of Midwestern University in Glendale, Arizona. Midwestern University's original campus is located in Downers Grove, Illinois, and the university was founded in 1900. The Glendale campus is situated on 146 acres 15 miles northwest of downtown Phoenix, and continues its growth and development from a single building in 1996 to a full-service university with over 20 buildings with 483,424 total square feet and over 1,300 students in 2006. Midwestern University's Glendale campus consists of more than nine colleges and programs offering a variety of graduate degrees, including doctoral degree programs. The four-year dental curriculum leads to a D.M.D. (Doctor of Dental Medicine) degree.

The greater Phoenix metropolitan area is one of the fastest-growing metropolitan areas in the United States. Glendale is home to both the NFL Arizona Cardinals professional football team as well as the NHL Phoenix Coyotes hockey team. The area offers an ideal climate and an abundance of social, cultural, and athletic activities, from concerts in Scottsdale and Phoenix to snow skiing in Flagstaff, just two hours north of the campus.

The residential Student Housing Complex comprises eight buildings with 216 studio, one-bedroom and two-bedroom units. The university has plans to build additional units as the campus community grows prior to fall 2008, which coincides with the matriculation date for the inaugural dental class. The campus is situated in a safe and secure environment for students and their families who live on the campus. Recreational facilities for the housing complex include a children's playground, a swimming pool, and a sand volleyball court.

The College of Dental Medicine plans to start its inaugural class in fall 2008 with 100 students. In order to accommodate the new dental school, the university is constructing new facilities and improving is existing facilities. The estimated cost of these projects is $140 million. Included in these projects are additional classrooms, auditoriums, and faculty offices. A new student recreational center is currently being constructed and an addition to the student services building will be completed prior to the arrival of the inaugural class. Funding for the $140 million expansion has been secured through a combination of existing university funds and external financing. In addition, a dental clinic will be constructed to meet the needs of the clinical portion of the students' education. Standard and Poor's has reviewed MWU financing plans and reaffirmed the university's long-term debt rating of A-.

ADMISSION REQUIREMENTS

NUMBER OF YEARS OF PREDENTAL EDUCATION: A general minimum of three years, but to be competitive an applicant is advised to have completed a bachelor's degree at an accredited North American college or university prior to matriculation. Applicants participating in special affiliated programs with the College and other exceptions to this policy will be considered on an individual basis.

LIMITATIONS ON COMMUNITY COLLEGE WORK: No more than 60 hours of college credit should be earned at a community college, and preference is given to candidates who complete the science prerequisites of a four-year institution.

REQUIRED COURSES:

With lab required	(semester/quarter hrs)
Biology	8/12
General Chemistry	8/12
Organic Chemistry	4/6
Anatomy	4/6
Microbiology	4/6

Other courses	
Physics	8/12
Physiology	4/6
Biochemistry	3/4.5
English composition/Technical writing	8/12

SUGGESTED ADDITIONAL PREPARATION: It is advantageous for applicants to have course credit in cellular and/or molecular biology and histology.

DAT: Mandatory. An Academic Average score of 18 or higher and a Perceptual Ability score of 17 or higher are desired. Test scores must not be older than three years.

GPA: Applicants should possess both a science and a total GPA over 2.50 on a 4.00 scale (although over 3.00 will be generally necessary to be competitive), as well as a bachelor's degree. A minimum science and an overall GPA of 2.50 on a 4.00 scale is required to receive a supplemental application.

ADVANCED STANDING: An advanced standing program is not available at this time for graduates of foreign dental schools. Transfer applicants from U.S. or Canadian dental schools can be considered only when vacancies occur. Normally, transfer applicants will be placed in the first or second year of study.

Timetable for the Class Entering Fall 2008

	Earliest Date	Latest Date	School Fee
Application Submission	6/1/07	2/1/08	
Supplemental Application	7/1/07	3/1/08	$75
Acceptance Notification	12/1/07	8/15/08	

Required Response:

30 days if accepted between 12/1 and 12/31
15 days if accepted between 1/1 and 1/31
10 days if accepted on or after 2/1
First nonrefundable $1,000 deposit with offer of place contract; second nonrefundable $1,000 deposit due 5/1. Both deposits credited toward first quarter tuition.

FOR FURTHER INFORMATION
Office of Admissions
James Walter
Director
623-572-3275 or 888-247-9277

Office of Financial Aid
Carol Dolan
Director
623-572-3321

Midwestern University
19555 N. 59th Avenue
Glendale, AZ 85308

www.midwestern.edu

MIDWESTERN UNIVERSITY COLLEGE OF DENTAL MEDICINE ARIZONA

THE DENTAL PROGRAM

The mission of the Midwestern University College of Dental Medicine is to educate competent clinical dentists of strong character and high ethical standards who serve the needs of the public and improve the health and well-being of society. The College promotes evidenced-based critical inquiry allowing for a preventive, minimally invasive orientation, with an emphasis on research and service in the practice of dentistry.

■ Degrees Offered

DENTAL DEGREE: D.M.D.

ALTERNATE DEGREES: Dual degree programs may be available for D.M.D. students. Under the College of Health Sciences, an M.A. degree in Bioethics and an M.P.H.E. (master's in health professions education) can be pursued concomitantly with the D.M.D. degree.

COSTS AND FINANCIAL AID

The Financial Aid Office is committed to employing every available means in assisting applicants to meet the needs of their education expense. In addition to federal loan programs, needs-based scholarships are available annually through the university's participation in the School-as-Lender program. For academic years 2007 and 2008, over $1 million per year is available for need-based aid. A pro-rata number of needy students in the College of Dental Medicine will receive these scholarships beginning with the entering class. Student employment is permitted, provided it does not impede academic performance or interfere with clinical activity. Entering students may request financial assistance information and application material any time after confirmation of acceptance by writing to the director of financial aid.

Estimated Total Expenses for Academic Year 2008-09

	YEAR 1*	YEAR 2	YEAR 3	YEAR 4	TOTAL
Tuition, resident	$48,881	$51,325	$53,891	$56,586	$210,683
Tuition, nonresident	$48,881	$51,325	$53,891	$56,586	$210,683
Fees	$9,000	$9,450	$9,923	$10,419	$38,792
TOTAL EXPENSES/RESIDENT	$57,881	$60,775	$63,814	$67,005	$249,475
TOTAL EXPENSES/NONRESIDENT	$57,881	$60,775	$63,814	$67,005	$249,475

* Note that Year 1 costs are for the academic year 2008-2009, which is the inaugural year for the Midwestern University College of Dental Medicine.

SELECTION FACTORS

If the undergraduate institution has a prehealth advisory committee, a committee evaluation is strongly recommended. Otherwise, three letters of evaluation are required, one of which should be from a predental advisor and two from health care or other professionals who know the applicant well and who can comment on the applicant's character, special abilities, and professional motivation.

The Admissions Committee carefully considers each applicant's scholastic record, scores on the DAT, AADSAS essay, letters of evaluation, evidence of manual dexterity (including the perceptual ability portion of the DAT), and other personal attributes and qualities, as well as demonstration of his or her understanding about a career in the dental profession.

Applicants who appear to meet the requirements will be invited to the dental school in Glendale for an interview with one or more of the Admissions Committee.

Midwestern University has established a firm policy of not discriminating against any applicant because of age, race, gender, creed, disability, or national origin. Established review procedures ensure applicants an equal opportunity to be considered for admission. The school has an affirmative action program with regard to admission of qualified ethnic minorities, females, and members of underrepresented groups.

ACADEMIC AND OTHER ASSISTANCE

Student Services interacts with students to develop and offer support programs and services that enrich students' experiences on campus. Examples of these programs include MWU Student Government, MWU Student Tutoring Program, student social and recreational activities including intramural sports, academic and personal counseling including general support and crisis intervention for spouses and significant others, stress and time management programs, multicultural, spiritual and diversity programming, and other professional development activities. The Department of Student Services has an open-door policy and is available to students on a continuing basis offering support, advice, and encouragement needed to meet student concerns and challenges. The student financial services staff serves the needs of students in all facets of financial aid counseling (debt management, financial literacy, and financial planning) and provides them with information regarding available private, state, institutional, and federal funding sources. In addition, the office provides electronic billing and payment services to all enrolled students. The office has an open-door policy regarding student counseling.

CALIFORNIA

LOMA LINDA UNIVERSITY
SCHOOL OF DENTISTRY

Dr. Charles J. Goodacre, Dean

GENERAL INFORMATION

Loma Linda University (LLU) represents distinction in quality Christian education. As a private university owned and operated by the Seventh-Day Adventist Church, the university has established a reputation for leadership in mission service, research, and advancements in the health-related sciences. Located 60 miles east of Los Angeles in one of the fastest growing areas in the United States, the university is comprised of seven health science schools including Schools of Dentistry, Medicine, Pharmacy, Nursing, Allied Health Professions, Public Health, and a Graduate School with an annual enrollment of over 3,000 students from over 100 countries. Each school is committed to diversity in both the student community and the distinguished faculty, which numbers over 1,800.

Since 1953, the School of Dentistry has sought to provide an educational environment in which students learn to provide high-quality dental care that is preventive in purpose, comprehensive in scope, and based on sound biological principles. Operating one of the largest dental clinics in the nation, the school affiliates with programs with the Loma Linda University Medical Center and the Pettis Memorial Veterans Medical Center. In addition to the D.D.S., the school offers a B.S. in dental hygiene, as well as advanced education programs in anesthesia, endodontics, oral and maxillofacial surgery, oral implantology, orthodontics, periodontics, prosthodontics, and pediatric dentistry. An International Dentist Program educates dentists trained in other countries to meet U.S. standards of care. In accordance with the university's focus on service, the School of Dentistry sponsors students on mission trips to clinics and extensive continuing education courses worldwide.

The school has full accreditation with the American Dental Association Commission on Dental Accreditation as well as the Western Association of Schools and Colleges. LLU participates in the Western Interstate Commission for Higher Education (WICHE) program and offers financial aid programs for eligible students through a financial aid advisor who is dedicated to assisting all students with financial planning and debt-management counseling.

ADMISSION REQUIREMENTS

NUMBER OF YEARS OF PREDENTAL EDUCATION: Three years; minimum of 96 semester or 144 quarter units; priority given to students with bachelor's degree.

REQUIRED COURSES: Science coursework must be completed within the five years prior to admission.

With lab required	(semester/quarter hrs)
General biology or zoology	8/12
General or inorganic chemistry	8/12
Organic chemistry	8/12
General physics	8/12

Other courses	
Composition and literature	3/4
Freshman English	3/4

SUGGESTED ADDITIONAL PREPARATION: Choose from upper-division biology courses including anatomy, histology, biochemistry, immunology, and physiology. Courses in psychology and sociology, principles of management, accounting, sculpture, and ceramics will contribute to a broad educational background.

DAT: Mandatory, minimum scores of 17 on academic average and PAT; recommended to be taken one year before entrance; a manual skills test may be included at time of interview.

GPA: Minimum of 2.7; grade of "C" or above in all required preentrance coursework.

RESIDENCY: No specific requirements.

ADVANCED STANDING: An international dentist program with limited space accepts students for a 21-month clinical program. Students from U.S. dental schools are eligible to transfer at the freshman level only.

Timetable for the Class Entering Fall 2008

	Earliest Date	Latest Date	School Fees
Regular Admission	6/1/07	12/1/07	$75
Acceptance Notification	12/1/07	4/1/08	

Required Response and Deposit:
$1,000

FOR FURTHER INFORMATION
Office of Admissions
Marlise Perry
Assistant Director of Admissions
909-558-4621; 800-422-4558

Esther Valenzuela
Director of Admissions
909-558-4621; 800-422-4558

Office of Financial Aid
Financial Aid Advisor
909-558-4509

Office of Diversity
Leslie Pollard
909-558-4787
Loma Linda University
Loma Linda, CA 92350

Housing
909-558-4510
Office of the Dean of Students
Loma Linda University
Loma Linda, CA 92350

www.dentistry.llu.edu

THE DENTAL PROGRAM

LLU's program is a traditional dental curriculum with emphasis in clinical training. Graduates are skilled in providing quality dental care that is comprehensive in its scope and preventive in its goals.

YEAR 1. Basic sciences with introduction to clinical sciences.

YEAR 2. Applied sciences and introduction to clinical practice.

YEAR 3. Clinical sciences with extensive patient contact.

YEAR 4. Delivery of comprehensive dental care with extramural programs in locations nationwide and worldwide.

■ Degrees Offered
DENTAL DEGREE: D.D.S.

ALTERNATE DEGREES: Combined D.D.S./Ph.D. or D.D.S./M.S. program in a biomedical science (available are anatomy, biochemistry, microbiology, pharmacology, and physiology).

■ Other Programs
RESEARCH: Excellent opportunities available in biomaterials, endodontics, and periodontics.

FELLOWSHIPS: Externships in the D.D.S./Ph.D. program. Available to fourth-year students only.

ETHICS: M.A. in Bioethics available through the University Center for Bioethics.

COSTS AND FINANCIAL AID

LLU offers financial aid programs for eligible students with documented needs. A financial aid advisor for all dental students is dedicated to assist each applicant with financial planning for dental educational costs.

Financial Aid Awards to First-Year Students in 2006-07
■ TOTAL NUMBER OF RECIPIENTS: 83 OUT OF 95 STUDENTS

Average Award	Range of Awards
$49,664	$0-$60,889

Estimated School-Related Expenses for Academic Year 2006-07

	YEAR 1	YEAR 2	YEAR 3	YEAR 4	TOTAL
Tuition	$37,377	$45,279	$45,279	$45,279	$173,214
University Fees	$1,395	$1,860	$1,860	$1,860	$6,475
Instruments and rental	$6,003	$3,995	$218	$88	$10,304
Supplies	$127	$452	$216	$404	$1,199
Lab fees	$135	$140	$120	$40	$435
Texts/manuals	$1,100	$1,260	$1,200	$300	$3,860
National Board exams	0	$220	0	$295	$515
Technical support fee	$450	$600	$600	$600	$2,250
ADA/CDA required fees	$72	$72	$72	$72	$288
Dental lab gold*	0	$360	$100	0	$460
Restorative dept. supplies	$253	$505	$116	$47	$921
Other dept. supplies	$95	$100	$330	0	$525
Computer	$2,200	0	0	0	$2,200
TOTAL	$49,207	$54,843	$50,111	$48,985	$203,146

Tuition and University Fees shown are actual figures for the 2006-07 school year. Students should plan on an annual tuition increase consistent with inflation in the education sector. Figures in all other categories are estimates based on the best information available at this time and are subject to change.
*Cost of gold is variable depending on actual usage and market value.

SELECTION FACTORS

Inasmuch as the School of Dentistry is owned by the Seventh-Day Adventist Church, some preference is shown to applicants from SDA universities and colleges. Priority is given to applicants from underrepresented minorities. Based on qualifications as revealed by the AADSAS application, a supplementary package is sent. After review of the supplementary material, transcripts, and recommendations, an applicant may be invited to the school for a personal interview. The Committee on Admissions bases its appraisal of an applicant on review of the completed AADSAS application, a supplementary application from LLU, transcripts that show strength in the predental science coursework, DAT scores with emphasis on the academic average and PAT, letters of recommendation with preprofessional committee reports if available, and a personal interview. Personal qualifications such as integrity and commitment to God and humankind, self-discipline, and self-direction are integral to an applicant's profile and are assessed by reviewing the essays written for both the AADSAS and supplementary applications as well as the personal interview.

See chapter 3 of this guide for information regarding numbers of applicants and enrollees to each dental school, along with their race, gender, age, type of predental education, mean DAT and GPA, and state of origin.

ACADEMIC AND OTHER ASSISTANCE

LLU sponsors a Careers in Dentistry workshop each summer that helps to prepare a student who is thinking of a dental career or provides an interested student an opportunity to see the school and participate in classes and labs. The admissions personnel advise at colleges throughout the United States, seeking to recruit and assist students from underrepresented populations.

CALIFORNIA

UNIVERSITY OF CALIFORNIA, LOS ANGELES
SCHOOL OF DENTISTRY

Dr. No-Hee Park, Dean

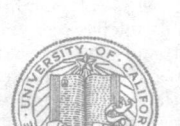

GENERAL INFORMATION

The UCLA School of Dentistry enrolled its first class in 1964 and is one of two public dental schools in California. It has an average enrollment of 88 dental students per class and 100 postgraduate residents. UCLA dental students traditionally have a pass rate in the top quintile for Parts I and II of the National Dental Boards and an average pass rate of 95 percent on the California State Board licensing examination. The vertical tier curriculum is competency-based with Pass/Not Pass grading.

The School of Dentistry, located in West Los Angeles, was established in 1960 by the Regents of the University of California. The school is located in the Center for Health Sciences on the UCLA campus. The center includes Schools of Medicine, Nursing, and Public Health and contains a 674-bed hospital, the Neuropsychiatric Institute, the Jules Stein Eye Institute, the Children's Health Center, and an outstanding biomedical library.

ADMISSION REQUIREMENTS

NUMBER OF YEARS OF PREDENTAL EDUCATION: Formal minimum of three; large majority have four; 90 semester or 135 quarter units.

LIMITATIONS ON COMMUNITY COLLEGE WORK: 70 semester or 105 quarter units.

REQUIRED COURSES:

With one year of lab required (2 semester/3 quarter hrs)

Inorganic chemistry	8/12
Organic chemistry	6/8
Physics	8/12
Biology	8/12

Other courses

English composition	6/8
Introductory psychology	3/4
Biochemistry	3/4

SUGGESTED ADDITIONAL PREPARATION: Choose from among histology, physiology, human or comparative anatomy, social sciences, microbiology, communication, business, composition, technical writing, fine arts, drafting, engineering, and learning skills.

DAT: Mandatory; must be taken no later than December 31 and within a three-year period. The Canadian DAT is not accepted.

GPA: Typical range: 2.7-4.0; typical median: 3.64

RESIDENCY: U.S. citizen or Permanent Resident. (Permanent Residents must be in possession of their resident alien card at time of application.)

ADVANCED STANDING: Graduates of foreign dental schools may apply for the Professional Program for International Dentists, which awards a D.D.S. degree after two years of study. The application deadline date is September 15.

Timetable for the Class Entering Fall 2008

	Earliest Date	Latest Date	School Fee
Application Submission	6/1/07	1/1/08	$60
Acceptance Notification	12/1/07	4/30/08*	

*Alternates may be accepted later.

Required Response:
30 days if accepted on or after December 1
15 days if accepted on or after January 1
7 days if accepted on or after February 1

FOR FURTHER INFORMATION

Office of Admissions
Noemi Benitez
Coordinator
310-794-7971; nbenitez@dent.ucla.edu
Office of Student Affairs and Outreach

Evelyn Marques
Office Manager
310-825-8311; emarques@dent.ucla.edu
Office of Student Affairs and Outreach

Professional Program for International Dentists
310-825-6218
Office of Student Affairs and Outreach

Office of Financial Aid
310-825-6994
Office of Student Affairs

10833 LeConte Avenue, Rm. A0-111
University of California, Los Angeles
Los Angeles, CA 90095-1762

Housing
Community Housing Office
310-825-4941
270 DeNeve Drive, 1st Floor Lobby
Business Enterprise Building
University of California, Los Angeles
Los Angeles, CA 90095-1495

www.dent.ucla.edu

UNIVERSITY OF CALIFORNIA, LOS ANGELES, SCHOOL OF DENTISTRY **CALIFORNIA**

THE DENTAL PROGRAM

The length of the program is 45 months with at least 34 in actual attendance. The program consists of 12 quarters of ten weeks each, plus three required nine-week summer sessions between years one and two, years two and three, and years three and four.

The goals of the program are to produce graduates who: 1) possess the preventive, diagnostic, and technical knowledge and skills necessary to provide patients with comprehensive dental health in a variety of health care delivery systems; 2) view their role in the profession from a humanitarian perspective, accepting patients' dental health as a right rather than a privilege, their patients' psychological and physical health being the prime focus of their practices; 3) are able to provide socially sensitive and responsible leadership in the community of their practice; and 4) continuously update their knowledge of dental health and oral diseases, their techniques, and their practices.

The basic sciences and preclinical laboratory courses are taught primarily in the first two years of the curriculum by the appropriate departments of the medical and dental school. The clinical experience in comprehensive patient care begins immediately in the first year. There are numerous selective programs covering a wide variety of experiences and topics, such as the clinical management of patients and hospital service rotations.

The off-campus clinical experiences that are an official part of the curriculum are at the Wilson-Jennings-Bloomfield UCLA Venice Dental Center in Venice, California, administered by the dental school in association with the local community; Harbor/UCLA Medical Center; Inglewood Children's Clinic.

■ Degrees Offered
DENTAL DEGREE: D.D.S.

ALTERNATE DEGREES: Combined D.D.S./M.S. or D.D.S./Ph.D. in Oral Biology or Ph.D., and a D.D.S./M.B.A.

■ Other Programs
RESEARCH: Students may choose a selective research project, normally completed at the end of their third year.

SELECTIVES: Twenty-six units are required for graduation of which at least eight units must be in service learning.

SELECTION FACTORS

The Admissions Committee takes into account: 1) scholastic record; 2) aptitude for science demonstrated by academic record and the DAT; 3) academic performance on DAT, in particular, the PMAT portion of the exam to determine spatial aptitude; 4) English composition performance on DAT, especially for English as a Second Language applicants; 5) manner in which scholastic record was achieved, i.e., course load, breadth of the courses of study, extracurricular activities, and work experience; and 6) substantive letters of recommendation.

The school participates in the Western Interstate Commission on Higher Education (WICHE).

COSTS AND FINANCIAL AID

UCLA School of Dentistry provides both need- and merit-based funds. The dental financial aid officer is available to ensure comprehensive, personal, and confidential counseling and servicing.

Financial Aid Awards to First-Year Students in 2006-07
■ TOTAL NUMBER OF RECIPIENTS: 82   ■ 94% OF CLASS

	Average Award	Range of Awards
Residents	$44,408	$1,000-$56,245
Nonresidents	$57,457	$41,500-$68,430

Estimated Total Expenses for Academic Year 2006-07

	YEAR 1	YEAR 2	YEAR 3	YEAR 4	TOTAL
Fees, Resident	$25,563	$27,873	$27,873	$27,873	$109,182
Fees and Tuition, Nonresidents	$35,826	$38,136	$38,136	$38,136	$150,234
Equipment/Books/Supplies/Instrument	$15,684	$10,128	$3,344	$3,909	$33,065
Living Expenses (off campus students: room/board, personal, transportation)	$18,027	$24,036	$24,036	$24,036	$90,135
TOTAL EXPENSES, RESIDENT	$59,274	$62,037	$55,253	$55,818	$232,382
TOTAL EXPENSES, NONRESIDENT	$69,537	$72,300	$65,516	$66,081	$273,434

Residents pay fees only. Nonresidents pay fees and tuition.
Tuition and fees listed above are estimates only.
NOTE: Fees subject to change without prior notice.

CALIFORNIA

UNIVERSITY OF CALIFORNIA, SAN FRANCISCO
SCHOOL OF DENTISTRY

Dr. Charles N. Bertolami, Dean

GENERAL INFORMATION

The University of California, San Francisco School of Dentistry (UCSF), located in what has been called America's favorite city, has been part of the University of California since 1881. UCSF is the only one of the nine UC campuses devoted solely to the health sciences. It consists of four professional schools: dentistry, medicine, nursing, and pharmacy; a graduate program in basic and behavioral sciences; two health policy institutes; a medical center with three hospitals; and the largest ambulatory care program in the state. UCSF also has one of the preeminent health sciences libraries in the world. Current enrollment at UCSF accommodates 80 dental students per entering class. As a major professional school campus, UCSF offers all of the amenities attendant to such an institution, such as a campus newspaper, bookstore, student union with handball courts, swimming pool, full court basketball gym, and state-of-the-art multifaceted exercise facility.

The UCSF School of Dentistry seeks to improve public health through excellence in teaching, research, patient care, and public service in the dental and craniofacial sciences. We foster an inspired environment where individuals identify themselves as scholars and realize their scholarship through service as clinicians, educators, and scientists.

In addition to the program leading to the D.D.S. degree, UCSF offers certification in most of the dental specialties, including oral and maxillofacial surgery, orthodontics, endodontics, prosthodontics, pediatric dentistry and public health dentistry. The Graduate Program in Oral and Craniofacial Sciences provides training at both the Ph.D. and M.S. levels. Postgraduate specialty training is available in dental public health, oral and maxillofacial surgery (including an M.D. option), endodontics, oral medicine, orthodontics, periodontology, pediatric dentistry, and prosthodontics as well as the General Practice Residency program. An integrated D.D.S.-Ph.D. program (Dental Scientist Training Program, DSTP) is also available for a small number of highly qualified students.

UCSF is state-supported and participates in the student exchange program provided by the Western Interstate Commission for Higher Education (WICHE), a program that supports students from western states without dental schools.

The faculty, students, and staff of the UCSF School of Dentistry are committed to fostering an environment of mutual trust and respect. UCSF believes this goal requires clear communication, compassion for others, and enthusiasm for the dental profession.

ADMISSION REQUIREMENTS

NUMBER OF YEARS OF PREDENTAL EDUCATION: Minimum three (93 semester or 139 quarter hours).

LIMITATIONS ON COMMUNITY COLLEGE WORK: 70 semester or 105 quarter hours.

REQUIRED COURSES: *(semester/quarter hrs)*

General chemistry with lab	8/12
Organic chemistry with lab	4/8
Physics with lab	8/12
Biology/zoology with lab*	8/12
Biochemistry	3/4
English composition and literature*	6/8
Psychology	3/4
Social sciences, humanities, and/or foreign language	11/16
Electives	42/63

* Anatomy and physiology do NOT fulfill this requirement
**ESL courses do NOT fulfill this requirement.

SUGGESTED ADDITIONAL PREPARATION: Recommended courses include embryology, comparative vertebrate anatomy, genetics, and statistics. At the same time, it is felt that the practice of dentistry is also a social science and an art, and well-rounded professionals need good verbal and liberal arts skills to be fully effective in the field. The school requires no specific undergraduate major or field of study, and candidates are urged to broaden their education with the inclusion of courses in the arts, humanities, and social sciences. Nonscience majors can be serious contenders for admission, although they should take at least one science course each quarter or semester.

DAT: Mandatory; no later than December 15, 2007.

GPA: California residents must have a minimum overall and science GPA of 2.4. Non-California residents must have a minimum overall and science GPA of 3.0. All required coursework *must* be finished by the end of spring of the year of intended enrollment. Foreign applicants must successfully complete *at least one year* of college work in the United States.

RESIDENCY: No specific requirements.

Foreign dental graduates should apply to the UCSF's International Dentist Program (IDP).

University of California
San Francisco

School of Dentistry

Timetable for the Class Entering Fall 2008

	Earliest Date	Latest Date
Application Submission	6/1/07	1/1/08
Acceptance Notification	12/1/07	4/15/08

Required Response and Deposit:
Acceptance card, along with $200 deposit fee.

FOR FURTHER INFORMATION
Office of Admissions
UCSF School of Dentistry
513 Parnassus Avenue, S619
San Francisco, CA 94143-0430
415-476-2737

Student Financial Services
Millberry Union, 520 Parnassus
University of California, San Francisco
San Francisco, CA 94143
415-476-4181

dentistry.ucsf.edu

THE DENTAL PROGRAM

Commencing with the summer 2004 quarter, an entirely new pre-doctoral curriculum was implemented at the School of Dentistry, affecting both the D.D.S. program and the International Dentist Program. The concept of the new curriculum is to organize material into five thematic streams that emphasize and reinforce the integration of basic sciences and clinical sciences in dental education. This will better enable graduates to provide the best patient care, to translate science into practice, and to follow a variety of career paths.

The dental curriculum is designed to prepare students to render comprehensive oral care of high quality. The curriculum emphasizes thorough understanding of diagnosis, prevention, and control of disease; recognition of social needs; and knowledge of general health problems. Students are evaluated by examination and clinical test cases or by the quality and quantity of procedures completed, depending on the requirements of the course. Courses are graded Passed/Not Passed/Passed with Honors. Tutorial services are available to all students.

Students from the health science schools on the UCSF campus share many facilities, faculty, and community experiences as well as a central library, which includes a complete self-instruction center. Audiovisual materials prepared by the campus's Educational Media Resources, faculty-prepared syllabuses, films, and videocassettes provide self-pacing opportunities for students, in addition to reinforcing health team concepts learned in satellite clinics and hospitals.

■ Degrees Offered

DENTAL DEGREE: D.D.S.

ALTERNATE DEGREES: B.S. in dental sciences integrated with the D.D.S. degree; M.S. in oral and craniofacial sciences integrated with the specialty certificate or D.D.S. degree; Ph.D. in oral and craniofacial sciences; Ph.D. (in bioengineering) integrated with the D.D.S. degree (DSTP). There is also a new clinical sciences Ph.D. program and a concurrent D.D.S./M.B.A. program, with the M.B.A. studies completed at the University of San Francisco.

■ Other Programs

A limited number of summer research fellowships are available to qualified entering students.

COSTS AND FINANCIAL AID

UCSF participates in all major federal and state financial aid programs, and eligible students receive federal Stafford, Perkins, and Health and Human Services loans, as well as grants and scholarships offered through both federal and institutional sources. Students can also apply for work-study funds. For students in the Ph.D. program, a number of support mechanisms are available, including institutional training grants and awards from the National Institute of Dental and Craniofacial Research. The campus also has a career services office.

Financial Aid Awards to First-Year Students in 2006-07
■ TOTAL NUMBER OF RECIPIENTS: 68   ■ 85% OF CLASS

	Average Award	Range of Awards
Residents	$50,457	$16,533-$67,933
Nonresidents	$50,690	$10,000-$71,202

SELECTION FACTORS

UCSF carefully reviews the perceptual ability portion of the required DAT to determine spatial aptitude. In addition, the Admissions Committee compares DAT academic scores with grades in the required courses to measure academic background and considers upward scholastic trends as evidence of motivation and goal direction. Along with competitive grades and DAT scores, the committee looks for evidence of interest in the dental profession, community service, research experience, probability of serving an underserved community, and the potential for future leadership within the dental profession.

Three letters of recommendation are required; two of them should be from college science professors or instructors. A single composite letter from a preprofessional advisory committee is also acceptable. A personal interview is required.

Applicants are encouraged to submit their AADSAS application early. The School will not accept applications that fail to meet the January 1 deadline. The school's selection process begins in October and continues until the entire class is selected usually around March.

See chapter 3 of this guide for information regarding numbers of applicants and enrollees to each dental school, along with their race, gender, age, type of predental education, mean DAT and GPA, and state of origin.

ACADEMIC AND OTHER ASSISTANCE

Several scholarships and other nonrepayable funds, as well as federal and university loans, are available to entering dental students with financial need.

Financial aid applications for entering students should be submitted to Student Financial Services at the time of the applicant's admission. A student's need for financial aid while in dental school may be reviewed at any time during the year.

Estimated Total Expenses for Academic Year 2006-07

	YEAR 1	YEAR 2	YEAR 3	YEAR 4	TOTAL
Fees, residents	$25,206	$25,206	$27,587	$27,587	$105,586
Fees, nonresidents	$37,451	$37,451	$39,832	$39,832	$154,566
Equipment cost	$11,472	$11,682	$8,415	$5,355	$36,924
Books and supplies	$2,158	$1,204	$1,529	$514	$5,405
Est. living expenses	$17,028	$17,028	$22,704	$22,704	$79,464
TOTAL EXPENSES, RESIDENT	**$55,864**	**$55,120**	**$60,235**	**$56,160**	**$227,379**
TOTAL EXPENSES, NONRESIDENT	**$68,109**	**$67,365**	**$72,480**	**$68,405**	**$276,359**

Tuition and fees are subject to change without notice.

CALIFORNIA

UNIVERSITY OF THE PACIFIC
ARTHUR A. DUGONI SCHOOL OF DENTISTRY

Dr. Patrick J. Ferrillo, Jr., Dean

GENERAL INFORMATION

One of the world's most distinctive metropolitan centers, San Francisco has been the home of the University of the Pacific Arthur A. Dugoni School of Dentistry since its incorporation in 1896 as the College of Physicians and Surgeons. The school has been recognized since its inception as a major resource of dental education in the western states and is the only dental school in which you can complete a four-academic year curriculum in just three calendar years. In 1962, the College of Physicians and Surgeons amalgamated with the University of the Pacific, and an eight-story building was completed in 1967 for functional teaching of clinical dentistry and to conduct dental research. Equipment and facilities are constantly updated, setting the pace for new and better methods of dental care delivery. In 1996 the school opened a state-of-the-art preclinical simulation laboratory.

The Alumni Association provided a 12 operatory dental clinic, which has served as the school's major extended campus in southern Alameda County since 1973. The university also purchased and renovated a building within seven blocks of the school to help meet student needs for reasonably priced housing. The facility houses 138 residents in 66 apartments and provides a contemporary dental technical laboratory, a fitness center, and study rooms.

The school as a community, its members, and its graduates are distinguished by continuous enhancement through professional development; humanistic values that respect the dignity of each individual and foster the potential for growth in all of us; application of theory and data for continuous improvement; and leadership in addressing the challenges facing the profession of dentistry, education, and our communities.

ADMISSION REQUIREMENTS

NUMBER OF YEARS OF PREDENTAL EDUCATION: General minimum of three years (90 semester or 135 quarter hours).

LIMITATIONS ON COMMUNITY COLLEGE WORK: Courses taken at a community college will be acceptable if they are equivalent to predental courses at a four-year college.

REQUIRED COURSES: *(semesters/quarters)*

Biological science*	4/6
Physics	2/3
Inorganic chemistry	2/3
Organic chemistry*	2/3
English, communications, or speech**	2/3

* Applicants should complete two semesters of organic chemistry or one semester each of organic chemistry and biochemistry, as well as one anatomical sciences course as part of the four required semesters of biological science.

**One course in composition or technical writing is required. Other courses should develop written or verbal communication skills. English as a Second Language (ESL) coursework does not meet this requirement.

SUGGESTED ADDITIONAL PREPARATION: Although we recommend that applicants have a baccalaureate degree, no specific major is required or preferred. Electives should be chosen from courses that extend the content of biomedical sciences (such as anatomy, physiology, histology) as well as subjects related to the art and practice of dentistry (such as accounting, business, economics, social sciences, fine arts, and humanities).

The Admissions Committee encourages every student to develop her or his course of study in conjunction with the college or university predental advisor. If a school does not have a predental advisor, the student should consult faculty members in the Departments of Chemistry and Biology to select courses that meet the intent of the predental requirements.

DAT: Preference is given to students who provide DAT scores no later than September.

GPA: Overall and science GPA, the schools attended, and the difficulty of the courseload are all assessed on an individual basis.

RESIDENCY: No specific requirements.

ADVANCED STANDING: Only under unusual and compelling circumstances does Pacific accept transfer students from other dental schools. No student will be admitted to advanced standing beyond the second year. Foreign dental graduates should apply to Pacific's International Dental Studies Program.

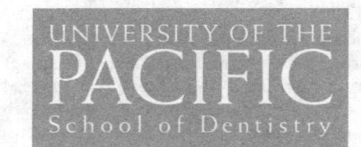

Timetable for the Class Entering Fall 2008

	Earliest Date	Latest Date	School Fee
Application Submission	5/07	12/1/07	$75
Acceptance Notification	12/1/07	7/1/08	

Required Response and Deposit:
$1,000 nonrefundable enrollment fee to hold place. Fee is applied to first-quarter tuition.

FOR FURTHER INFORMATION

Office of Admissions
Kathy Candito
Director
415-929-6491

Office of Financial Aid
Marco Castellanos
Director
415-929-6496

Office of Student Services & Housing
Kathy Candito
Director
415-929-6491

University of the Pacific
Arthur A. Dugoni School of Dentistry
2155 Webster Street
San Francisco, CA 94115

www.dental.pacific.edu

UNIVERSITY OF THE PACIFIC ARTHUR A. DUGONI SCHOOL OF DENTISTRY **CALIFORNIA**

THE DENTAL PROGRAM

The mission of the School of Dentistry is to educate individuals who, upon completion of the program, will be professionally competent to provide quality dental care in an evolving profession; provide patient-centered, comprehensive, quality care in an efficient clinical model that demonstrates the highest standards of service achievable; conduct research and disseminate findings that promote the scientific practice of dentistry; and assist dental professionals with their diverse needs for continuous professional growth through information, formal advanced training, and other services.

The curriculum emphasizes early initiation of clinical experience, integration of biomedical and clinical science, problem solving, and clinical excellence. Students with research interests and ability are encouraged to undertake projects under the guidance of experienced faculty members.

Student progress in the program is evaluated by academic performance committees and carefully monitored by the Academic Advisory Committees that serve to identify any problems (such as undiagnosed learning disabilities) and recommend tutorial and other support. The highest standards are maintained in preparation for National Dental Examining Boards and licensure for practice. Very few students are delayed in their progress toward graduation.

Basic biomedical, preclinical, clinical arts, and science subjects are combined with applied behavioral sciences in a program that prepares graduates to provide excellent quality dental care to the public. Our curriculum equips graduates to enter a changing world that will require them to supplement and adapt existing knowledge and skills. The 36-month curriculum begins in July and is divided into 12 quarters.

Preclinical instruction is concentrated in the first four quarters. During the first quarter, students practice use of dental instructions and materials, working position and posture using direct and indirect vision, and basic dental laboratory procedures. They are introduced to study and test-taking skills and methods of time management. Biomedical science instruction is offered in the first eight quarters, followed by multidisciplinary presentations of basic science foundations for clinical topics.

Clinical work with patients is initiated in the fourth quarter of the first year. Students are assigned to comprehensive care clinics for approximately 500 hours during their second year and 1,000 hours during their third, in addition to specialty clinical rotations. The school's comprehensive patient care program is based on the concept of private dental practice where the student assumes responsibility for assigned patients' treatment, consultation, and referral for specialty care. The school is a pioneer in competency-based dental education—an approach that replaces the traditional system of "clinical requirements" with experiences that ensure that graduates possess the skills, understanding, and professional values needed for the independent practice of general dentistry. The school is also known for its humanistic approach to dental education, stressing the dignity of each individual and his or her value as a person.

Advanced clinical dentistry and new developments and topics that involve several disciplines are learned in the senior year in conjunction with patient care. Rotation to extramural clinics provides management training as well. Behavioral science aspects of human resource and practice management, ethics, and personal productivity, along with dental jurisprudence, are presented throughout the curriculum.

■ Degrees Offered
DENTAL DEGREE: D.D.S.

■ Dental Honor Programs
The university offers three accelerated dental programs, which combine undergraduate preparation with the only three-year D.D.S. program in the country. Students will complete two (2+3), three (3+3), or four (4+3) years of undergraduate work at the University of the Pacific's main campus in Stockton, followed by three years of professional courses at the School of Dentistry in San Francisco. For additional information, contact our Stockton campus at 3601 Pacific Avenue, Stockton, CA 95211, 209-946-2701.

The School of Dentistry also offers an honors program with Grand Canyon University (GCU) in Arizona. This program entails three or four years of undergraduate work at GCU followed by three years of professional education at Pacific. For additional information contact GCU, 3300 West Camelback Road, Phoenix, AZ 85017, 602-249-3300.

SELECTION FACTORS

If the undergraduate institution has a prehealth advisory committee, a committee evaluation is strongly recommended. Otherwise, three letters of evaluation are required, one of which should be from a predental advisor and two from predental or upper division science course professors. At the applicant's discretion, additional letters of evaluation beyond the stated requirements may be submitted regarding the applicant's character, special abilities, and professional motivation. Evaluations from health care professionals who know the applicant well are encouraged.

The Admissions Committee carefully considers each applicant's scholastic record, scores on the DAT, AADSAS essay, letters of evaluation, evidence of manual dexterity (including the perceptual ability portion of the DAT), and other personal attributes and qualities, as well as demonstration of his or her understanding about a career in the dental profession.

Applicants who appear to meet the requirements will be invited to the dental school in San Francisco for an extended orientation and interview with one or more members of the Admissions Committee.

Pacific has established a firm policy of not discriminating against any applicant because of age, race, gender, creed, disability, or national origin. Established review procedures ensure applicants an equal opportunity to be considered for admission. The school has an affirmative action program with regard to admission of qualified ethnic minorities, females, and members of underrepresented groups.

See chapter 3 of this guide for information regarding numbers of applicants and enrollees to each dental school, along with their race, gender, age, type of predental education, mean DAT and GPA, and state of origin.

COSTS AND FINANCIAL AID

All applicants are considered for admission regardless of their financial circumstances. Financial aid is awarded on the basis of need as long as the student is a U.S. citizen or an eligible noncitizen. The Financial Aid Office assists students in managing their financial resources and their indebtedness. All students are encouraged to apply for assistance. The Financial Aid Office will mail materials beginning in early January to all students who apply for admission.

Financial Aid Awards to First-Year Students in 2006-07
■ TOTAL NUMBER OF RECIPIENTS: 136 ■ 96% OF CLASS

Average Award	Range of Awards
NA	NA

Estimated Total Expenses for Academic Year 2006-07
Pacific's curriculum is structured to complete four academic years over three calendar years. Estimated expenses are listed by academic year.

	YEAR 1	YEAR 2	YEAR 3	YEAR 4	TOTAL
Tuition, resident or nonresident	$48,889	$50,778	$52,723	$54,723	$207,113
Other expenses					
Fees					
IMF	$387	$550	$550	0	$1,487
Disability/health insurance	$528	$528	$528	$420	$2,004
Memberships	$70	$70	$70	0	$210
Boards	0	$220	0	$295	$515
Miscellaneous	$25	$150	0	$205	$380
Equipment	$15,203	$4,173	$691	0	$20,067
Estimated living expenses					
Rent & board, personal expenses, transportation	$14,715	$14,715	$14,715	$14,715	$58,860
TOTAL EXPENSES	**$79,817**	**$71,184**	**$69,277**	**$70,358**	**$290,636**

CALIFORNIA

UNIVERSITY OF SOUTHERN CALIFORNIA
SCHOOL OF DENTISTRY

Dr. Harold C. Slavkin, Dean

GENERAL INFORMATION

The School of Dentistry of the University of Southern California (USC) is a private institution founded in 1897. Over the years, the school has become recognized for the excellence of its faculty in the clinical disciplines. This recognition is attested to by the fact that many procedures and techniques used in everyday dental practice were originated by USC faculty members. This heritage continues today, and the school's fundamental goal continues to be the education and development of sophisticated general practitioners of dentistry. When the USC College of Dentistry became a school of the university in 1947, it received an allocation of land on campus for a permanent building to replace the rented quarters it had previously occupied. In 1952 a clinic building was completed, to which a wing was added in 1958. Three additional floors, totaling 115,000 square feet, were added in 1969, and the building was named after its principal donors as the Eileen and Kenneth T. Norris Dental Science Center.

In more recent years, the faculty's efforts in research have attracted national recognition. For example, active research programs currently include fundamental investigations of the mechanisms of the growth and development of the craniofacial structures and of the immune mechanism. These efforts are complemented by clinically related investigations in semiprecious metal alloys, anterior tooth restorative materials, and the use of vitreous carbon as a dental implant.

Programs of the school include those leading to the degree of D.D.S. and B.S. in dental hygiene, certificate programs in advanced (specialty) education and continuing education for the practicing dentist, the Advanced Standing Program for International Dentists for foreign dental school graduates, and the graduate program in craniofacial biology leading to the M.S. or Ph.D. degrees. The requirements for each are given in the appropriate section of the University of Southern California Bulletin. For the latest updated information, applicants should contact the Office of Admissions and Student Affairs.

ADMISSION REQUIREMENTS

NUMBER OF YEARS OF PREDENTAL EDUCATION: Formal minimum of two completed at time of application (60 semester hours) from an accredited college or university in the United States or Canada; no foreign coursework accepted.

LIMITATIONS ON COMMUNITY COLLEGE WORK: None.

REQUIRED COURSES:

With lab required	(semester hrs*)
General biology (zoology)	8
Inorganic chemistry	8
Organic chemistry	8
Physics	8

Other courses	
English composition	8
Philosophy, history, or fine arts	8

*Credit must conform to full academic year's work and must represent a terminal course. All requirements must be taken in sequential order.

SUGGESTED ADDITIONAL PREPARATION: It is strongly suggested that students take additional upper division courses, such as biochemistry, human or comparative anatomy, embryology, histology, genetics, physiology, psychology, sociology, and economics.

DAT: Mandatory; must be taken no later than March 1, 2007; suggested test date is October 2006. Applications are not considered without official DAT scores; therefore, it is advised that applicants take earliest possible DAT exam.

GPA: No specific requirements.

RESIDENCY: No specific requirements.

INTERNATIONAL GRADUATES: Graduates of foreign dental schools may apply for the Advanced Standing Program for International Dentists, which awards the D.D.S. degree after two years of study. Deadline for application is September 15.

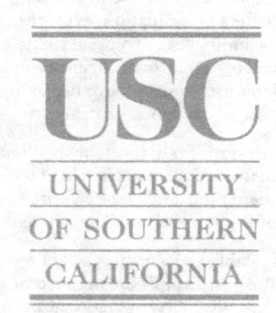

Timetable for the Class Entering Fall 2008

	Earliest Date	Latest Date	Processing Fee
Application Submission	6/1/07*	3/1/08	
Acceptance Notification	12/1/07	4/30/08**	$65/$145***

* Early filing is recommended for students desiring an off-site interview.
** Alternates may be called up to one week after class has begun.
*** Domestic applicants must submit a nonrefundable $65 processing fee. Canadian applicants or those requiring an I-20 student visa must pay a nonrefundable processing fee of $145. Send directly to USC Processing Center, File Number 12154, Los Angeles, CA 90074-2145. USC Fee Receipt Form should accompany fee. A list of other required documentation can be obtained from the Office of Admissions.

Required Response and Deposit:
45 days if accepted on or after 12/1
30 days if accepted on or after 1/1
15 days if accepted on or after 2/1 (preferred time, 10 days)

$1,500 ($500 due on acceptance, $1,000 due on 5/1/07); $1,500 due on 7/15/07; all applied toward tuition.

FOR FURTHER INFORMATION

Office of Admissions and Student Affairs
Eva Yen
Assistant Director
213-740-2841; uscsdadm@usc.edu

Office of Financial Aid
Sergio Estavillo
Director
213-740-2841; uscsdadm@usc.edu

University of Southern California
School of Dentistry
925 W. 34th Street, Room 201
Los Angeles, CA 90089-0641

To order the USC catalogue, call 800-447-8620 or view it online at www.usc.edu.

www.usc.edu/hsc/dental

UNIVERSITY OF SOUTHERN CALIFORNIA SCHOOL OF DENTISTRY **CALIFORNIA**

THE DENTAL PROGRAM

USC's educational philosophy is to provide an educational environment that fosters lifelong learning. Central to this environment is a curriculum that is student-centered and inquiry-based, which integrates all aspects of the fundamental basic and clinical sciences from the onset of the education. Students work in small groups together with faculty facilitators in sessions designed to achieve the learning outcomes of the curriculum. This integration is achieved through the teaching methodology of problem-based learning (PBL). This methodology has been proven to result in greater retention of material by students and an increased appreciation of the clinical relevance of that material. The curriculum is organized to empower each student to learn and evaluate new information through the use of numerous types of educational resources and thus make decisions regarding diagnosis and treatment based on critical analysis.

The goals of this curricular approach are as follows: 1) to use student-centered, inquiry-based methods in all aspects of basic science, preclinical science, and clinical science instruction throughout the four years of study that will encourage students to develop lifelong problem-solving and group learning skills; 2) to encourage students to question materials presented and develop a collegial interaction with the faculty—all areas of instruction occur in a professional atmosphere, and there is no activity that demeans students or creates an atmosphere in which student inquiry is repressed; 3) to vertically integrate the curriculum over four years so that the basic sciences, preclinical sciences, clinical sciences, and clinical skills are organized into a cohesive program to emphasize the direct relevance of basic science learning outcomes to clinical problems; and 4) to develop dental graduates who are dedicated to lifelong, self-motivated learning, accomplished in the methods required to solve problems in a clinical setting, and able to effectively understand and respond to multiple changes in the nature of dental practice that will occur during their careers.

Patient treatment continues as a dominant theme in the dental curriculum and begins during the first trimester. This segment of the curriculum increases until the fourth year, when the students' total efforts are spent in this activity. In addition, there are formal and informal opportunities for research available through collaboration with the faculty on a variety of clinical and basic science research activities in the biomedical science area.

The School of Dentistry takes advantage of the teaching resources in the Los Angeles basin, such as at affiliated hospitals (Los Angeles County/USC Medical Center, Rancho Los Amigos Hospital, John Wesley Hospital, and Children's Hospital), other schools at the university (such as the schools of Medicine, Pharmacy, Allied Health, Business Law, Education, and Gerontology), and extramural settings such as the Mobile Clinic Program and the Downtown Union Rescue Mission.

■ Degrees Offered
DENTAL DEGREE: D.D.S.

ALTERNATE DEGREES: D.D.S./M.B.A. in five years; M.S. or Ph.D. through the Graduate School (a master's or Ph.D. in craniofacial biology and other fields such as education, experimental pathology, and cellular molecular biology); D.D.S./M.S. in gerontology in five years.

SELECTION FACTORS

Students are selected by the Committee on Admissions, which bases its decisions on consideration of an applicant's personal qualities, aptitudes, and superior scholarship necessary for the successful study and practice of dentistry. Applicants must have completed 60, preferably 90, units. A strong biological, chemical, or physical science background is advantageous. An interview at the School of Dentistry may be required of all applicants who appear qualified for consideration, as determined by the Office of Admissions and Student Affairs. As a private institution, USC actively seeks a culturally and geographically diverse population. Therefore, out-of-state applicants are evaluated and selected based on the same criteria as California residents.

The school encourages the application of qualified minority applicants and is committed to a policy of nondiscrimination on the basis of race, color, creed, religion, gender, age, sexual orientation, or national origin. An otherwise qualified individual shall not be excluded from admission solely by reason of his or her disability, medical condition, or marital status. Tutorials and academic, personal, and financial counseling are available to students requiring assistance.

See chapter 3 of this guide for information regarding numbers of applicants and enrollees to each dental school, along with their race, gender, age, type of predental education, mean DAT and GPA, and state of origin.

COSTS AND FINANCIAL AID

The school maintains a financial aid office to assist students in obtaining a variety of aid. Currently, 90 percent of the student body receives some form of financial assistance. The School of Dentistry itself provides institutional aid in various forms and provides individual financial counseling.

Estimated Total Expenses for Academic Year 2006-07

	YEAR 1	YEAR 2	YEAR 3	YEAR 4	TOTAL
Tuition, resident or nonresident	$53,347	$53,347	$53347	$42805	202,846
Fees	$1,599	$1,599	$1,599	$1,599	$6,396
Estimated living expenses*	$17,500	$17,500	$17,500	$17,500	$70,000
TOTAL EXPENSES	**$72,446**	**$72,446**	**$72,446**	**$61,904**	**279,242**

*Estimate includes transportation, room and board, and other personal expenses for single students.

COLORADO

UNIVERSITY OF COLORADO AT DENVER AND HEALTH SCIENCES CENTER
SCHOOL OF DENTISTRY

Dr. Denise K. Kassebaum, Dean

GENERAL INFORMATION

Creation of the University of Colorado School of Dentistry (UCSD) was authorized in 1922 by an amendment to the state constitution. In the spring of 1967, the Colorado Legislature authorized initial capital construction and operating funds for the School of Dentistry, and in August the Board of Regents appointed a dean. The School of Dentistry enrolled its first class of 25 in 1973, which graduated in May 1977. Presently the school enrolls 50 dental and 18 dental hygiene students annually. The small class size is an asset to the teaching and learning process.

UCSD has established a growing reputation for the personalized quality of its educational experience and for its accomplished, successful graduates. To provide dental and dental hygiene students with practice-oriented training, the school operates a clinic for a closed population selected for educational purposes. It also maintains close working relations with the University of Colorado Hospital and has implemented a nationally recognized service learning program. The Advanced Clinical Training and Service (ACTS) program emphasizes external programs in clinics, dental offices, and hospitals across the state, to care for Colorado's underserved populations.

While the school seeks primarily to produce competent general practitioners and puts the emphasis on giving students hands-on experiences in a variety of settings, it also has a growing research program. In addition to the dental curriculum, the school offers a B.S. degree in dental hygiene; a postgraduate residency in general dentistry, pediatric dentistry, and orthodontics; and an international student program. The continuing education program has been in existence since the inception of the school.

This is an exciting time for UCSD and the entire University of Colorado Health Science Center as the educational, research, and patient care activities are in the process of being relocated to a new state-of-the-art academic health center on the Fitzsimons campus. In spring 2004, a major research building, Research Complex 1, opened approximately 600,000 square feet of high technology research laboratories to campus investigators. Educational facilities to house all of the academic programs of the Health Science Center are presently under construction. The overriding vision for this new academic health center is interprofessional collaboration in education, research, and patient care/service. The School of Dentistry moved into its new comprehensive oral health center equipped with the highest technology clinical and educational facilities, the Lazzara Center for Oral Facial Health, in August 2005.

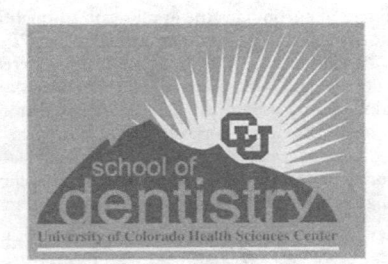

Timetable for the Class Entering Fall 2008

	Earliest Date	Latest Date	School Fee
Application Submission	6/1/07*	1/1/08	$50**
Acceptance Notification	12/1/07	8/16/08	$200***

* Early application (prior to 8/06) highly recommended.
** Due on school's request.
***Due on acceptance; applies toward tuition.

FOR FURTHER INFORMATION

Admissions Committee and Student Affairs
Brad J. Potter
Chair
303-724-7120
University of Colorado at Denver
School of Dentistry
Admissions and Student Affairs
Lazara Center for Oral-Facial Health
13065 E. 17th Avenue, Room 310
Mail Stop F833
P.O. Box 6508
Aurora, CO 80045
www.uchsc.edu/sod

Office of Diversity
303-315-8558
University of Colorado at Denver
Health Sciences Center
4200 E. Ninth Avenue, A-049
Denver, CO 80262

Student Financial Aid Office
303-315-8364
University of Colorado at Denver
Health Sciences Center
4200 E. Ninth Avenue, A-088
Denver, CO 80262
www.uchsc.edu/finaid/

www.uchsc.edu/sod

ADMISSION REQUIREMENTS

NUMBER OF YEARS OF PREDENTAL EDUCATION: The majority of students accepted to the School of Dentistry have completed at least four years of undergraduate work and have received an undergraduate degree. The basic requirement for admission is the completion of at least 90 semester hours (135 quarter hours) with at least 30 hours of upper division courses for a letter grade.

LIMITATIONS ON COMMUNITY COLLEGE WORK: Not more than 60 semester hours/90 quarter hours will count toward the 90 semester hour minimum.

REQUIRED COURSES: *(semesters)*

General chemistry with laboratory*	2
Organic chemistry with laboratory*	2
General biology/zoology with laboratory*	2
General physics with laboratory*	2
Humanities	2
English composition	1

Must receive a letter grade for the required courses.

*Science courses must have associated laboratories.

HIGHLY RECOMMENDED COURSES: Biochemistry, microbiology, human anatomy, physiology.

SUGGESTED ADDITIONAL COURSES: Business management/finance, psychology, communications, studio art, cell biology, immunology, and histology are possible electives to consider.

DAT: Mandatory; taken no later than October the year preceding admission.

GPA: No specific requirements.

RESIDENCY: No specific requirement; however, see Selection Factors.

ADVANCED STANDING: Granting of advanced standing will be considered on an individual basis.

OTHER: Documentation of immunization and Basic Life Support CPR required for matriculation. Background investigation will also be required.

THE DENTAL PROGRAM

The goal of the dental curriculum is to graduate a dentist in four years who is capable of entering into dental practice. Graduates of this program will be able to do the following: 1) prevent, diagnose, and treat oral disease; 2) understand biological, physical, and social sciences and apply that knowledge in performing appropriate prevention, diagnosis, and treatment; 3) develop and apply personal and professional skills to practice effectively and relate to patients and colleagues; 4) recognize professional capabilities and judiciously refer patients for specialty care; and 5) continue to acquire knowledge through patterns of lifelong study.

The dental curriculum begins by teaching the student to understand health and to differentiate between conditions of general health and disease. It then proceeds to teach concepts of oral health and oral disease. Subsequently, the curriculum teaches dental diagnostic procedures and therapeutic techniques. Prevention is also taught throughout the curriculum. Behavioral sciences, auxiliary utilization, and practice management courses round out the predoctoral curriculum.

The philosophical design of the dental curriculum is based upon progression of learning from health to disease and from that to a mastery of skills essential in therapy and development of interpersonal and professional skills in support of the delivery of oral health care.

Basic science instruction occurs in the first and second years of the program. Basic science information is reinforced by clinical faculty in such courses as systemic disease and oral and organ pathology and traditional clinical disciplines as appropriate. Clinical experiences are a part of the entire program, although patient care experiences take place primarily in the later two years of the program. Some scheduled time is available for elective coursework in the last years, and these courses may be of a research orientation.

A unique feature of the curriculum is the Advanced Clinical Training and Service Program. The student will spend much of his or her last eight months outside the School of Dentistry in hospitals, geriatric centers, children's care centers, public clinics, and private practices in both urban and rural communities. These extramural rotations may be mixed with intramural rotations in which a student gains experience in specialty areas of his or her choosing. This program will provide a significant amount and variety of experience and will serve as a transition to private practice.

■ Degrees Offered
DENTAL DEGREE: D.D.S.

ALTERNATE DEGREES: Bachelor of Science through participating universities.

COSTS AND FINANCIAL AID

The school policy is to accept students on the basis of their potential as dentists. Financial aid is available on the basis of need to the extent possible. However, limited sources of funds for financial aid make it necessary for the student to have an acceptable plan for meeting his or her financial obligations while in school. Applications for aid may be made only after acceptance into the school.

Financial Aid Awards to First-Year Students in 2006-07
■ TOTAL NUMBER OF RECIPIENTS: 49   ■ 98% OF CLASS

	Average Award	Range of Awards
Residents	$37,801	$18,500-$43,800
Nonresidents	$53,133	$18,500-$57,000

Estimated Total Expenses for Academic Year 2006-07*

	YEAR 1	YEAR 2	YEAR 3	YEAR 4	TOTAL
Tuition, resident	$17,134	$17,134	$17,134	$17,134	$68,536
Tuition, nonresident	$17,134	$17,134	$17,134	$17,134	$68,536
Accountable Student Fee	$23,108	$23,108	$23,108	$23,108	$150,968
Other expenses					
Fees					
Textbooks	$1,300	$1,300	$1,300	$435	$4,335
Magnification kit	$800	0	0	0	$800
Other	$2,510	$2,295	$2,295	$2,295	$9,395
Equipment	$6,325	$3,575	$1,800	$400	$12,100
Estimated living expenses	$13,640	$13,640	$13,640	$12,000	$52,920
TOTAL EXPENSES, RESIDENT	$41,709	$37,944	$36,169	$32,264	$148,086
TOTAL EXPENSES, NONRESIDENT	$64,817	$61,052	$59,277	$55,372	$240,518

*These estimates are subject to change at any time prior to the beginning of the academic year.

SELECTION FACTORS

Applicants are evaluated on their ability to complete academic work successfully, their performance on the DAT, letters of evaluation, and other evidence of personal characteristics. Applications are encouraged from members of groups underrepresented in the profession, specifically members of ethnic minority groups and women. The school does not discriminate on the basis of race, creed, national origin, or gender and encourages ethnic minority groups, the disadvantaged, and women to apply.

The average GPA of those admitted during the past three years is 3.7 (A = 4.0). The average DAT scores of those same students has been above 19.5. Personal interviews at the request of the Admissions Committee are required before final acceptance. Students must also have acceptable plans for meeting their financial obligations while in school.

Letters of evaluation are required from the student's undergraduate faculty predental advisory committee. If there is no such committee, letters from two instructors who have taught him or her science courses and one who has taught him or her a nonscience course will be acceptable.

The UCSD actively accepts both residents and non-residents for its dental program. The CU School of Dentistry is also a member of the Western Interstate Commission for Higher Education (WICHE) program. For nonresident applicants, the Colorado State Legislature recently implemented a law concerning tuition for professional schools. All nonresident students will be required to pay an Accountable Student Fee along with their tuition. Nonresidents will be responsible for the Accountable Student Fee for each of the four years of enrollment at the Dental School. You must be a legal Colorado resident at the time of acceptance in order to qualify for in-state tuition.

See chapter 3 of this guide for information regarding numbers of applicants and enrollees to each dental school, along with their race, gender, age, type of predental education, mean DAT and GPA, and state of origin.

ACADEMIC AND OTHER ASSISTANCE

A Health Career Opportunity Program for ethnic minorities is available through the Office of Diversity.

CONNECTICUT

UNIVERSITY OF CONNECTICUT
SCHOOL OF DENTAL MEDICINE

Dr. R. Lamont MacNeil, Dean

GENERAL INFORMATION

Since its inception in 1968, the University of Connecticut School of Dental Medicine has become a prominent leader in dental education and dental research. The school is an integral member of the University of Connecticut Health Center complex, which is home to the School of Medicine, the John Dempsey Hospital, and the Graduate School, which offers degree programs in the biomedical sciences. The Health Center encompasses 200 acres in the historic New England town of Farmington, seven miles from the state capital at Hartford and midway between Boston and New York. As the only public dental program in New England, the school participates in the New England Regional Student Program that offers significant tuition savings to all Maine, Massachusetts, New Hampshire, Rhode Island, and Vermont residents.

The predoctoral curriculum focuses on the biological and epidemiological bases of disease and provides strong preparation in the diagnostic and technical skills required for the practice of dentistry in the 21st century. The school shares an award-winning basic medical science curriculum with the School of Medicine that emphasizes an integrative approach to understanding the dynamics of the human body. As a result of its innovative and demanding curriculum, the school typically places in the top 10 percent of dental schools on both sections of the National Board Examinations. Upon graduation, up to 80 percent of the students pursue advanced education in the clinical specialties and general dentistry residency programs.

The advancement of knowledge is an integral part of our mission, and students are encouraged to participate in research opportunities in basic science, behavioral science, and clinical research. The University of Connecticut has been designated a Research I University by the Carnegie Foundation and is ranked by the National Science Foundation in the top 10 percent of institutions of higher learning in research and development funding. The dental school is the recipient of an NIDCR Institutional National Research Service Award, which encourages dental students to engage in research during their undergraduate dental education, and an NIDCR Institutional Dentist Scientist Training Program Award, which offers students interested in an academic career the opportunity to pursue a combined D.M.D./Ph.D.

In addition to its outstanding academic programs, the School of Dental Medicine provides an array of cultural, social, and recreational opportunities designed to complement and enhance the educational experience. Community and volunteer service play an important role in the school's culture, and students are involved in activities such as the Special Olympics and providing care to the homeless, migrant workers, and the underserved, including residents of impoverished villages in Peru, Haiti and Belize. As a member of Connecticut's premier flagship university, students are provided state-of-the-art facilities and enjoy the benefits derived from the presence of nationally renowned sports teams and other traditions that serve to enrich the overall experience.

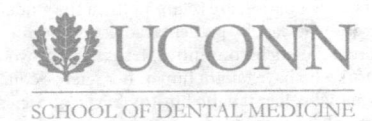

ADMISSION REQUIREMENTS

NUMBER OF YEARS OF PREDENTAL EDUCATION: Generally acceptable minimum, four; exceptional three-year applicants considered.

LIMITATIONS ON COMMUNITY COLLEGE WORK: None.

REQUIRED COURSES:

With lab required	(years)
Inorganic chemistry	1
Organic chemistry	1
Physics	1
Biology	1

All required courses must be at least equal to introductory courses for students majoring in the respective disciplines.

SUGGESTED ADDITIONAL PREPARATION: Courses in biochemistry, cell biology, and molecular biology are strongly recommended, but not required. Students should have a strong facility in English and be able to handle quantitative concepts.

DAT: Mandatory; no later than October 1, 2007, preferred.

GPA: No specific requirements; 3.2 or above science GPA recommended.

RESIDENCY: Out-of-state residents are encouraged to apply. UCSDM participates in the New England Regional Student Program, which bestows preferred status on New England residents and offers a reduced tuition rate for students from the New England states.

ADVANCED STANDING: Foreign dental graduates may be considered for entry at the second-year level.

Timetable for the Class Entering Fall 2008

	Earliest Date	Latest Date	School Fees
Application Submission	6/1/07	2/1/08	$75*
Acceptance Notification	12/1/07	8/1/08	

*May be waived if it causes undue hardship.

Required Response and Deposit:
45 days after notification if received between 12/1 and 12/31
15 days after notification if received between 1/1 and 1/31
7 days after notification if received on or after 2/1

$400 due with acceptance letter; applies toward tuition and is nonrefundable.

FOR FURTHER INFORMATION
Office of Admissions/Student Affairs
Edward A. Thibodeau
Assistant Dean for Admissions
860-679-2175
University of Connecticut, MC 3905
School of Dental Medicine
Farmington, CT 06030-3905

sdm.uchc.edu

THE DENTAL PROGRAM

The curriculum is designed to provide students with a comprehensive educational experience that allows them to master the knowledge and requisite skills associated with the practice of general dentistry.

The goals of the curriculum are to help students accomplish the following:

- gain an understanding of the basic sciences related to structures, functions, and interrelationships among body systems in both health and disease;
- develop competency in clinical skills, which include but are not limited to patient assessment, treatment planning, patient education, prevention of oral disease, control of pain and anxiety, prevention and management of dental and medical emergencies, and the diagnosis, management, and treatment of the major oral diseases and conditions; and
- gain an understanding of behavioral science concepts from the fields of psychology, sociology, public health, and administration applied to the delivery of care and to the management of a dental practice.

Students are evaluated in a series of examinations at the conclusion of each course. Evaluation is by written and practical examinations in the medical, dental, and clinical sciences, along with observation of students' development in patient oral health care delivery. Performance in clinical care is partially based on proficiency so that students may progress at an optimal rate. The grading system is on a pass/fail basis.

YEARS 1 AND 2. During the first two years, dental and medical students follow an integrated course of study in the basic sciences. At the same time, dental students devote a gradually increasing amount of time to the dental sciences curriculum, which builds on the basic sciences in those areas directly relevant to dental diseases and prepares students for their clinical experiences. First patient contact occurs during the first year of dental school.

YEARS 3 AND 4. The third- and fourth-year clinical program extends for 22 months. Students study the principles of oral disease prevention and their application to clinical practice and treat patients in outpatient clinics in the various clinical departments. The clinical program emphasizes comprehensive care, prevention, and the emerging epidemiologic patterns of dental diseases.

The clinical practicum for third- and fourth-year students is conducted via practice groups (teams) in which there is a vertical integration of students, a horizontal integration of faculty, and a dedicated staff. Delivery of care is the responsibility of the team. Patients are assigned to students for examination and the development of a treatment plan. Student performance and competency are evaluated on an ongoing basis using standard competency criteria.

The School of Dental Medicine maintains ten onsite dental clinics with 14-16 individual operatories in each. Patients represent a full age range and are of varied socioeconomic status. Clinical training is also provided at the John Dempsey (University) Hospital, UConn Head and Neck Cancer Unit, Hartford Hospital, St. Francis Hospital, Connecticut Children's Medical Center, Burgdorf Dental Clinic, and the Veterans' Administration Medical Center.

■ Degrees Offered

DENTAL DEGREE: D.M.D.

ALTERNATE DEGREES: B.S./D.M.D. with University of Connecticut, Spelman College, and Morehouse College; combined D.M.D./Ph.D. program; combined D.M.D./M.P.H. program.

■ Other Programs

RESEARCH AND FELLOWSHIPS: Available on a competitive basis prior to matriculation and throughout the D.M.D. program.

EXTERNSHIPS AND ELECTIVES: Available throughout the D.M.D. program.

SELECTION FACTORS

Men and women of any color, race, or creed residing in any state or country are equally eligible to apply for admission. Criteria used to select applicants for admission are college grades, science GPA, DAT scores, evidence of inquiring independent thought, an interest in continued education, motivation toward a dental career, good interpersonal skills, and a record of accomplishment that shows an applicant's leadership qualities and interest in the community. These may vary in emphasis, depending on individual applicants. A letter of recommendation from a preprofessional committee, or three faculty members if such a committee does not exist, is required. Financial need will not be a factor in the selection process. Personal interviews will be arranged at the discretion of the Admissions Committee.

See chapter 3 of this guide for information regarding numbers of applicants and enrollees to each dental school, along with their race, gender, age, type of predental education, mean DAT and GPA, and state of origin.

ADDITIONAL INFORMATION

The university encourages applications from women and minorities. All applications are evaluated according to a single set of standards. Free tutorial assistance is available to all students. Information regarding budgets and financial aid is available to all applicants; however, financial need is not considered in the admission process. Discussions with each student about financial assistance will be held following admission. Every effort will be made to meet a student's minimum financial requirements. Each case is considered on an individual basis.

FINANCIAL AID

The intent of our financial aid program is to minimize the costs of financing education. Each case is considered according to information reflected in the application for aid. UCSDM uses the Free Application for Federal Student Aid (FAFSA) as the means of determining eligibility for aid. All students seeking financial aid must file a FAFSA application and institutional application. The Board of Trustees of the university allots a portion of the dental school fees for scholarships and loans. There are other school scholarships awarded each year.

Financial Aid Awards to First-Year Students in 2006-07
■ TOTAL NUMBER OF RECIPIENTS: 35/39   ■ 95% OF CLASS

	Average Award	Range of Awards
Residents	$38,442	$19,500-$52,864
New England Resident	$51,178	$38,500-$62,261
Nonresidents	$63,053	$44,587-$74,187

Estimated Total Expenses for Academic Year 2008-09

	YEAR 1	YEAR 2	YEAR 3	YEAR 4	TOTAL
Tuition, resident	$16,853	$16,853	$16,853	$16,853	$67,412
Tuition, NE*	$29,514	$29,514	$29,514	$29,514	$118,056
Tuition, nonresident	$43,225	$43,225	$43,225	$43,225	$172,900
Fees: professional schools fee, student activity fee, student health insurance	$7,000	$7,000	$7,000	$7,000	$28,000
Equipment: supplies, books, instruments	$8,547	$3,497	$4,065	$2,550	$18,659
Estimated living expenses: food, clothing, rent, utilities, travel, auto	$22,000	$24,000	$24,000	$24,000	$94,000
TOTAL EXPENSES, RESIDENT	$54,400	$51,350	$51,918	$50,403	$208,071
TOTAL EXPENSES, NE*	$67,061	$64,011	$64,579	$63,064	$258,715
TOTAL EXPENSES, NONRESIDENT	$80,772	$77,722	$78,290	$76,775	$313,559

Estimated tuition and fees do not reflect anticipated university-mandated annual increases and purchase of a laptop computer.
* New England residents

HOWARD UNIVERSITY
COLLEGE OF DENTISTRY

Dr. Leo E. Rouse, Dean

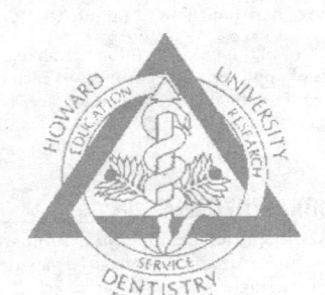

GENERAL INFORMATION

The College of Dentistry at Howard University was established in 1881. It is the fifth oldest dental school in the United States. As a teaching and patient care institution, the college has trained thousands of highly skilled dental professionals to serve their communities, particularly the underserved. Our graduates are currently serving communities in 40 states and 53 foreign countries.

Our more than 80 faculty members constitute one of the best-trained dental faculties in the world, thus making our institution the capstone for transforming competent students into leaders for America and the world.

Our mission includes the philosophy that education, research, and service are inseparable constituents of a modern dental education. The college's primary goal is to remain a national resource for dental leaders and a comprehensive education and research institution that attracts highly motivated and academically accomplished students from culturally diverse backgrounds.

Howard University College of Dentistry offers postdoctoral programs in the fields of oral and maxillofacial surgery, orthodontics, pediatric dentistry, general practice residency, and an advanced education program in general dentistry. These programs meet the educational requirements necessary for certification by the respective specialty boards. The five existing programs fulfill the accreditation requirements for postdoctoralspecialty programs in dentistry as determined by the Council on Dental Education of the American Dental Association and the Commission on Accreditation.

The newly renovated state-of-the-art orthodontic clinic and new simulated preclinical laboratory are some of the innovative additions to the college. In addition, the multimedia center allows students to access the Internet, Patient Automated Management Systems (PAMS), and their email accounts. Currently, first- and second-year dental students are equipped with their personal laptop computers.

The university's new Louis Stokes Health Science Library, a four-story, state-of-the-art information technology facility, houses 400,000 volumes, periodicals, and electroncially formatted material and is wired with data ports to support Internet connectivity. The information lab (i-Lab), a technology center lab, houses several hundred computer workstations. Each workstation is voice, data, and video capable to support full communication, including videoconferencing. The i-Lab hosts "smart classrooms" with full network capabilities, one of which is housed in the College of Dentistry.

Howard University College of Dentistry has long been a leader in graduating women, African Americans, and other underrepresented and disadvantaged groups.

ADMISSION REQUIREMENTS

NUMBER OF YEARS OF PREDENTAL EDUCATION: A bachelor's degree from an accredited four-year college.

LIMITATIONS ON COMMUNITY COLLEGE WORK: Considered if academic average is 3.0 or better and if DAT scores are above the national norm. Additionally, all prerequisites must be from an accredited four-year college.

REQUIRED COURSES:

With lab required	(semester/quarter hrs)
Inorganic chemistry	8/12
Organic chemistry	8/12
Biology*	8/12

Other courses	
English/literature	6/9
Electives	22/33

*Zoology and botany are acceptable alternatives.

SUGGESTED ADDITIONAL PREPARATION: Biochemistry, human gross anatomy, physiology, microbiology, and histology.

DAT: Mandatory; 17 minimum score in all areas. (Must be taken within two years of application.)

GPA: 2.7 or above required.

RESIDENCY: No requirement.

ADVANCED STANDING: Consideration is given to students transferring from other U.S. dental schools, provided they are in good academic standing and the approved request does not place the student beyond the beginning of the third year of the dental program.

Timetable for the Class Entering Fall 2008

	Earliest Date	Latest Date	Application School Fees
Application Submission	7/1/07	2/1/08	$45 (money orders only)
Acceptance Notification	12/1/07	7/15/08	

Required Response and Deposit:
45 days after notification if received between 12/1 and 12/31
30 days after notification if received between 1/1 and 1/31
15 days after notification if received after 2/1

$400 for new students; $100 for students previously enrolled at Howard. $100 applied toward tuition and is nonrefundable.

FOR FURTHER INFORMATION

Office of Admissions
202-806-0400
Room 126

Office of Financial Aid
202-806-0375
Room 508

Office of Student Affairs
202-806-0443
Room 128

Howard University College of Dentistry
600 W Street, NW
Washington, DC 20059

www.howard.edu/collegedentistry

THE DENTAL PROGRAM

The primary objective of the curriculum is to educate individuals for the practice of general dentistry. Specific objectives are as follows: 1) to provide comprehensive undergraduate dental education such that the dental graduate will be competent in the prevention, diagnosis, and treatment of oral diseases and disorders and knowledgeable about the interrelationship of oral and systemic health; and 2) to inculcate in our graduates the highest standards of ethical and moral responsibility to the dental profession and to the communities they serve.

The Foundation courses in the basic sciences are taught during the first two years in the preclinical science area of the medical school. Although clinical experience begins in the second year of dental training, the basic and clinical sciences are integrated by the participation of clinical and basic science faculty in both areas of instruction. The current curriculum contains some special features: DAU (Dental Auxiliary Utilization); CIAP (Chronically Ill and Aged Program), an extramural program which involves an offsite clinical rotation as part of a National Dental Pipeline initiative funded by the Robert Wood Johnson Foundation to increase access to oral health care for underserved communities. The college has installed an efficient learning resource facility and is developing the necessary software for instructional support.

■ Degrees Offered

DENTAL DEGREE: D.D.S.

ALTERNATE DEGREES: B.S./D.D.S. with Howard University.

COSTS AND FINANCIAL AID

Financial aid resources are available at the college in the form of both scholarships and loans. The Office of Financial Aid strives to assist as many needy qualified students as possible in meeting some of their university-related expenses such as tuition, books, and instruments.

Because of the college's limited financial aid resources, students are strongly advised not to depend solely on receiving financial aid from the university. Students should be prepared to finance their expenses through federal student scholarships or loans, loans from local dental societies, private organizations, parents, and other relatives. As a last resort, students may wish to seek permission to work part time.

All students should apply for federal financial aid by completing a FAFSA or Electronic FAFSA. You may contact any financial aid office to receive a FAFSA, or you may submit an Electronic FAFSA to the Federal Processor via the Internet. The college has a February 15 priority consideration date for first-year students and a March 15 date for continuing students.

Financial Aid Awards to First-Year Students in 2006-07

■ TOTAL NUMBER OF RECIPIENTS: 76   ■ 93% OF CLASS

Average Award	Range of Awards
$38,500	$8,500-$44,357

Financial aid is awarded on a first-come, first-served need basis.

Estimated Total Expenses for Academic Year 2007-08

	YEAR 1	YEAR 2	YEAR 3	YEAR 4	TOTAL
Tuition, resident or nonresident	$19,415	$19,415	$19,415	$19,415	$77,660
Fees: matriculation, self-help, endowment, liability, books and instruments, DN Assoc., board exam	$12,367	$6,958	$3,633	$2,308	$25,266
Equipment: microscope rental	$35	0	0	0	$35
Estimated living expenses: room/board, incidentals, transportation	$14,804	$17,757	$17,757	$18,657	$68,875
TOTAL EXPENSES	**$46,622**	**$44,130**	**$40,705**	**$40,380**	**$171,837**

SELECTION FACTORS

Selection is competitive, based on both cognitive and noncognitive factors, e.g., grade point averages, DAT scores, community service, and overall demonstration of interest in dentistry. The college requires personal interviews and three letters of recommendation or a committee evaluation from science instructors or from individuals who have personal knowledge of the applicant.

See chapter 3 of this guide for information regarding numbers of applicants and enrollees to each dental school, along with their race, gender, age, type of predental education, mean DAT and GPA, and state of origin.

ACADEMIC AND OTHER ASSISTANCE

Howard University has devoted many of its activities to the education of minorities, the educationally disadvantaged, women, etc. The College of Dentistry strongly supports this university policy and has made many efforts to identify and retain such students with potential.

The College of Dentistry offers the Academic Reinforcement Program, a pre-entrance enrichment program with tutorial assistance, to applicants who may be deficient in some of the prerequisites. If applicants successfully complete the program, they are recommended to the Admissions Committee and may be eligible for admission to the first-year dental class. Participants in this program must be U.S. citizens.

The college has no optional decelerated program; however, every consideration is given to the slow learner who demonstrates potential, and extra time may be added to his or her curriculum if recommended and approved by the faculty of the college.

FLORIDA

NOVA SOUTHEASTERN UNIVERSITY
COLLEGE OF DENTAL MEDICINE

Dr. Robert A. Uchin, Dean

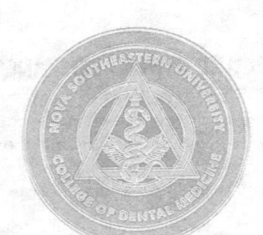

GENERAL INFORMATION

The College of Dental Medicine, the newest of six schools in the university's Health Professions Division, was established in 1996. It joins the Colleges of Osteopathic Medicine, Pharmacy, Optometry, Allied Health, and Medical Sciences. Basic science courses (anatomy, microbiology, pathology, pharmacology, and physiology) are taught by the College of Medical Sciences, and students have the opportunity to interact with students of the other schools.

Nova Southeastern University, the largest independent institution of higher learning in the state of Florida, is the product of the merger of Nova University and Southeastern University of the Health Sciences in January 1994. As a result of the merger, the Health Professions Division relocated to the Ft. Lauderdale campus of Nova Southeastern University and moved into a newly constructed complex of seven buildings that house all of the colleges. This $60 million complex consists of over 975,000 square feet of serviceable space at the western margin of the campus and is centrally located in South Florida's tri-county area. The major structures include a five-story Administration Building and an Assembly Building consisting of a 500-seat auditorium/classroom, a 250-seat auditorium/classroom, and eight 125-seat auditorium/classrooms. The new Assembly Building II houses a 312-seat auditorium, 50-station computer science laboratory, and 37 seminar rooms. All of the clinic, research, and basic science laboratories for all of the colleges, along with the library, are conveniently located in the library/laboratory building. The adjacent Clinical Services Building consists of primary medical care services on the first floor, primary eye care operated by the College of Optometry on the second floor, a medical specialty care faculty practice on the third floor, and a fully functional pharmacy. A 2,000-car garage is a short walk away from these facilities.

The main structure for the College of Dental Medicine is a 72,000-square foot building. The first floor consists of 105 operatories for comprehensive dental care, as well as four oral surgery operatories and four radiology operatories. The second floor houses a 116-chair technique laboratory, seminar rooms, a faculty practice facility, and postgraduate practice facilities in pediatric dentistry, orthodontics, endodontics, periodontics, and prosthodontics and oral and maxillofacial surgery. Laboratory facilities support all the units on the first and second floors. The third floor includes administrative and faculty offices, research laboratories, and seminar rooms.

The Health Professions Division facilities occupy 21 acres on the spacious 232-acre Nova Southeastern University campus. A new 55 million dollar state-of-the-art library and buildings for administration and the Center for Psychological Studies have been added to an already spacious campus that included, among others, an undergraduate college, law school, student center, family center, athletic facilities, student dormitories, and training facility for the Miami Dolphins football team. Only a short drive from the Ft. Lauderdale Airport, the campus is conveniently located with nearby housing, restaurants, recreational facilities, and major thoroughfares.

ADMISSION REQUIREMENTS

NUMBER OF YEARS OF PREDENTAL EDUCATION: Prior to matriculation, applicants must have completed a minimum of 90 semester hours of coursework from a regionally accredited college or university.

LIMITATIONS ON COMMUNITY COLLEGE WORK: Not more than 60 semester hours will be applied toward the 90-semester hour minimum requirements.

REQUIRED COURSES: The college requires students to earn a grade of 2.0 or better in the designated number of semester hours in each of the following required subjects:

With lab required	(semester hrs)
General biology	8
General chemistry	8
Organic chemistry	8
Physics	8
English composition	3
English literature	3
A choice of two of the following science courses	
Biochemistry	3
Cell or molecular biology	3
Microbiology	3
Physiology	3
Histology	3
Genetics	3
Human or comparative anatomy	3

SUGGESTED ADDITIONAL PREPARATION: Additional courses in the advanced biological sciences and courses in social sciences, principles of management, accounting, communication, foreign languages, art, and sculpture will contribute to a broad educational background.

DAT: All students are required to take the Dental Admission Test (DAT) and submit their scores. There are no minimum score requirements for entrance into the college. It should be noted, however, that the mean DAT Academic Average score for entering first-year students is 19.

GPA: Students should have a cumulative grade point average of 3.0 or higher on a four-point scale. Students must earn a grade of 2.0 or better in each required course.

Timetable for the Class Entering Fall 2008

	Earliest Date	Latest Date	School Fees
Application Submission*	6/1/07	2/1/08	$50
Acceptance Notification**	12/1/07	5/15/08	

*Notice of acceptance is on a rolling or periodic schedule, so early completion of application is in the student's best interest.
**Alternates may be called up to two weeks after classes begin.

Required Response and Deposit:
30 days if accepted on or after 12/1
Two weeks if accepted on or after 1/1

Acceptance Fee: $1,000. This fee is payable on January 1 for applicants accepted December 1. For applicants accepted after January 1, this fee is payable within two weeks of acceptance.

Preregistration Fee: $1,000, due April 15, under the same terms as the acceptance fee. These nonrefundable fees and deposits are subtracted from the tuition due the first semester.

FOR FURTHER INFORMATION
Office of Admissions
Marla Frohlinger
Vice Chancellor for Student Services and Professional Coordination
954-262-1101

Hal R. Lippman, D.D.S.
Associate Dean of Admissions and Student Affairs
954-262-1796

Su-Ann Zarrett
Associate Director of Admissions and Student Affairs
954-262-1101

Office of Student Financial Aid
Pemra Cetin
Student Financial Aid Coordinator
954-262-1130

College of Dental Medicine
Nova Southeastern University
3200 South University Drive
Ft. Lauderdale, FL 33328

Housing
Office of Residential Life
Rick Mayfield
Director of Housing
954-262-7052

Nova Southeastern University
3301 College Avenue
Ft. Lauderdale, FL 33314

dental.nova.edu

THE DENTAL PROGRAM

The College of Dental Medicine's mission is to educate and train students to ensure their competency to practice the art and science of the dental profession. This requires graduates to be biologically knowledgeable, technically skilled, compassionate, and sensitive to the needs of all patients and the community. The college fosters excellence in dental education through innovative teaching, research, and community service.

YEAR 1. The fall semester of 18 weeks will include courses in Human Anatomy, Dental Anatomy and Lab, Biochemistry, Histology/Embryology, Cariology, Introduction to Periodontics, Introduction to the Dental Profession, and Dental Biomaterials. The winter semester consists of 18 weeks of coursework with Microbiology/Immunology, Physiology, Neuroanatomy, Applied and Clinical Oral Histology, Pathology and Operative Dentistry lectures and labs.

YEAR 2. The fall semester of 18 weeks will continue studies of Restorative Dentistry, Periodontics, Pharmacology, Diagnostic Radiology, Endodontics, Anesthesia, and Fixed and Removable Prosthodontics. The winter semester of 18 weeks will include Oral Medicine, Endodontics, Radiology, Pediatric Dentistry, Oral Surgery, and Orthodontics.

YEAR 3. The fall semester of 18 weeks will include courses in Oral Pathology, Ethics, and Jurisprudence. Periodontics, Cosmetic Dentistry, Restorative Dentistry, and Treatment Planning will complete the didactic program. Patient care and patient behavioral techniques will be enhanced along with development of clinical skills through clinical practice. The winter semester of 18 weeks will consist of clinical practice and the following academic program: Internal Medicine, Behavioral Science, Periodontics, Practice Management, Community Dentistry, Implantology, Cosmetic Dentistry, Oral Pathology, Forensic Dentistry, and Behavioral Sciences.

YEAR 4. The fall and winter semester of 36 weeks will be devoted to expanding clinical expertise in patient care. Community health-based programs for care of the aging population and disabled children will be conducted in various affiliated hospitals and clinical facilities. Remaining didactic courses will include Advanced Treatment Planning, Periodontics, and Oral Manifestations of Systemic Disease. Additionally, optional academic and clinical programs utilizing visiting professors and guest lecturers will be offered.

■ Degree Offered
DENTAL DEGREE: D.M.D.

SELECTION FACTORS

The College of Dental Medicine selects students based on preprofessional academic performance, DAT scores, personal interviews, written application, and letters of evaluation.

Nova Southeastern University College of Dental Medicine encourages the application of qualified minority applicants and admits students of any race, color, gender, age, non-disqualifying disability, religion or creed, or national or ethnic origin to all the rights, privileges, programs, and activities generally accorded or made available to students at the school, and does not discriminate in administration of its educational policies, admissions policies, scholarships and loan programs, and athletic and other school-administered programs.

See chapter 3 of this guide for information regarding numbers of applicants and enrollees to each dental school, along with their race, gender, age, type of predental education, mean DAT and GPA, and state of origin.

COSTS AND FINANCIAL AID

The school maintains a financial aid office to assist students in obtaining a variety of aid. The majority of the student body receives some form of financial assistance.

Estimated Total Expenses for Academic Year 2007-08

	YEAR 1	YEAR 2	YEAR 3	YEAR 4	TOTAL
Tuition, resident	$37,585	$37,585	$37,585	$37,585	$150,340
Tuition, nonresident	$39,585	$39,585	$39,585	$39,585	$158,340
Other expenses charged by school	$12,440	$9,350	$3,550	$2,550	$27,890
Estimated living expenses	$21,000	$21,000	$21,000	$21,000	$84,000
TOTAL EXPENSES, RESIDENT	**$71,025**	**$67,935**	**$62,135**	**$61,135**	**$263,030**
TOTAL EXPENSES, NONRESIDENT	**$73,025**	**$69,935**	**$64,135**	**$63,135**	**$270,230**

UNIVERSITY OF FLORIDA
COLLEGE OF DENTISTRY

Dr. Teresa A. Dolan, Dean

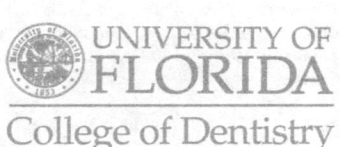

GENERAL INFORMATION

The University of Florida is one of only 17 public, land grant universities granted membership in the Association of American Universities (AAU), the prestigious organization comprised of the top higher education institutions in this country. Located in one of America's most livable cities, the University of Florida College of Dentistry is in an area rich with opportunities for outdoor sports and cultural activities year round. The College of Dentistry is located on the main campus of the University of Florida in the J. Hillis Miller Health Science Center, which also houses the Colleges of Medicine, Nursing, Pharmacy, Veterinary Medicine, and Public Health and Health Professions in a state-of-the-art facility.

Florida ranks among the leading research institutions nationally, and the College of Dentistry is a leader in dental research among dental schools. UF's more than 47,000 students are among the best in the nation, ranking Florida second among public universities and fifth among all universities in the number of National Freshman Merit Scholars.

The health-oriented professions exchange information within the Health Science Center and draw upon other university resources in their educational, research, and service efforts. A strong affiliation exists between the colleges of the Health Science Center, Shands Hospital, the Veterans Administration Medical Center, and University Hospital in Jacksonville, Florida. The College of Dentistry maintains an active continuing education program, programs in almost all dental specialties, and a broad research program.

ADMISSION REQUIREMENTS

NUMBER OF YEARS OF PREDENTAL EDUCATION: Minimum of three; usual minimum of four. Bachelor's degree strongly recommended.

LIMITATIONS ON COMMUNITY COLLEGE WORK: None.

REQUIRED COURSES:

With lab required hrs)	(semester/quarter)
Inorganic chemistry	8/12
Organic chemistry	8/12
Biology*	8/12
Physics	8/12
Biochemistry	4/6
Microbiology	4/6
Molecular biology/genetics	4/6
English grammar and composition	6/8
General psychology	3/5

*Zoology is an acceptable alternative.

SUGGESTED ADDITIONAL PREPARATION: Courses in immunology, calculus, statistics, sociology/cultural diversity, business management, conversational Spanish, and speech are suggested.

DAT: Must be taken by mid November of application year; minimum acceptable score is 15/15.

GPA: 3.2 or above recommended.

RESIDENCY: Preference given to Florida residents.

ADVANCED STANDING: Transfer students from U.S. dental schools will be considered on an individual basis, providing space is available. A limited number of foreign dental graduates may be admitted to the first-year D.M.D. program and must apply through the Four Year Internationally Educated Dentist Program (IEDP). Candidates must present evidence of completion of an approved dental education program and must have passed the TOEFL (213) examination and Part I of the National Board Examination (75). Candidates must be U.S. citizens or possess a permanent residency visa. The application process must be completed by November 1 to be eligible for admission the following August. Preference will be given to Florida residents.

Foreign dental graduates may also apply for a two-year IEDP certificate program. Candidates must present evidence of completing an approved educational program and must have passed the TOEFL (213) examination and Parts I and II of the National Board Examination (75). Candidates must be U.S. citizens or possess a permanent residency visa. The application process must be completed by November 1 to be eligible for admission the following June.

Timetable for the Class Entering Fall 2008

	Earliest Date	Latest Date	School Fee
Application Submission	5/1/07	12/1/07	$30
Acceptance Notification	12/1/07	Flexible	

Required Response and Deposit:
45 days after notification received between 12/1 and 12/31
30 days after notification received between 1/1 and 1/31
15 days after notification received after 2/1

$200 to reserve a place in the class. Nonrefundable deposit is credited to first semester tuition upon enrollment.

FOR FURTHER INFORMATION

Office of Admissions
Venita J. Sposetti
352-273-5955

Office of Financial Aid
Tom Kolb
352-846-1384

Office of Multicultural Affairs
Patricia Xirau-Probert
352-273-5954

College of Dentistry
Office of Dental Admissions
University of Florida
P.O. Box 100445
Gainesville, FL 32610-0445

Housing
Housing and Residence Education
SW 13th Street and Museum Road
P.O. Box 112100
University of Florida Housing Office
Gainesville, FL 32611-2100
352-392-2161

www.dental.ufl.edu

THE DENTAL PROGRAM

The College of Dentistry has a dynamic curriculum relevant to the educational needs of the present and adaptable to those of the future. This curriculum applies instructional technology to enhance learning effectiveness. Graduates will be well prepared to practice competently, implement current dental concepts, guide the work of others, and manage a dental office.

The curriculum is organized as follows:

YEAR 1. Basic science, preclinical technique, and introduction to clinics.

YEAR 2. Completion of basic sciences, preclinical technical courses, and beginning of comprehensive patient care.

YEAR 3. Clinical rotations and comprehensive patient care.

YEAR 4. Comprehensive patient care, extramural rotations, and experience in private practice concepts.

■ Degrees Offered
DENTAL DEGREE: D.M.D.

ALTERNATE DEGREES: B.S./D.M.D. with the following schools:
- University of Florida
- University of South Florida
- Florida International University
- University of North Florida
- University of West Florida
- Florida A&M University
- Edward Waters College
- Bethune Cookman College
- Florida Memorial College

■ Other Programs
UF offers an Honors Combined B.S./D.M.D. Program and two programs for graduates of non-accredited dental schools.

COSTS AND FINANCIAL AID

The financial obligations for completing the dental program are the direct responsibility of the student. The College of Dentistry and UF will make every effort to help the student obtain available financial aid. Present financial aid is almost entirely restricted to loan programs.

SELECTION FACTORS

Each applicant is evaluated on the basis of previous academic records, DAT scores, personal interview, recommendations, and experience in the field. A personal interview with members of the Admissions Committee in Gainesville, Florida, is required.

Students applying for admission should plan to complete the requirements for a bachelor's degree. Applicants with a strong "B" average (>3.2), as a minimum, will receive strongest consideration. Non-Florida resident applicants are admitted. The College of Dentistry attracts students possessing high standards of scholastic achievements and moral character, maturity, integrity, intellectual honesty, and a sense of responsibility.

See chapter 3 of this guide for information regarding numbers of applicants and enrollees to each dental school, along with their race, gender, age, type of predental education, mean DAT and GPA, and state of origin.

Financial Aid Awards to First-Year Students in 2005-06
■ TOTAL NUMBER OF RECIPIENTS: 71　　■ 86% OF CLASS

	Average Award	Range of Awards
Residents	$33,133	$1,038-$40,531
Nonresidents	$54,364	$16,385-$71,245

Estimated Total Expenses for Academic Year 2006-07

	YEAR 1	YEAR 2	YEAR 3	YEAR 4	TOTAL
Tuition, resident	$19,276	18,452	$16,950	$16,950	$71,628
Tuition, nonresident*	$46,454	$45,630	$44,128	$44,128	$180,340
Equipment					
Instruments	$4,422	$4,212	$3,102	$1,968	$13,704
Books, supplies	$1,203	$1,865	$1,680	$1,420	$6,168
Estimated living expenses	$14,800	$14,800	$14,800	$11,170	$55,570
Food, rent, personal insurance, transportation, clothing, maintenance					
TOTAL EXPENSES, RESIDENT	$39,701	$39,329	$36,532	$31,508	$147,070
TOTAL EXPENSES, NONRESIDENT	$66,879	$66,507	$63,710	$58,686	$255,782

*In some cases, nonresident students may qualify for resident status after one year.

MEDICAL COLLEGE OF GEORGIA
SCHOOL OF DENTISTRY

Dr. Connie L. Drisko, Dean

GENERAL INFORMATION

Since enrolling its first class in 1969, the Medical College of Georgia School of Dentistry has had as its primary mission the improvement of the oral health of the citizens of Georgia. The school remains committed to this goal with programs for education, research, and public service through patient care. Students are limited to residents of the state of Georgia.

The School of Dentistry is part of the Medical College of Georgia, one of 34 autonomous institutions within the University System of Georgia. In addition to dentistry, the institution includes schools of allied health, graduate studies, medicine, and nursing and is adjacent to a large complex of health care facilities, providing a diverse and stimulating environment for its students on the fringe of downtown Augusta, Georgia.

ADMISSION REQUIREMENTS

NUMBER OF YEARS OF PREDENTAL EDUCATION: The minimum is three years of college (135 quarter or 90 semester hours). Most students complete a degree (120 semester or 180 quarter hours) prior to matriculation. All college-level preparation, including required courses listed below, must be completed at an accredited U.S. college or university.

LIMITATIONS ON COMMUNITY COLLEGE WORK: None.

REQUIRED COURSES:

With lab required
General biology—1 academic year*
General or inorganic chemistry—1 academic year*
Advanced chemistry**—1 academic year*
Physics—1 semester or 2 quarters

Other courses
English—1 academic year or the amount required by the applicant's undergraduate institution to earn a bachelor's degree

* One academic year equals two semesters or three quarters or one semester plus two quarters.
** Advanced chemistry must include either 1) one semester of organic chemistry with lab followed by a second semester of organic chemistry or a semester of biochemistry or 2) two quarters of organic chemistry with lab followed by a third quarter of organic chemistry or a quarter of biochemistry. For the advanced chemistry requirement, a second semester of lab or third quarter of lab is not required but should be taken if available.

SUGGESTED ADDITIONAL PREPARATION: The Student Admissions and Recruitment Committee suggests that applicants take a course or courses in biochemistry, comparative anatomy with lab, microbiology, marketing, personnel management, psychology, and art (requiring drawing or sculpting). Applicants should seek additional learning experiences in areas where their preparation is weak.

DAT: Mandatory; no later than September 2007 and within three years of expected first enrollment. Applicants for 2008 must take the computerized DAT by September 30, 2007.

ENGLISH LANGUAGE REQUIREMENTS: The combined Test of English as a Foreign Language (TOEFL) and the Test of Spoken English (TSE-P) is required of all applicants whose native language is not English. Applicants taking the combined test must register for the combined exam; results of the TSE-A category exam will not be accepted. For admission to the School of Dentistry, students must score the equivalent of at least 600 on the TOEFL and at least 50 on the TSE-P. Applicants must take the combined examination no later than September 2007 in order to be considered for admission for the class admitted in August 2008.

GPA: A minimum overall GPA and science GPA of 3.0 is required.

RESIDENCY: Admission for 2008 is limited to Georgia residents. Individuals from other countries who are in the United States only temporarily are not considered for admission.

ADVANCED STANDING: No students are admitted with advanced standing.

Timetable for the Class Entering Fall 2008

	Earliest Date	Latest Date	School Fee
Application Submission	6/1/07	10/15/07	$30
Acceptance Notification	12/1/07	8/14/08	$100

The Medical College of Georgia does not participate in the Associated American Dental Schools Application Service (AADSAS).

Required Response and Deposit:
$100 deposit, applied to tuition for first semester. Refunded if student withdraws no later than 90 days prior to registration.

FOR FURTHER INFORMATION

Office of Admissions
Carole M. Hanes
Associate Dean for Students, Admissions, and Alumni
706-721-3587; chanes@mail.mcg.edu

Office of Student Financial Aid
Rhonda Johnson
Assistant Director
706-721-4901

Office of Student Diversity
Beverly Y. Tarver
Director
706-721-2821

Housing
Tom Fitts
Director of Housing
706-721-3471

Medical College of Georgia
Augusta, GA 30912

To obtain an application, visit www.mcg.edu/careers/dentistry.htm. The application will be available June 1, 2007.

www.mcg.edu/sod

THE DENTAL PROGRAM

The School of Dentistry awards the D.M.D. degree. The program of study consists of 11 semesters spread over approximately 45 months. Students are enrolled for eight regular semesters (fall and spring) of 15 weeks and for summer semesters of eight, 13, and 14 weeks after the first, second, and third years, respectively. Clinical and basic science courses are taught throughout the eight regular semesters, and elementary clinical treatment of patients, including restorative dentistry, begins in the first year. The placement of clinical experiences in the first year shifts some basic science courses to the third year.

The basic science faculty are all full-time faculty within the school of dentistry. The high percentage of dual-degree basic science faculty contributes significantly to the integration of basic and clinical sciences. The unique basic science faculty and its impressive array of research equipment and facilities provide ample opportunities for research. Students who are clinically proficient and in good academic standing may participate in elective research experiences. Student clinical progress is determined more by demonstrated competency than by the number of hours in class or completion of numerical units, and graduation depends on reaching an established level of competency.

The clinical curriculum employs a comprehensive care approach to patient treatment rather than block assignments. This provides students with experiences that more closely resemble the private practice of dentistry and encourages personalized service for the patients. Classes are scheduled from 8 a.m. to 5 p.m. five days a week with few scheduled breaks. Students participate in off-campus clinical experiences during the summer between the third and fourth years, and all students must spend at least three weeks in an off-campus clinical setting. Students may select areas of service, including public health clinics, charitable health programs, and government and private institutions.

Percentage of curriculum time by area

	Biol. Sci.	Clin. Sci.	Patient Care Clinic	Behav. Sci.
Year 1	41%	50%	1%	28%
Year 2	25%	58%	17%	0%
Year 3	18%	30%	51%	1%
Year 4	2%	14%	83%	1%

■ Degrees Offered

DENTAL DEGREE: D.M.D.

ALTERNATE DEGREES: D.M.D./M.S. or D.M.D./Ph.D. in oral biology. For information, contact the Graduate Program Director, Department of Oral Biology, School of Dentistry, Medical College of Georgia, Augusta, GA 30912-1122; phone 706-721-2526; fax 706-721-6276.

COSTS AND FINANCIAL AID

The innovative and well-staffed Office of Student Financial Aid has been extremely successful in assisting students in acquiring assistance. Need- and merit-based awards are available. Applications for aid should be made between January 1 and March 31 of the desired year of entry. Applications for financial aid are distributed to students who are invited to campus for interviews.

Financial Aid Awards to First-Year Students in 2006-07

■ TOTAL NUMBER OF RECIPIENTS: 57   ■ 92% OF CLASS

	Average Award	Range of Awards
Residents	$34,287	$500 - $41,606

Estimated School-Related Expenses for Academic Year 2006-07

	YEAR 1	YEAR 2	YEAR 3	YEAR 4	TOTAL
Tuition, resident	$14,151	$14,151	$14,151	$9,434	$51,877
Total other fees	$8,769	$6,654	$6,834	$5,066	$27,323
TOTAL EXPENSES, RESIDENT	$22,920	$20,805	$20,985	$14,500	$79,200

SELECTION FACTORS

The Student Admissions and Recruitment Committee consists of School of Dentistry faculty members, students, and at least one private practitioner. Admission is granted by the dean following a recommendation from the committee. Selection is based on merit and perceptions of the applicant's potential for success as a health care practitioner. The committee strives to accept the best applicants from those who present their credentials for review. The school seeks applicants who have demonstrated excellence in their academic preparation and have the personal qualities requisite for successful patient management and leadership. Although all references are evaluated, more credence is given to the recommendation from the predental advisor. If the applicant has attended a college or university that does not have a predental advisor, the applicant should substitute a report from a faculty member who knows the applicant well. A minimum of three references is required. Applicants should have recommendations submitted from the predental advisor of their undergraduate college, their family dentist, and at least one other individual. Reference forms are included in the admission application packet available at the school's website.

The committee is eager to review applications from all qualified applicants, and women and members of underrepresented minority groups are encouraged to apply. The school strives to admit and enroll classes containing a cross section of talents and skills. Race, gender, age, creed, color, national origin, nor disability is a basis for discrimination among qualified applicants.

While the committee has no preference for undergraduate major, it recognizes that a program of study containing many science courses will contribute to a better performance on the DAT. Students seeking admission should carry a full academic load, maintain good grades, and participate in campus social, cultural, and athletic activities. Applicants who work should advise the committee of this fact. The committee recognizes that some students flounder academically until they have selected a career, when their performance often improves significantly. These "late bloomers" can be admitted after several years of strong academic performance and good DAT scores. However, due to increasing competition for admission, these students are finding it more and more difficult to gain acceptance. The preferred approach is to start well and maintain a high level of achievement throughout college. No attempt is made to weigh the academic reputation of any college or university. Performance on the DAT is taken by the committee to be a measure of each applicant's undergraduate preparation.

Interviews are by invitation of the Student Admissions and Recruitment Committee. Only applicants who have visited the campus for an admission interview can be recommended for admission. For accepted students with recognized academic deficiencies, a special pre-enrollment summer session is offered to improve study skills. Students who encounter difficulties in the regular curriculum are provided with tutors as indicated by the severity and nature of the student's difficulties. There is little attrition.

See chapter 3 of this guide for information regarding numbers of applicants and enrollees to each dental school, along with their race, gender, age, type of predental education, mean DAT and GPA, and state of origin.

ILLINOIS

UNIVERSITY OF ILLINOIS AT CHICAGO
COLLEGE OF DENTISTRY

Dr. Bruce S. Graham, Dean

GENERAL INFORMATION

The University of Illinois at Chicago (UIC) College of Dentistry confers over half of the D.D.S./ D.M.D. degrees awarded by Illinois schools. The college offers postgraduate programs in endodontics, oral and maxillofacial surgery, orthodontics, pediatric dentistry, periodontics, and prosthodontics. Programs leading to the M.S. and Ph.D. degrees are also available through the Graduate College.

The UIC College of Dentistry's vision for the future is to become a pre-eminent academic center for oral and craniofacial health. Located on the urban academic health center campus of the University of Illinois at Chicago in the home city of organized dentistry, the college collaborates with America's largest medical college and nationally recognized Colleges of Nursing, Pharmacy, Engineering, and Public Health.

The college is educating dentists who will graduate with new professional competencies needed in the 21st century. In addition to the knowledge and skills requisite for clinical practice in traditional private dental office practice settings, the college is preparing dentists for leadership roles in addressing the silent epidemic of oral diseases afflicting 160 million Americans who today have no access to a dentist's care. Our students' clinical patient care education occurs in a real world-based group practice environment that employs a computer-based electronic patient record technology and links faculty and students in mentorship relationships. Our students explore the scientific evidence basis for clinical patient care and have the opportunity to participate in the discovery of new knowledge in collaboration with faculty conducting original research. These scientifically oriented educational experiences provide exceptional preparation for the student who wishes to pursue a career as dental educator and provide a solid foundation for practicing the profession of dentistry in a rapidly changing world.

With a faculty dedicated to excellence and innovation in education and research, and the strong support of the University of Illinois, the UIC College of Dentistry is preparing its graduates for leadership roles in every aspect of their chosen profession.

ADMISSION REQUIREMENTS

NUMBER OF YEARS OF PREDENTAL EDUCATION: Formal minimum of three (90 semester hours or 135 quarter hours), but the baccalaureate degree is strongly preferred.

LIMITATIONS ON COMMUNITY COLLEGE WORK: None, but four-year colleges/universities are preferred.

REQUIRED COURSES: All course credits must be from accredited U.S. colleges or universities.

With lab required	(semester/quarter hrs)
Chemistry	14/21
Biological science	6/9
Physics	6/9

Other courses	
English	6/9
Electives	58/87

SUGGESTED ADDITIONAL PREPARATION: In addition to the required science courses, strong preference is given to applicants who have completed coursework in four of the following science courses: biochemistry, physiology, histology, human anatomy, microbiology, and cell and molecular biology. AP credit from high school can be applied toward electives only.

GPA AND DAT SCORES: Each applicant must present a minimum cumulative GPA of 2.5/4.0 and a minimum science GPA of 2.5/4.0. The academic average score and perceptual ability score on the DAT cannot be less than 15 and 14, respectively. Generally, applicants must present credentials well above the minimum for their application to be competitive.

RESIDENCY: The University of Illinois is a state-supported institution and, therefore, strong preference is given to residents of the state of Illinois.

INTERVIEWS: Interviews are mandatory.

ADVANCED STANDING: The College does not admit D.D.S. students with advanced standing. The College does consider transfer students who are currently attending a U.S. dental school. Opportunities for transfer are dependent on whether there is space available in the class to which the student is requesting transfer. No student will be considered for transfer if he/she has been dismissed from another dental school for poor academic performance or dishonorable conduct.

Timetable for the Class Entering Fall 2008

	Earliest Date	Latest Date	School Fee
Application Submission	6/1/07	12/1/07	$65
Acceptance Notification	12/1/07	5/15/08	

Required Response and Deposit:
$300 resident nonrefundable fee
$1,500 nonresident nonrefundable fee

FOR FURTHER INFORMATION

Office of Admissions
Ann Shorrock
Director of Admissions
312-996-2873

Office of Admissions
Jill Hofmeister
Admissions and Student Affairs Coordinator
312-355-0350

Student and Diversity Affairs
Darryl Pendleton
Associate Dean for Student and Diversity Affairs
312-355-1670

College of Dentistry
University of Illinois at Chicago
801 S. Paulina Street
Chicago, IL 60612-7211

dentistry.uic.edu

UNIVERSITY OF ILLINOIS AT CHICAGO COLLEGE OF DENTISTRY ILLINOIS

THE DENTAL PROGRAM

The curriculum in dentistry comprises 11 semesters of instruction over four calendar years. The first- and second-year curriculum is designed to provide foundational knowledge of biomedical sciences integrated with clinical care preparation. During the third and fourth years, the majority of coursework is devoted to providing oral health care in a variety of settings designed to expose students to a wide array of experiences. Emphasis is also placed on developing a practitioner with a strong sense of community values.

The college has adopted a list of competencies that must be attained prior to graduation. Competencies are those levels of knowledge, skills, and values expected of the beginning dental practitioner.

The curriculum extends over four academic years. Summer sessions are required between freshman and sophomore years, sophomore and junior years, and junior and senior years.

Most required courses follow the UIC grading system of A, B, C, D, and E, with some courses being pass/fail. Examinations include: written tests; on occasion, oral examinations; practical and mock-board examinations; and station-type examinations. The college also conducts an interdisciplinary exam simulating clinical practice to aid in determining competence. To graduate, a student must have a grade point average of at least 2.0 on a 4.0 scale. No student is graduated who has a failing grade in any required course; all failures must be made up.

■ Degrees Offered
DENTAL DEGREE: D.D.S.

ALTERNATE DEGREES:

- B.S.D. program: some predental institutions will accept credits earned in the basic medical sciences at the College of Dentistry and apply these toward the baccalaureate degree, which is then awarded by the school of origin.
- D.D.S./M.S. programs: can usually be completed within four years.
- D.D.S./Ph.D. programs: can usually be completed within seven or eight years.

COSTS AND FINANCIAL AID

The UIC College of Dentistry currently accepts financially needy students and is committed to helping those students secure financial aid. Due to the rigorous academic program, students are strongly discouraged from working during their first and second years. Scholarships and other nonrepayable grants will be available on a very limited level to entering students. All students who may qualify are encouraged to apply for guaranteed student loans. These loans are available to most students who apply.

Financial Aid Awards to First-Year Students in 2006-07
■ TOTAL NUMBER OF RECIPIENTS: 273   ■ 100% OF CLASS

Average Award	Range of Awards
$23,812	$200-$42,000

Average for residents (fall/spring semesters): $42,000
Average for nonresidents (fall/spring semesters): $62,975

Estimated Total Expenses for Academic Year 2006-07

	YEAR 1	YEAR 2	YEAR 3	YEAR 4	TOTAL
	(2 semesters)	(3 semesters)	(3 semesters)	(3 semesters)	
Tuition, resident	$20,412	$27,216	$27,216	$27,216	
Tuition, nonresident	$46,910	$62,547	$62,547	$62,547	
Fees	$2,962	$3,383	$3,383	$3,383	
Textbooks (estimate)	$900	$700	$500	$300	
Dentistry Instrument Leasing	$5,470	$5,665	$4,350	$4,230	
TOTAL, RESIDENT	$29,744	$36,964	$35,449	$35,129	
TOTAL, NONRESIDENT	$56,242	$72,295	$70,780	$70,460	

SELECTION FACTORS

The capacity of the College of Dentistry is limited, and thus selection is based upon the quality of data presented by each applicant and upon the changing needs of society. To meet these societal needs, the college encourages students with an interest in practicing in underserved communities. Students of the following minority backgrounds are strongly encouraged to submit applications: Native American, African-American, and Americans of Hispanic origin.

No student will be considered who is on scholastic probation or who has been dropped for poor scholarship from the last institution attended prior to seeking admission to UIC. In selecting applicants, the Committee on Admissions takes into consideration such factors as scholastic records, the schools and colleges previously attended, letters of recommendation (especially from professors in the laboratory sciences), DAT scores, and information collected during the interview process. Preference is given to applicants who complete their bachelor's degree.

It is the policy of UIC not to engage in discrimination or harassment against any person because of race, color, religion, gender, national origin, ancestry, age, marital status, disability, sexual orientation, unfavorable discharge from the military, or status as a disabled veteran or a veteran of the Vietnam era. In addition, UIC complies with all federal and state nondiscrimination, equal opportunity, and affirmative action laws, orders, and regulations.

See chapter 3 of this guide for information regarding numbers of applicants and enrollees to each dental school along with their race, gender, age, type of predental education, mean DAT and GPA, and state of origin.

ACADEMIC AND OTHER ASSISTANCE

The Office of Student and Diversity Affairs aims to assist individuals from underrepresented minority groups (African-American, Hispanic, and Native American) aspiring to become dentists and to increase the number of underrepresented minority enrollees at the College of Dentistry. Program services include the following: academic counseling (advice for predental course planning and selection and interpretation of dental school eligibility requirements), academic retention (prematriculation summer sessions, tutorial services, and nonclinical dental practice workshops), application assistance (advice on application management and procedures), and financial aid. These services are available to all applicants.

ILLINOIS

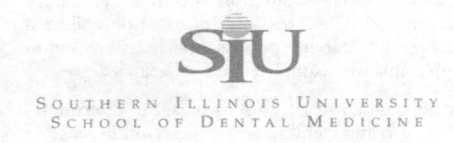

SOUTHERN ILLINOIS UNIVERSITY
SCHOOL OF DENTAL MEDICINE

Dr. Ann M. Boyle, Dean

GENERAL INFORMATION

Southern Illinois University (SIU), a state-supported institution, established the School of Dental Medicine (SDM) in 1969. The dental school is located on the campus of the former Shurtleff College in Alton, 15 miles from the Edwardsville campus. Situated within the metropolitan St. Louis area, SIU-SDM offers the social and cultural attractions of an urban environment while it identifies with predominantly rural southern Illinois. This unique circumstance enables application of the theoretical knowledge of formal education to the broadest spectrum of oral health care needs.

ADMISSION REQUIREMENTS

NUMBER OF YEARS OF PREDENTAL EDUCATION: Formal minimum of two; usual minimum of three.

LIMITATIONS ON COMMUNITY COLLEGE WORK: Maximum of 60 semester hours.

REQUIRED COURSES:

With lab required	(semester/quarter hrs)
Inorganic chemistry	6/9
Organic chemistry	6/9
Biology	6/9
Physics	6/9

Other courses
English   6/9

SUGGESTED ADDITIONAL PREPARATION: Choose from among biochemistry, upper division biology, quantitative analysis, calculus, literature, art, and sculpting.

DAT: Mandatory.

GPA: 3.0 or above recommended.

RESIDENCY: No specific requirements; see Selection Factors.

ADVANCED STANDING: The School of Dental Medicine accepts transfer students only under exceptional circumstances. The school does not offer a program for foreign-trained dentists.

Timetable for the Class Entering Fall 2008

	Earliest Date	Latest Date	School Fee
Application Submission	5/5/08	2/1/08*	$20**
Acceptance Notification	12/1/07	8/14/08	

*Applicants should apply well before 11/1/07 in order to receive full consideration.

**To have your AADSAS application processed, send fee directly to the Southern Illinois University School of Dental Medicine at the time you return your AADSAS application and no later than 2/1/08. (Fee is subject to change prior to the next applicant cycle.)

Required Response and Deposit:
45 days after notification if received between 12/1 and 12/31
30 days after notification if received between 1/1 and 1/31
15 days after notification if received between 2/1 and 6/1
7 days after notification or as specified if received 6/1–7/15
$80 to hold place.

FOR FURTHER INFORMATION
Admissions Office
618-474-7170

Financial Aid, Housing
Office of Student Services
618-474-7175

Minority Affairs
Office of Multicultural Issues and Recruitment
618-474-7170

Southern Illinois University
School of Dental Medicine
2800 College Avenue
Alton, IL 62002

www.siue.edu/sdm

THE DENTAL PROGRAM

SIU-SDM combines educational tradition and innovation in the curriculum. As a result, students are able to develop the appropriate fund of knowledge and skills that allows them to become the best in their fields.

The curriculum incorporates biomedical, clinical, behavioral, and social sciences to provide the knowledge and experience necessary for comprehensive oral health care. Emphasis is focused on the reciprocal aspects of dentistry and medicine in total patient health management.

Contemporary trends have shaped the approach—an unqualified commitment to the use of auxiliaries and the techniques of "four-handed, sit-down" dentistry. Initially, classmates enact patient/practitioner relationships; ultimately, each student acquires a "family" of patients from the outpatient clinic register. Thus, through simulation, a natural climate is introduced that parallels the professional's patient load and affords the student practical and technical diagnoses and treatment situations demanding all the skills of the art and science of clinical dentistry. Training is available in a variety of settings in addition to the school's own patient care center-hospital dental programs, private practices, and community health centers.

YEAR 1. Introduction to dental medicine.

YEAR 2. Concepts of patient health management.

YEAR 3. Basic patient care.

YEAR 4. Comprehensive patient care.

■ Degrees Offered

DENTAL DEGREE: D.M.D.

ALTERNATE DEGREES: Students entering without a degree may earn their bachelor's degree while completing the dental curriculum, if the institution at which preprofessional coursework was taken offers such a program.

B.S./D.M.D. THROUGH SOUTHERN ILLINOIS UNIVERSITY AT EDWARDSVILLE: The preprofessional part of this curriculum is completed within three years on the Edwardsville campus, and the professional part in the School of Dental Medicine, Alton, Illinois. Upon successful completion of the first year in the SDM and recommendation of the dean, this student will be granted the degree of Bachelor of Science by the Southern Illinois University at Edwardsville.

B.A./D.M.D. THROUGH AUGUSTANA COLLEGE: Southern Illinois University School of Dental Medicine offers a special program leading to the degrees of Bachelor of Arts and Doctor of Dental Medicine. The preprofessional part of this curriculum is completed in three years at Augustana College in Rock Island, Illinois, and the professional part at the School of Dental Medicine in Alton, Illinois.

SELECTION FACTORS

All applicants are given consideration without regard to race, gender, creed, national origin, or disability status as defined by Section 504 of the Rehabilitation Act of 1973. Each applicant is evaluated in terms of the composite scholastic record, calculation of the required science courses credit point average, quality of preprofessional education, DAT performance, academic recommendations, and other special elements as determined by the school. Preference is given to Illinois residents. Applicant interviews are by invitation only and are required for acceptance consideration. The School of Dental Medicine actively encourages applications from persons in those segments of society currently underrepresented in the dental profession.

See chapter 3 of this guide for information regarding numbers of applicants and enrollees to each dental school, along with their race, gender, age, type of predental education, mean DAT and GPA, and state of origin.

COSTS AND FINANCIAL AID

SIU-SDM provides need-based and alternative loan funds. For more information, contact the Financial Aid Office.

Financial Aid Awards to First-Year Students in 2006-07

■ TOTAL NUMBER OF RECIPIENTS: 49   ■ 96% OF CLASS

	Average Award	Range of Awards
Residents	$38,678	$0-$45,778
Nonresidents	$42,979	

Estimated Total Expenses for Academic Year 2005-06

	YEAR 1	YEAR 2	YEAR 3	YEAR 4	TOTAL
Tuition, resident	$18,150	$18,150	$18,150	$18,150	$72,600
Tuition, nonresident	$54,450	$54,450	$54,450	$54,450	$217,800
Fees	$4,394	$4,394	$4,394	$4,394	$17,576
Student activity, athletics, fitness center, university center, instrument rental					
Equipment	$5,635	$3,375	$155	$83	$9,248
Living expenses	$14,619	$14,619	$14,619	$14,619	$58,476
Lodging, transportation, personal expenses					
TOTAL, RESIDENT	$42,798	$40,538	$37,318	$37,246	$157,900
TOTAL, NONRESIDENT	$79,098	$76,838	$73,618	$73,546	$303,100

INDIANA UNIVERSITY
SCHOOL OF DENTISTRY

Dr. Lawrence I. Goldblatt, Dean

GENERAL INFORMATION

The School of Dentistry is an integral part of Indiana University's Medical Center in Indianapolis, which includes a medical school, a school of nursing, and a complex of hospitals with a total of over 600 beds. Clinical facilities are excellent, and patients are drawn from a population area of more than one million persons. The school maintains dental clinics in the James Whitcomb Riley Hospital for Children, Regenstrief Health Center, and the University Hospital on the Medical Center Campus. The School of Dentistry was established as a private school in 1879 and has been a part of Indiana University since 1925. Approximately 100 students are accepted for each freshman class. Graduate students are candidates for either M.S. or M.S.D. degrees in most departments in the dental school; a limited number of Ph.D. programs are offered. Dental auxiliary programs in dental hygiene and dental assisting are offered at Indianapolis and four other campuses in the state. Dental laboratory technology is offered at the Fort Wayne campus.

ADMISSION REQUIREMENTS

NUMBER OF YEARS OF PREDENTAL EDUCATION: Minimum requirement of three years (90 semester or 135 quarter hours); most students enter with four years (120 semester or 180 quarter hours).

LIMITATIONS ON COMMUNITY COLLEGE WORK: No more than 60 semester hours.

REQUIRED COURSES:

With lab required (semester/quarter hrs)
Biology or zoology	8/12
Inorganic chemistry	8/12
Physics	8/12
Organic chemistry	4/6
Anatomy	4/6
Physiology (lecture only)	4/6
Biochemistry (lecture only)	3/4.5

Other courses
English composition	2/3
Introductory psychology	2/3

SUGGESTED ADDITIONAL PREPARATION: Minor in foreign language or social science; business management, cell biology, genetics, histology, molecular biology, microbiology, physical chemistry, solid art.

DAT: IU School of Dentistry must receive your DAT scores before you will be considered for an interview.

GPA: Preferential consideration will be given to those whose overall, science, and BCP GPAs exceed 3.2.

RESIDENCY: Nonresidents are encouraged to apply.

Timetable for the Class Entering Fall 2008

	Earliest Date	Latest Date	School Fee
Application Submission	5/15/07	12/1/07	$50
Acceptance Notification	12/1/07		

Required Response and Deposit:
Applicants must respond within 45 days if they are notified of their acceptance on December 1. A $500 nonrefundable deposit is required to hold their place in the class.

FOR FURTHER INFORMATION

Office of Records and Admissions
Robert H. Kasberg, Jr.
Director of Admissions
317-274-8173; rkasberg@iupui.edu
Indiana University School of Dentistry
1121 W. Michigan St.
Indianapolis, IN 46202

Office of Student Financial Aid
Paul Koch
Assistant Director of Graduate/Professional Financial Aid
317-278-8477; gradaid@iupui.edu
Cavanaugh Hall, Room 103
425 University Blvd.
Indianapolis, IN 46202

Director of Student Diversity Support
Traci Adams
317-274-7052; tadams@iupui.edu
Indiana University School of Dentistry
1121 W. Michigan Street
Indianapolis, IN 46202

Housing
Associate Director of Housing & Residence Life
317-274-5159
Indiana University
Purdue University at Indianapolis
1226 W. Michigan Street, BR 107
Indianapolis, IN 46202
www.housing.iupui.edu

www.iusd.iupui.edu

THE DENTAL PROGRAM

The school has implemented a new curriculum that promotes critical thinking and problem-solving skills and places more responsibility for learning on the students. It integrates biological, clinical, and behavioral sciences and employs block scheduling. This means that courses meet several times per week for several hours instead of only once or twice per week. The larger blocks of time allow faculty to use innovative methods of classroom instruction instead of relying solely on a traditional lecture format. In addition, the block scheduling reduces the number of courses running simultaneously so that there is less competition for the students' time. The curriculum is based on a two-term year, and the terms are approximately 23 weeks in length.

In the first year, the students are introduced to the profession and take courses that lay the foundations of biological and preclinical dental sciences and begin their hand skills development. In the second year, the biomedical sciences are presented along with more advanced dental sciences, and the students begin delivering patient care in comprehensive care clinics. While classroom courses are offered in the third and fourth years, the focus is primarily on all aspects of patient care in a variety of clinical settings in the school's comprehensive care clinics, in community-based clinics, and in hospital-based clinics.

Research is strongly encouraged for all students. Students' individual interests can be met through elective courses in the fourth year.

■ Degrees Offered
DENTAL DEGREE: D.D.S.

ALTERNATE DEGREES: Students entering without a degree may earn a bachelor's and a dental degree concurrently if such an undergraduate degree is awarded by their undergraduate institution.

COSTS AND FINANCIAL AID

Students accepted to IUSD are encouraged to have firm plans to support the entire expense of their dental education. At the same time, the university's Office of Financial Aid is committed to employing every available means of aiding prospective students in meeting their financial obligations through student loans. Approximately 92 percent of students borrow money through the financial aid office to cover their education expenses.

Financial Aid Awards to First-Year Students in 2006-07

This information pertains to student loans as the primary financial aid resource:

■ **TOTAL NUMBER OF RECIPIENTS: 93 out of 100 students** (93% of D.D.S. program)

	Average Award
Residents	$39,259
Nonresidents	$53,271

Estimated School-Related Expenses for Academic Year 2006-07

	YEAR 1	YEAR 2	YEAR 3	YEAR 4	TOTAL
Tuition, resident	$19,244	$19,244	$19,244	$19,244	$76,976
Tuition, nonresident	$45,980	$45,980	$45,980	$45,980	$183,920
Mandatory general fees:	$246	$246	$246	$246	$984
Instrument purchase	$4,804	$5,414	$392	0	$10,610
Instrument rental	$2,700	$2,700	$2,700	$2,700	$10,800
Books and supplies	$1396	$1362	$242	0	$3,000
Living expenses (housing, transportation, personal):	$18,756	$18,756	$18,756	$18,756	$75,024
TOTAL, RESIDENT	**$47,146**	**$47,772**	**$41,580**	**$40,946**	**$177,444**
TOTAL, NONRESIDENT	**$73,882**	**$74,508**	**$68,316**	**$67,682**	**$284,388**

IUSD requires no fee for health services, but all students must acquire health insurance on their own. The school provides malpractice insurance for the students.

SELECTION FACTORS

Selection criteria include, but are not limited to the following: overall GPA, science GPA, DAT scores, interview, recommendations, years and hours of college credit, degrees received, motivation, exploration of dentistry, manual and artistic skills, character, personality, and ethics.

Although applications from all underrepresented groups are encouraged, the IUSD Admissions Committee reviews all applications without discriminating in favor of or against any applicant because of age, gender, race, creed, religion, disability, or national origin. Selections are made on an individual basis upon appraisal of the applicant's established record and potential for development. Selected applicants will be contacted for an interview with members of the Admissions Committee. Applications should be submitted one year prior to expected enrollment.

The selection process consists of a thorough review of all credentials supplied by every applicant. Through this means, the class positions are filled and a group of alternate candidates selected and ranked.

See chapter 3 of this guide for information regarding numbers of applicants and enrollees to each dental school, along with their race, gender, age, type of predental education, mean DAT and GPA, and state of origin.

THE UNIVERSITY OF IOWA
COLLEGE OF DENTISTRY

Dr. David C. Johnsen, Dean

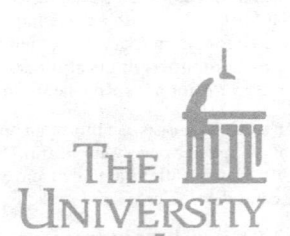

GENERAL INFORMATION

The University of Iowa (UI) is a state-supported institution with an enrollment of over 29,000, located on a 900-acre campus spanning the Iowa River Valley and merging with the business center of Iowa City, a community of 60,000. The College of Dentistry, founded in 1882, has an enrollment of about 300 dental students and a faculty of 96. The College of Dentistry is part of the university's health sciences campus that includes the Colleges of Dentistry, Nursing, Medicine, Public Health, and Pharmacy, as well as a new Medical Education and Biomedical Research Facility, the Eckstein Medical Research Building, the University Hospitals, the Bowen Science Building (basic sciences), and the Hardin Library for the Health Sciences. The Dental Science Building includes patient care clinics, academic classrooms, a simulation clinic, and preclinical research laboratories. In addition to the D.D.S. program, the College of Dentistry offers advanced education programs in all dental specialties recognized by the American Dental Association. The college also offers additional outstanding programs and residencies with study toward master's and Ph.D. degrees.

ADMISSION REQUIREMENTS

NUMBER OF YEARS OF PREDENTAL EDUCATION: Formal minimum of three (90 semester hours); usual and recommended, four.

LIMITATIONS ON COMMUNITY COLLEGE WORK: Maximum of 60 semester hours accepted.

REQUIRED COURSES:

With lab required	(semester hrs)
Inorganic chemistry	8
Organic chemistry	8
Physics	8
Biology*	8

Other courses
Satisfaction of the English composition, rhetoric, and speech requirements for a bachelor's degree at the college attended.

*Must take a complete introductory biology course as required by school attended; zoology combined with other courses such as microscopic anatomy, cell biology, etc. makes an acceptable program.

SUGGESTED ADDITIONAL PREPARATION: Additional hours (to reach the required minimum total of 90) chosen to ensure a well-rounded background can be selected from among the following: biochemistry, upper division biology, anatomy, physiology, quantitative analysis, calculus, literature, arts, and the social sciences.

INTERVIEW: An on-site interview is required.

DAT: Mandatory; taken no later than August of the year in which the application is made.

GPA: A 3.0 or above is preferred.

RESIDENCY: No specific requirements; classes average 20–25 percent non-Iowa residents.

ADVANCED STANDING: The college does not have a formal advanced standing program.

Timetable for the Class Entering Fall 2008

	Earliest Date	Latest Date	School Fee
Application Submission	6/1/07	11/1/07*	$60
Acceptance Notification	12/1/07	8/15/08	

*Early application is strongly encouraged.

Required Response and Deposit:
45 days after notification if received 12/1
30 days after notification if received between 12/15 and 1/31
15 days after notification if received after 2/1

$500 deposit required to hold place in class.

FOR FURTHER INFORMATION
Office of Admissions
B. Elaine Brown
Coordinator for Student Admissions
319-335-7157; elaine-brown@uiowa.edu
The University of Iowa
College of Dentistry
Iowa City, IA 52242-1010

Office of Student Financial Aid
Mark S. Warner
Director
319-335-1450
The University of Iowa
Calvin Hall
Iowa City, IA 52242

Minority Affairs/Financial Aid/Admissions
Yvonne M. Chalkley
Associate Dean for Student Affairs
319-335-7164
The University of Iowa
College of Dentistry
Iowa City, IA 52242-1010

Housing
Family Housing Office
319-335-9199
Housing Service Building
The University of Iowa
Iowa City, IA 52242

www.dentistry.uiowa.edu

THE DENTAL PROGRAM

The University of Iowa College of Dentistry is committed to providing a high-quality dental education to aspiring dentists to help them meet the health needs of a large and diverse population.

YEAR 1. Basic sciences, laboratory and technique courses, and an introduction to clinical experiences.

YEAR 2. Continuation of basic sciences and technical courses, plus definitive clinical patient treatment.

YEAR 3. Students rotate through a series of clerkships in each of the seven clinical disciplines.

YEAR 4. Delivery of comprehensive dental care under conditions approximating those in private practice; seniors will also participate in extramural programs in locations primarily throughout the Midwest.

■ Degrees Offered

DENTAL DEGREE: D.D.S.

ALTERNATE DEGREES: Students entering without a degree may be able to earn a bachelor's degree by the transfer of course credits back to their undergraduate institution to satisfy elective hours. Applicants must check with their advisors on the specific requirements for the baccalaureate degree at their university, including transfer of credits.

■ Other Programs

HONORS RESEARCH: For interested and qualified students, there are opportunities to participate in dental research with faculty.

DEFERRED ADMIT PROGRAM: The College of Dentistry has a Deferred Admit Program (DAP) that allows academically motivated, Iowa resident students who are interested in a dental career to be admitted as early as the first year of their undergraduate college education. DAP students must complete the equivalent number of hours required for a degree at their undergraduate university prior to enrolling in the College of Dentistry. Students selected for the DAP must maintain a specified GPA and present competitive DAT scores to assure matriculation at the College of Dentistry.

COSTS AND FINANCIAL AID

Students eligible for dental school are considered for enrollment regardless of financial need. Students accepted for admission may apply for financial aid by completing and submitting the Free Application for Federal Student Aid (FAFSA), which is sent to each incoming student. Every effort is made to fund students to the documented need level, depending upon the availability of federal and state funds. Limited loan funds are available on a short-term or emergency basis from the financial aid officer of the college. A college work-study program is available at UI but is generally not appropriate for freshman and sophomore dental students. Financial aid is available to all classes; yearly reapplication is necessary. Scholarships may be provided to applicants with outstanding academic records.

DENTAL RESEARCH/TEACHING AWARDS: Scholarships will be awarded each year to qualified entering dental students. The scholarships provide financial support for as many as four years if the student maintains an appropriate level of performance. Dental research awards are based upon demonstrated academic excellence. The minimum review standards are a 3.5 GPA for all previous college coursework and an 18 on the individual science portions of the DAT. Applicants must submit all other regular application materials including an official transcript from each undergraduate and graduate institution attended, DAT scores, letters of recommendation, and an on-campus interview. In order to accommodate interviews, it is advisable to have the application process completed as early as possible.

Financial Aid Awards to First-Year Students in 2006-07

■ TOTAL NUMBER OF RECIPIENTS: 78   ■ 100% OF CLASS

	Average Award	Range of Awards
Residents	$47,395	Up to cost of attendance
Nonresidents	$64,149	Up to cost of attendance

Estimated Total Expenses for Academic Year 2006-07

	YEAR 1	YEAR 2	YEAR 3	YEAR 4	TOTAL
Tuition, resident	$21,927	$21,927	$21,927	$21,927	$87,708
Tuition, nonresident	$38,681	$38,681	$38,681	$38,681	$154,724
Other expenses	$4,981	$3,337	$1,387	$1,255	$10,960
Student health, computer fees, expendable supplies, breakage deposit, textbooks, activities fees, health insurance					
Equipment	$7,138	$4,000	$3,000	$1,000	$15,138
Instrument rental and sterilization, microscopes, dissection kits					
Estimated living expenses	$14,573	$14,573	$16,029	$16,029	$61,204
Room and board, personal, transportation					
TOTAL EXPENSES, RESIDENT	$48,619	$43,837	$42,343	$40,211	$175,010
TOTAL EXPENSES, NONRESIDENT	$65,373	$60,591	$59,097	$56,965	$242,026

SELECTION FACTORS

The Admissions Committee reviews the total GPA, science GPA, DAT scores, interview, and letters of recommendation. Also considered are the college attended, year in school, any trend in grades, degrees attained, awards, and such personality characteristics as social awareness. Applicants will be considered regardless of the applicant's gender, race, creed, national origin, or disability. Applications from women and members of minority groups are encouraged.

See chapter 3 of this guide for information regarding numbers of applicants and enrollees to each dental school, along with their race, gender, age, type of predental education, mean DAT and GPA, and state of origin.

ACADEMIC AND OTHER ASSISTANCE

UI has a long-established Educational Opportunity Program that provides financial and counseling services to students from economically and educationally disadvantaged or culturally different backgrounds who have special educational or economic needs. A summer enrichment program prior to matriculation into the College of Dentistry that helps students acclimate to the college and an orientation to the dental curriculum are also provided. Educational Opportunity Program eligibility must be formally requested and documented by the applicant.

UNIVERSITY OF KENTUCKY
COLLEGE OF DENTISTRY

Dr. Sharon P. Turner, Dean

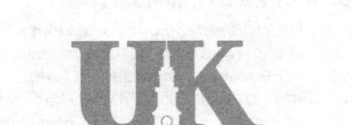

GENERAL INFORMATION

The College of Dentistry, a public institution with a statewide mission, is located on the main campus of the University of Kentucky. The university has a suburban setting in Lexington, a city with a population of 260,000 situated in the heart of the scenic bluegrass region of Kentucky. Along with the Doctor of Dental Medicine (D.M.D.) program, postdoctoral education programs are offered in oral and maxillofacial surgery, orthodontics, pediatric dentistry, periodontics, general practice dentistry, and orofacial pain. In addition to strong research and continuing education programs, the college conducts many public service activities throughout Kentucky, especially with pediatric patients.

The college is an integral part of the Chandler Medical Center at the University of Kentucky. The other colleges and facilities of this academic health science center are the Colleges of Medicine, Pharmacy, Nursing, Health Sciences and Public Health; the Sanders-Brown Center on Aging; the Markey Cancer Center; the University Hospital; and the Kentucky Clinic.

The College of Dentistry admitted its first class in 1962. Today it has an enrollment of 218 student dentists and 47 postdoctoral students. There are 77 full-time faculty in the college for an excellent student/faculty ratio of three to one.

ADMISSION REQUIREMENTS

NUMBER OF YEARS OF PREDENTAL EDUCATION: Usual minimum of four years; bachelor's degree desired.

LIMITATIONS ON COMMUNITY COLLEGE WORK: 60 semester hours.

REQUIRED COURSES: Students should pursue a major in a discipline of greatest interest to them. However, competitive applicants are expected to have a solid predental preparation, which includes the following:

Two courses in English composition*

With lab required
Two courses in general biology*
Two courses in general chemistry*
Two courses in organic chemistry*
One courses in general physics*

*Or equivalent.

SUGGESTED ADDITIONAL PREPARATION: Students should have a well-rounded curriculum. Each candidate must present evidence of potential for success in all phases of the dental curriculum, especially the basic sciences. Along with the required courses, the college recommends that students consider additional preparation from among possibilities such as cell biology, microbiology, immunology, physiology, biochemistry, genetics, and molecular biology.

DAT: Applicants should plan to take the DAT in the spring of their junior year with a retake, if needed, in the early fall of their senior year; prefer scores of 17 or higher.

CANADIAN DAT: Accepted.

GPA: Competitive applicants should have a GPA of 3.0 or higher.

RESIDENCY: Forty Kentucky residents and 10-14 nonresidents enroll annually. As in most states, the tuition guidelines for in-state residency are strict. Students who enroll as nonresidents often retain this status throughout their enrollment.

ADVANCED STANDING: The college does not have an established advanced standing program for transfer students or graduates of foreign dental schools.

Timetable for the Class Entering Fall 2008

	Earliest Date	Latest Date	School Fee
Application Submission	6/1/07	12/15/07	Nonres. $50*
Acceptance Notification	12/1/07	2/15/08	Res. $50*

Applicants should apply well before December 1, 2007 in order to receive full consideration. The 2006 entering class was filled by February 15, 2006.

*Due upon request

Required Response and Deposit:
45 days after notification if received between 12/1 and 12/31
30 days after notification if received between 1/1 and 1/31
15 days after notification if received after 2/1

$50 application processing fee; $250 due with confirmation of acceptance for Kentucky residents; $1,000 deposit for out-of-state students; applies toward tuition; nonrefundable.

FOR FURTHER INFORMATION
Office of Admissions and Student Affairs
Kim Bryan
Assistant Dean
859-323-6072

Melissa Lockard
Admissions Coordinator
859-323-6071; mlock@email.uky.edu

Don Brown
Financial Aid Coordinator
859-323-5280

Brenda Hays
Administrative Asistant
859-326-6071; blhays2@email.uky.edu

University of Kentucky
College of Dentistry
D-155 Chandler Medical Center
Lexington, KY 40536-0297

www.mc.uky.edu/dentistry

THE DENTAL PROGRAM

The College of Dentistry's program integrates basic science, preclinical lab, technique, clinical, and related courses throughout the curriculum. Basic science courses begin at enrollment. Clinical course time and patient contact start early in the first year and expand as the basic science and preclinical curriculum decreases. The curriculum is evaluated annually and courses are continuously improved to ensure that students have the best learning experience possible.

The dental curriculum has four primary areas of study: basic sciences, behavioral sciences, preclinical dentistry, and clinical dentistry. The basic sciences, such as anatomy, biochemistry, and pharmacology, and the didactic portion of the preclinical courses are taught mainly by lecture, seminar, some self-instruction, or by any combination of these teaching methods. The technical skills of the preclinical subjects, such as restorations, denture construction, and periodontal therapy, are taught in laboratory and clinical settings.

The student dentist learns clinical dentistry by treating patients in modern clinics under the supervision of the clinical faculty. Comprehensive dental care for the patient is emphasized and, because of the different needs of individual patients, the clinical cases of each student dentist will vary. The concept of comprehensive care permits learning experiences in all of the clinical disciplines of dentistry. The dental education program focuses on learning, competency-building, and the development of critical thinking and problem-solving skills in a dynamic, student-centered environment. The University of Kentucky has an excellent reputation in dental education stemming from its innovative and progressive programs and also its dedication to the excellent preparation of dental practitioners, specialists, and other future leaders in the profession. The college is committed to making the student dentist's experience a positive and very satisfying one.

■ Degree Offered
DENTAL DEGREE: D.M.D.

■ Other Programs
Research fellowships are offered to selected student dentists through the Center for Oral Health Research. A summer research program and federal work-study opportunities are also available.

EXTERNSHIP EXPERIENCES: Required of all student dentists in the summer prior to the fourth year. Six-week assignments may be arranged in private practice, U.S. Public Health Service, specialty program, military, and other settings.

COSTS AND FINANCIAL AID

The college works with all candidates to obtain the resources needed to help meet documented financial need. Loans and scholarships vary, depending on both private and public funding agencies and student eligibility. Approximately 90 percent of the student population receives some type of financial assistance. Student dentists may apply for research scholarships and work/study employment at the completion of the first year.

Financial Aid Awards to First-Year Students in 2006-07
■ TOTAL NUMBER OF RECIPIENTS: 50   ■ 87% OF CLASS

	Average Award	Range of Awards
Residents	$38,938	$8,500-$46,209
Nonresidents	$51,023	$8,500-$68,789

Estimated Total Expenses for Academic Year 2006-07

	YEAR 1	YEAR 2	YEAR 3	YEAR 4	TOTAL
Tuition/fees, resident	$19,534	$19,534	$19,018	$19,018	$77,104
Tuition/fees, nonresident	$42,114	$42,114	$41,388	$41,388	$167,004
Other expenses					
Fees					
PTS & Sterilization	$1,200	$1,200	$1,200	$1,200	$4,800
Immunizations	$75	0	0	0	$75
National Board Exams (Computer Test)	0	$295	0	$295	$590
CPR	$36	0	$36	0	$72
Course fees	$125	$115	$160	$115	$515
Equipment					
Instruments	$4,165	$4,852	$136	0	$9,153
Books & Supplies	$2,821	$3,636	$2,853	$826	$10,136
Estimated living expenses	$18,328	$18,328	$18,328	$18,328	$73,312
Housing, utilities, transportation, food/household, clothing/personal, insurance (car, health, renters)					
TOTAL EXPENSES, RESIDENT	$46,209	$47,960	$41,731	$39,782	$175,682
TOTAL EXPENSES, NONRESIDENT	$68,789	$70,540	$64,101	$62,152	$265,582

SELECTION FACTORS

Applicants should present strong GPAs, DAT scores, and predental course preparation to be viable candidates. The level of academic performance, difficulty of curriculum followed, academic loads carried, record of improved performance, and other factors are of more significance than a simple GPA. Although candidates should have demonstrated an ability to perform in the basic sciences, students who have not followed a traditional type of preparation will be considered and are encouraged to apply. Five factors are given greatest consideration: quality of preprofessional preparation, DAT scores, knowledge of and exposure to the dental profession, letters of evaluation, and interview results.

A well-rounded candidate (with a solid record in academics, extracurricular activities, leadership roles, and other life experiences) tends to be more competitive than one whose background is more limited. Involvement in college and community activities is frequently an advantage.

On-site interviews are required for admission consideration. Interviews are scheduled only for candidates presenting competitive credentials. Informal visits to the college may be arranged easily, and prospective applicants are always welcome. Three letters of evaluation (or a preprofessional committee letter) must be submitted along with other admission documents. These letters should be written by faculty, dentists, and others who are aware of the applicant's academic potential, interest in dentistry, initiative, integrity, concern for people, and social awareness. The college is committed to a policy of considering for admission all qualified students regardless of their race, creed, gender, national origin, or disability.

See chapter 3 of this guide for information regarding numbers of applicants and enrollees to each dental school, along with their race, gender, age, type of predental education, mean DAT and GPA, and state of origin.

ACADEMIC AND OTHER ASSISTANCE

The University of Kentucky seeks to attract highly qualified applicants to the dental education program including individuals from underrepresented populations and underserved areas. Women represent over 40 percent of the student population. The college offers a broad range of support programs, including annual orientations, a pre-enrollment workshop, counseling, free tutorial assistance, planning seminars for postdoctoral program applicants, college financial aid/debt management assistance, minority student services, and others designed to promote student success and satisfaction.

KENTUCKY

UNIVERSITY OF LOUISVILLE
SCHOOL OF DENTISTRY

Dr. Wood E. Currens, Acting Dean

GENERAL INFORMATION

Offering outstanding clinical education, pioneering simulation education and technology, and leading biomedical research, the University of Louisville School of Dentistry (ULSD) continues its quest to provide quality education and unique opportunities. The philosophy of the school is to consider students partners in learning and to provide them with the knowledge and skills to meet the challenges of today's dental profession. Many ULSD graduates choose to practice general dentistry, while others continue their education in a specialty, engage in dental research, or prepare for a career in education.

The School is a state-supported institution located within the University Health Sciences Center (HSC) in downtown Louisville (metropolitan area population of more than one million). Founded in 1887, the school is housed in a building that opened in 1970 as part of the HSC. The Schools of Medicine, Nursing, and Public Health are also located on the campus. Adjacent hospitals, the Ambulatory Care Building of U of L Hospital, and the Brown Cancer Center contribute to academic, clinical, and research experiences.

ADMISSION REQUIREMENTS

NUMBER OF YEARS OF PREDENTAL EDUCATION: Minimum of three (90 semester hours); preference given to applicants with bachelor's degrees.

LIMITATIONS ON COMMUNITY COLLEGE WORK: Maximum of 60 hours.

REQUIRED COURSES:

General chemistry: 2 semesters
Organic chemistry (1 semester) and Biochemistry (1 semester) or Organic chemistry (2 semesters)
Physics: 1 semester

Recommended courses are:
Human anatomy or comparative anatomy (strongly recommended)
Biochemistry (strongly recommended)
Cellular biology
Microbiology
Histology
Immunology
Other upper-level animal biology courses

It is expected that all applicants have completed college general education requirements including English composition and courses in the humanities and social sciences. Additional courses that students have found helpful are fine arts, personal and business finance, psychology, and communications.

DAT: It is recommended that the DAT be taken late in the junior year. Applications are encouraged as early as possible, even before taking the DAT, but with the understanding that acceptance decisions will **not** be made until official DAT scores are received.

GPA: Competitive applicants should have a 3.0 GPA or higher.

RESIDENCY: 44 Kentucky residents; 36 out-of-state.

ADVANCED STANDING: Transfer students are considered for placement on a case-by-case basis. Students must demonstrate that they were in good academic and ethical standing at their previous institution. Foreign dental graduates are **not** considered for advanced standing.

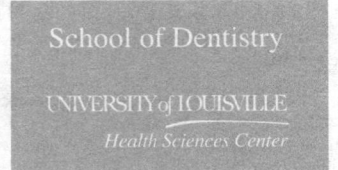

Timetable for the Class Entering Fall 2008

	Earliest Date	Latest Date	School Fee
Application Submission	5/15/07	1/1/08*	$50
Acceptance Notification	starts 12/1/07		

*Applicants are strongly encouraged to apply early.

Required Response and Deposit:
$200 tuition deposit for Kentucky residents; $500 for out-of-state students

FOR FURTHER INFORMATION

Admissions
Dianne Foster
Director of Student Services and Admissions
502-852-5081 or 800-334-8635, ext. 5081
Office of Student Affairs, Room 231
School of Dentistry

Financial Aid
Laurie A. O'Hare
Financial Aid Coordinator
502-852-5081 or 800-334-8635, ext. 5081
Office of Student Affairs, Room 234
School of Dentistry

Minority Affairs/Student Affairs
Sherry Babbage
Coordinator of Minority Recruitment
502-852-5081 or 800-334-8635, ext. 5081

Housing
502-852-6636
Office of Residence Life

University of Louisville
Louisville, KY 40292-0001

www.dental.louisville.edu/dental

UNIVERSITY OF LOUISVILLE SCHOOL OF DENTISTRY **KENTUCKY**

THE DENTAL PROGRAM

The ULSD offers a balance of didactic, clinical, student research, and postgraduate programs. Academic courses consist of instruction in the basic, behavioral, and clinical sciences. Instruction occurs in lectures, laboratories, and clinics. The Simulation Clinic is a state-of-the-art setting that closely replicates the comprehensive care patient treatment setting. It is the site of all the preclinical technique courses. The labs supporting the Simulation Clinic are used for all basic science courses except gross anatomy.

YEAR 1. Basic science and preclinical technique courses; clinical experiences in diagnosis, periodontics, and complete dentures; clinical observation/assisting.

YEAR 2. Continuation of basic science and more advanced preclinical technique courses; patient treatment begins during fall semester.

YEARS 3 AND 4. Completion of advanced basic science and clinical courses; extensive clinical patient treatment in comprehensive care setting; rotations in pediatric dentistry and oral surgery. Clinical experience emphasizes demonstration of competency, using critical thinking and problem solving skills. Practice management courses teach the business aspect of dental practice; senior electives permit students to explore many different aspects of the profession, e.g., zoo dentistry or forensic dentistry.

■ Degrees Offered

DENTAL DEGREE: D.M.D.

ALTERNATE DEGREES: D.M.D./M.S. in Oral Biology through participation in optional research program.

Students admitted after three years of predental study wanting to earn a bachelor's degree may do so if their undergraduate institution accepts the credits of the student's dental studies and it awards the degree.

■ Other Programs

SUMMER RESEARCH PROGRAM: Each summer 10 to 12 D.M.D. students are funded with awards of approximately $3,000. Students are paired with a faculty mentor and design and conduct projects in a variety of areas—basic, clinical, and social sciences. Academic credit toward an M.S. in Oral Biology may be received with no additional tuition charge.

EXTERNSHIPS: Fourth-year students participate in an extramural experience. Externships can be arranged in many different practice settings—rural, urban, public health clinic, various private practices, etc. Opportunities are available through the Public Health Services and the military, also.

SELECTION FACTORS

The Admissions Committee uses an "Admissions Index" to identify and select qualified applicants. Overall GPA, biology/chemistry/physics GPA, and DAT scores comprise 60 percent of the criteria. Letters of recommendation and required "on-site" interviews comprise 40 percent. Committee impressions supplement these scores. Applicants from rural areas and underrepresented minorities in dentistry are encouraged to apply. The ULSD does not discriminate on the basis of race, gender, creed, national origin, or disability.

See chapter 3 of this guide for information regarding numbers of applicants and enrollees to each dental school, along with their race, gender, age, type of predental education, mean DAT and GPA, and state of origin.

ACADEMIC AND OTHER ASSISTANCE

The Professional Education Preparation Program (PEPP) offers summer academic workshops for precollege minority and rural Kentucky students. The Summer Medical and Dental Education Program (SMDEP) is offered to students from underrepresented groups or disadvantaged backgrounds who have completed their freshman or sophomore years of college. The MCAT/DAT Review Workshop is offerd to prepare underrepresented students and rural students for taking the Medical College Admissions Test or the Dental Admissions Test. The goal of these programs is increasing students' chances for acceptance. Support programs for admitted students include counseling, tutoring services, assistance with study skills, and assistance with career and financial planning. Services are provided at no additional charge.

COSTS AND FINANCIAL AID

The ULSD offers both need- and merit-based funds. For more information, contact the Office of Student Affairs.

Financial Aid Awards to First-Year Students in 2006-07

■ TOTAL NUMBER OF RECIPIENTS: 80   ■ 100% OF CLASS

	Average Award	Range of Awards
Residents	$42,000	$500-$44,878
Nonresidents	$64,000	$1,000-$68,758

Estimated Total Expenses for Academic Year 2006-07

	YEAR 1	YEAR 2	YEAR 3	YEAR 4	TOTAL
Tuition, resident	$17,088	$17,088	$17,088	$17,088	$68,352
Tuition, nonresident	$40,968	$40,968	$40,968	$40,968	$163,872
Equipment and instrument rental	$5,000	$5,000	$5,000	$5,000	$20,000
Living expenses: room/board	$8,580	$8,580	$8,580	$7,146	$32,886
	(12 mos.)	(12 mos.)	(12 mos.)	(9 mos.)	
TOTAL EXPENSES, RESIDENT	**$30,668**	**$30,668**	**$30,668**	**$29,234**	**$121,238**
TOTAL EXPENSES, NONRESIDENT	**$54,548**	**$54,548**	**$54,548**	**$53,114**	**$216,758**

LOUISIANA STATE UNIVERSITY HEALTH SCIENCES CENTER
SCHOOL OF DENTISTRY

Dr. Eric J. Hovland, Dean

GENERAL INFORMATION

The Louisiana State University School of Dentistry (LSUSD) admitted its first class in September 1968. In 1972, the $16 million dental school buildings were dedicated. The dental school complex provides excellent basic sciences, preclinical, and clinical facilities. The School of Dentistry is a public, state-supported institution and is an integral part of the LSU Health Sciences Center in New Orleans. The school serves as a center for education, research, and service related to oral health for the state of Louisiana and as such offers a variety of educational opportunities, including advanced education, continuing education, and programs in dental hygiene and laboratory technology.

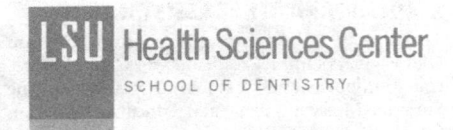

ADMISSION REQUIREMENTS

NUMBER OF YEARS OF PREDENTAL EDUCATION: Formal minimum of three (90 semester hours).

LIMITATIONS ON COMMUNITY COLLEGE WORK: None.

REQUIRED COURSES:

With lab required	(semester hrs)
Inorganic chemistry	8
Organic chemistry	8
Physics	8
Biology	12

Other courses	
English	9

SUGGESTED ADDITIONAL PREPARATION: Applicants are urged to acquire a strong background in the biological sciences. Courses such as histology, comparative anatomy, cell and molecular biology, and embryology are strongly recommended. In addition, courses that develop a social awareness and aid in interpersonal relationships are recommended. These include psychology, sociology, philosophy, and history. Courses that assist in the development of manual skills, such as basic art, sculpture, and ceramics, are also strongly recommended.

DAT: Mandatory; scores must be received by the application deadline.

GPA: No specific requirements; however, a GPA of 3.5 or higher is strongly recommended.

RESIDENCY: Admission preference is given to residents of Louisiana and Arkansas. A limited number of non-Louisiana, non-Arkansas applicants may be admitted.

ADVANCED STANDING: Selected students in good standing at an accredited U.S. dental school may be admitted with advanced standing. Louisiana residency is required for admittance.

Timetable for the Class Entering Fall 2008

	Earliest Date	Latest Date	School Fee
Application Submission	9/1/07	3/31/08	$50
Acceptance Notification	12/1/07	6/1/08	

Required Response and Deposit:
30 days if accepted on or after 12/1
15 days if accepted on or after 1/1
15 days if accepted on or after 2/1
Preferred time: 2 weeks

$200 due on acceptance; applied toward tuition and nonrefundable.

FOR FURTHER INFORMATION

Office of Admissions
Jim Weir
Assistant Dean
225-334-1864

Office of Financial Aid
Kim Bruno
Associate Director
504-568-4820

Louisiana State University
Health Sciences Center
New Orleans, LA 70119

lsusd.lsuhsc.edu

THE DENTAL PROGRAM

LSUSD follows a diagonal curriculum providing a blend of basic, clinical, and behavioral sciences and practice management. This approach allows early introduction to clinical experience and integration of basic science material into the clinical curriculum.

YEAR 1. Basic sciences, preclinical technical courses, and behavioral science with limited clinical experience.

YEAR 2. Continuation of basic sciences and preclinical technical courses with clinical patient treatment in operative dentistry, oral diagnosis, and removable prosthodontics.

YEAR 3. Clinical patient treatment in operative dentistry, fixed and removable prosthodontics, pediatric dentistry, oral and maxillofacial surgery, orthodontics, oral diagnosis, and endodontics.

YEAR 4. Total patient care in general dentistry; selective courses are available in all departments.

■ Degrees Offered

DENTAL DEGREE: D.D.S.

ALTERNATE DEGREES: A student entering without a degree may earn a bachelor's degree while in dental school, provided the student makes appropriate arrangements with his or her undergraduate college or university. A program leading to a combined D.D.S./Ph.D. is available.

SELECTION FACTORS

Admission is on a competitive basis. Selection is based primarily on: 1) scholastic records; 2) DAT scores; 3) recommendations from predental faculty; 4) a personal interview; and 5) manual dexterity. Applicants are expected to provide evidence of ability to successfully complete the school's biologically oriented dental curriculum. The LSU School of Dentistry does not in any way discriminate on the basis of race, gender, color, religion, age, disability, marital status, veteran's status, or national origin.

See chapter 3 of this guide for information regarding numbers of applicants and enrollees to each dental school, along with their race, gender, age, type of predental education, mean DAT and GPA, and state of origin.

COSTS AND FINANCIAL AID

LSU provides federally funded financial aid. For more information, contact the Office of Financial Aid.

Financial Aid Awards to First-Year Students in 2006-07
■ TOTAL NUMBER OF RECIPIENTS: 51   ■ 84% OF CLASS

	Average Award	Range of Awards
Residents	$33,933	$3,811-$38,222
Nonresidents	$52,222	$52,222

Estimated Total Expenses for Academic Year 2006-07

	YEAR 1	YEAR 2	YEAR 3	YEAR 4	TOTAL
Tuition, resident	$10,041	$10,041	$10,041	$10,041	$40,164
Tuition, nonresident	$22,415	$22,415	$22,415	$22,415	$89,660
Other expenses					
Fees, books, supplies, instrument rental, insurance	$7,685	$5,404	$3,882	$4,411	$21,382
Equipment	$4,293	$1,262	$550	0	$6,105
Estimated living expenses	$16,317	$19,943	$14,504	$12,691	$63,455
TOTAL EXPENSES, RESIDENT	**$38,336**	**$36,650**	**$28,977**	**$27,143**	**$131,106**
TOTAL EXPENSES, NONRESIDENT	**$50,710**	**$49,024**	**$41,351**	**$39,517**	**$180,602**

Due to the damage caused by Hurricane Katrina, the School of Dentistry has temporarily relocated to Baton Rouge and is continuing the education of its students there. The School will return to its home in New Orleans in 2007.

UNIVERSITY OF MARYLAND
BALTIMORE COLLEGE OF DENTAL SURGERY

Dr. Christian S. Stohler, Dean

GENERAL INFORMATION

The Baltimore College of Dental Surgery, Dental School, University of Maryland, Baltimore is a public institution that began as the first school in history to offer a course in dental education. Founded in 1840, the college was later consolidated with the Maryland Dental College and in 1923 merged with the Dental Department of the University of Maryland.

The first dental college in the world, the Baltimore College of Dental Surgery has maintained its position as a leader in dental education. The school offers a very strong curriculum, supported by well-trained, highly committed faculty. Faculty in the biological and clinical sciences are recognized as leaders in education, research, and service.

During early phases of instruction, students develop skills using Clinical Simulation before applying those skills in direct patient care. Each student is assigned to a group general practice within a state-of-the-art clinical facility. The school also offers programs in dental hygiene, advanced dental education, graduate studies in the biological sciences, research, and continuing education; instructional facilities such as an independent learning center; and an innovative facility for the treatment of patients with disabilities.

The dental school enjoys the advantages of sharing an urban campus with the Schools of Medicine, Law, Pharmacy, Nursing, Social Work, and the Veterans Administration and University Medical Centers. The school is located in Baltimore's famous revitalized downtown center.

ADMISSION REQUIREMENTS

NUMBER OF YEARS OF PREDENTAL EDUCATION: Baccalaureate degree strongly preferred; formal minimum of 90 credits.

LIMITATIONS ON COMMUNITY COLLEGE WORK: Maximum of 60 semester hours validated by an accredited college of arts and sciences.

REQUIRED COURSES: Applicants are strongly urged to complete the required courses (see below) at an accredited four-year university.

With lab required	(semester hrs)
Inorganic chemistry	8
General biology	8
Organic chemistry	8
General physics	8

Other courses	
English composition	6
Biochemistry	3

SUGGESTED ADDITIONAL PREPARATION: Advanced science courses such as physiology, genetics, cell biology, and molecular biology.

INTERVIEW: Scheduled at the discretion of the Committee on Dental Recruitment and Admissions.

DAT: Mandatory; should be taken no later than December of year prior to desired matriculation.

GPA: GPA competitive within applicant pool.

RESIDENCY: No specific requirements; preference to Maryland residents.

ADVANCED STANDING: There is no formal advanced standing program. In rare instances, consideration is given to students requesting to transfer from U.S./Canadian dental schools. Also in rare instances, graduates of non-U.S./non-Canadian dental schools may be considered for admission at an advanced level, generally at the second-year level.

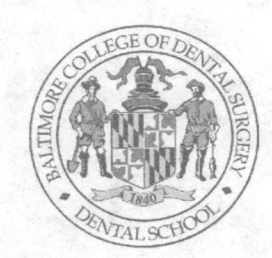

Timetable for the Class Entering Fall 2008

	Earliest Date	Latest Date	School Fee
Application Submission	6/1/07	1/1/08	$75
Acceptance Notification	12/1/07	8/08	

Required Response and Deposit:
45 days after notification if received between 12/1 and 12/31
30 days after notification if received between 1/1 and 1/31
15 days after notification if received after 2/1

$500 to hold place; additional $500 required by 4/1.

FOR FURTHER INFORMATION
Office of Admissions
410-706-7472
Baltimore College of Dental Surgery, Dental School
University of Maryland, Baltimore
650 W. Baltimore Street, 6-South
Room 6410
Baltimore, MD 21201

Office of Financial Aid
410-706-7347
110 S. Paca Street
Second floor
Baltimore, MD 21201

www.dental.umaryland.edu

THE DENTAL PROGRAM

The Baltimore College of Dental Surgery continually strives to build on its tradition as the world's first dental school in achieving excellence in education, science, and practice. As a result, graduates are capable of functioning competently at the fullest breadth and depth of their professional areas of expertise.

YEAR 1. Basic and behavioral sciences with introduction to clinical situations and clinical skills building.

YEAR 2. Basic and clinical sciences, plus definitive clinical patient treatment.

YEARS 3 AND 4. Delivery of comprehensive patient care within group general practices; clerkships, and externships.

■ Degrees Offered

DENTAL DEGREE: D.D.S.

ALTERNATE DEGREES: B.S./D.D.S. with schools within the University of Maryland system. Combined D.D.S./Ph.D. program.

■ Other Offerings

EXTERNSHIPS: Clinical experiences at a wide range of remote sites; generally available to senior students only.

CLERKSHIPS: Opportunities to devote a significant amount of clinical time to a specific discipline.

ELECTIVES: Students may choose from a variety of courses in topics specific to their interests.

RESEARCH: Opportunities available for predoctoral students and postgraduate residents in basic, behavioral, and clinical sciences.

COSTS AND FINANCIAL AID

A wide range of need-based and merit-based funds are available through the Baltimore College of Dental Surgery and federal and state agencies.

Financial Aid Awards to First-Year Students in 2006

■ TOTAL NUMBER OF RECIPIENTS: 118   ■ TOTAL $5,406,366

	Average Award
Average Award	$45,816
Residents (64)	$41,429
Nonresidents (54)	$51,016

Estimated Total Expenses for Academic Year 2006-07

	YEAR 1	YEAR 2	YEAR 3	YEAR 4	TOTAL
Tuition, resident	$17,913	$17,913	$17,913	$17,913	$71,652
Tuition, nonresident	$37,536	$37,536	$37,536	$37,536	$150,144
University/dental school fees	$5,378	$4,661	$2,726	$2,631	$15,396
Estimated living expenses	$17,200	$17,200	$20,640	$17,200	$72,240
TOTAL EXPENSES, RESIDENT	$40,491	$39,774	$41,279	$37,774	$159,288
TOTAL EXPENSES, NONRESIDENT	$60,114	$59,397	$60,902	$57,367	$237,780

SELECTION FACTORS

The University of Maryland strives to enroll the highest caliber students who will become exemplary health care professionals. In considering applicants, the Admissions Committee carefully considers scholastic records, previously attended postsecondary schools, letters of recommendation (from a preprofessional committee or from professors in laboratory sciences), DAT scores, research experience, and motivation toward a career in dentistry. Based on preliminary review of AADSAS applications, potentially qualified candidates are invited for interviews. The Admissions Committee reserves the right to modify the prerequisites in exceptional cases where an applicant's background supplants the need for such courses or in cases when additional courses are necessary to improve an applicant's preparation for dental school. The University of Maryland encourages applications from individuals with a strong interest in academics and research, as well as individuals from nonscience backgrounds who have demonstrated excellence in challenging baccalaureate programs in their respective disciplines. The dental school encourages applications from members of underrepresented minorities in dentistry.

See chapter 3 of this guide for information regarding numbers of applicants and enrollees to each dental school along with their race, gender, age, type of predental education, mean DAT and GPA, and state of origin.

ACADEMIC AND OTHER ASSISTANCE

The University of Maryland sponsors recruitment and retention programs for all students, including students who are members of underrepresented populations in dentistry. These programs include a summertime Dentistry Today program and individual assistance upon request. Upon matriculation, students also benefit from a wide range of academic and personal support services.

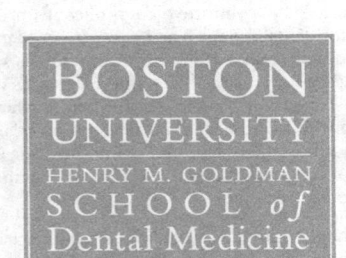

BOSTON UNIVERSITY
GOLDMAN SCHOOL OF DENTAL MEDICINE

Dr. Spencer N. Frankl, Dean

GENERAL INFORMATION

The Boston University School of Dental Medicine (BUSDM) is a forward-thinking educational institution that produces a highly competent dentist in a challenging and exciting environment. A comfortable class size combined with a dedicated, talented faculty provides an exceptionally stimulating educational experience. The curriculum successfully integrates the basic sciences with the clinical care of patients both within the school and in selected private practice sites. The Extramural Program comprised of a both an APEX Program (Applied Professional EXperience) in the first and second academic years and an Externship during the fourth year provides the students with practical clinical experience in preparation for their professional careers upon graduation. In addition, dental students can work with graduate dentists in the eight specialties of dentistry during their clinical years and benefit from the graduate dentists' advanced knowledge and skills. About 20 percent of graduating seniors choose to remain at Boston University to complete a program of specialty study.

The vibrant city of Boston offers students an abundance of social, cultural, and athletic activities—from the Boston Symphony Orchestra to the Boston Marathon. The youthful ambiance of the city is reflected in the school's motto: "Boston University, where the future of dentistry is being made every day."

ADMISSION REQUIREMENTS

NUMBER OF YEARS OF PREDENTAL EDUCATION: The successful completion of a minimum of three years in an accredited four-year college or university is a requirement for admission to Boston University School of Dental Medicine. The Admissions Committee gives preference to candidates who have completed at least a baccalaureate degree.

LIMITATIONS ON COMMUNITY COLLEGE WORK: 30 credit hours. Prerequisite coursework should be completed at an accredited, four-year North American institution.

REQUIRED COURSES:

With lab required	(semester/quarter hrs)
Inorganic chemistry	8/12
Organic chemistry	8/12
Physics	8/12
Biology	12/18

Other courses	
English	8/12
Mathematics with calculus	6/9

SUGGESTED ADDITIONAL PREPARATION: The Committee on Admissions strongly recommends that applicants take courses in biochemistry, cell biology, anatomy, genetics, and physiology. Additionally, the committee recommends that applicants include in their predental curriculum courses in the humanities and social sciences, such as psychology, sociology, anthropology, and economics.

DAT: Mandatory; preferably no later than September. DAT score should be from a test taken within the past two years.

GPA: 3.2 or above recommended in both science and overall GPAs.

INTERVIEW: Mandatory; invitations are issued to selected applicants by the Admissions Committee.

RESIDENCY: No specific requirements.

ADVANCED STANDING: Graduates of foreign dental schools are eligible for a two-year program. Information on the application process for the Advanced Standing program is on the Boston University School of Dental Medicine website at dentalschool.bu.edu.

MASSACHUSETTS

Timetable for the Class Entering Fall 2008

	Earliest Date	Latest Date	School Fee
Application Submission	6/1/07	3/1/08	$65/$95*
Acceptance Notification	12/1/07	after 12/1, rolling admissions	

*School application fee of $65 for U.S. citizens and permanent residents; $95 for non-U.S. citizens and non-permanent residents. Authorized requests for fee waivers are honored.

Required Response and Deposit:
45 days if admitted between 12/1 and 12/31
30 days if admitted between 1/1 and 1/31
15 days if admitted on or after 2/1

$3,000 nonrefundable deposit to accompany applicant's acceptance of admission.

FOR FURTHER INFORMATION

Office of Admissions
Sydell Shaw
Associate Dean of Admissions and Student Services
617-638-4787; sshawdds@bu.edu

Office of Student Financial Services
Kathy Stavropoulos
Executive Director of Student Financial Services
617-638-5130; osfm-sdm@bumc.bu.edu

Minority Affairs
Dr. Gregory Stoute
Director of Minority Affairs, Goldman School of Dental Medicine
617-638-4787; gastoute@bu.edu

Boston University Goldman School of Dental Medicine
Office of Admissions
100 East Newton Street, Room G-305
Boston, MA 02118
617-638-4787

dentalschool.bu.edu

THE DENTAL PROGRAM

The mission of the School of Dental Medicine is to educate dentists who can apply the biomedical sciences to the practice of contemporary patient-oriented oral health care. To this end, the curriculum combines a rigorous didactic program with a series of practical learning experiences in private dental offices, community dental health centers, and clinical experience within the school's modern patient treatment centers. In addition, students are given the opportunity to participate in extensive research activities.

Development of clinical skills and competence has been strengthened with the opening of our Simulation Learning Center in the Evans Research Center. The simulation center supports the preclinical courses in which students practice and learn clinical skills in preparation for the provision of oral health care for patients. State-of-the-art electronics and audiovisual equipment support individual and group teaching and evaluation. The Simulation Learning Center provides students with an optimum virtual patient care experience in a completely nonclinical setting.

Another technological advance supports learning as well as the development of critical thinking and self-directed, lifelong learning skills. Students may select an electronic library containing over 100 complete dental and biomedical textbooks along with internally generated materials on a single DVD computer disk, replacing previously required textbooks. As one of the first schools of dental medicine to use an entirely digital presentation of curriculum materials, BUSDM provides students with a unique personalized learning experience. With this electronic library and the laptop computer, students have fingertip access to a wealth of material, including the most recent innovations in dental medicine.

The entire four-year curriculum is based on carefully integrated learning experiences designed to provide the student with the ability to ultimately provide the highest level of oral health care. The curriculum makes use of the School of Medicine, affiliated hospitals and health centers, private dental offices, and the school's own modern facilities in order to integrate the education opportunities.

YEAR 1. The program begins with biomedical science courses oriented toward dentistry as well as an accelerated program in oral radiology and dental assisting techniques designed to give the student the essential skills to function in the dental office environment. The year continues with simulated dental experiences and culminates with a supervised rotation in a private dental office, working as a dental intern (APEX).

YEAR 2. The second year of the curriculum continues with the biomedical and behavioral sciences; APEX rotations; simulated dental experiences and the clinical sciences. During this year, an emphasis is placed on integrating the biomedical and behavioral sciences with the clinical sciences. Alternating APEX rotations with the didactic and simulated clinic courses permits the student to gain additional experiences with which to integrate formal instruction with actual relevant dental office practice.

YEARS 3 AND 4. The third and fourth years are designed to allow for maximum opportunity for patient care. The school's patient treatment centers lay the foundation for dental practice by emphasizing total patient care. A faculty group practice leader oversees and coordinates the clinical activities of assigned students. These faculty stimulate learning and encourage students to deal with the problems and questions that arise in any dental practice. The students, with assistance from additional clinical faculty, provide oral health care to groups of patients as in a private practice. Faculty work closely with students and provide practice management guidance as well as supervision. Faculty supervisors help students identify areas where competencies need improvement and, when appropriate, design activities to address those competencies. Through seminars and a computer laboratory, students learn to organize and administer a dental practice, including the application of data management systems. In addition students have an externship experience at either local or distant sites. The externship program allows students to choose one of more than 20 different sites from Boston to Hawaii for a rewarding clinical experience.

■ Degrees Offered

DENTAL DEGREE: D.M.D.

ALTERNATE DEGREES: B.A./D.M.D. or B.S./D.M.D. High school graduates may apply for a combined seven-year baccalaureate degree with the College of Arts and Sciences at Boston University-D.M.D. degree program initiated at the university in 1978. For additional information contact Glen B. Zamansky, Ph.D., Assistant Dean for Premedical Advising, Room B-2, Boston University, 725 Commonwealth Avenue, Boston, MA 02215; gzamansk@acs.bu.edu.

POSTDOCTORAL PROGRAMS: Boston University School of Dental Medicine offers postdoctoral programs leading to: C.A.G.S. (Certificate of Advanced Graduate Study), M.S.D. (Master of Science in Dentistry), D.Sc.D. (Doctor of Science in Dentistry), and M.S. (Master of Science) in Dental Public Health, as well as D.Sc. (Doctor of Science) and Ph.D. (Doctor of Philosophy) in Oral Biology. Programs are offered in the following areas of specialization: Dental Public Health, General Dentistry, Endodontics, Implantology, Operative Dentistry, Oral and Maxillofacial Pathology, Oral and Maxillofacial Surgery, Oral Biology, Orthodontics and Dentofacial Orthopedics, Pediatric Dentistry, Periodontology, and Prosthodontics.

COSTS AND FINANCIAL AID

Boston University acknowledges a commitment to assist financially needy students. The Office of Student Financial Services administers institutional and federal aid programs, certifies private loan applications, and counsels students regarding funding opportunities and debt management. Requests for financial information should be forwarded only after the applicant has been accepted for admission.

SELECTION FACTORS

There are no geographic restrictions on admission. Applications from minorities and women are encouraged. All candidates must submit the AADSAS application and supplemental application materials as indicated on the website and in the AADSAS application. Scores from the DAT taken before September 1 are preferred. The committee takes into account the applicant's scores on the Dental Admissions Test, as well as factors such as previous scholastic performance, the quality and difficulty of courses taken, demonstrated leadership ability, and motivation for the study of dentistry. Applicants' personal statements submitted as part of the AADSAS application and letters of recommendation are important elements in the evaluation. The Admissions Committee may request additional information from an applicant to enable a complete assessment of the applicant's suitability. No applicant is admitted without a personal interview. Qualified applicants are invited by the Admissions Committee for a personal interview and to visit the school's facilities. Some regional interview locations may be available.

See chapter 3 of this guide for information regarding numbers of applicants and enrollees to each dental school, along with their race, gender, age, type of predental education, mean DAT and GPA, and state of origin.

Financial Aid Awards to First-Year Students in 2006-07
■ TOTAL NUMBER OF RECIPIENTS: 92   ■ 80% OF CLASS

Typical Award	Range of Awards
$43,000	$4,000-$50,167

Estimated Total Expenses for Academic Year 2006-07

	YEAR 1	YEAR 2	YEAR 3	YEAR 4	TOTAL
Tuition	$46,265	$48,115	$50,041	$52,043	$196,465
School fees	$904	$1,109	$1,129	$1,094	$4,236
Instruments	$5,274	$4,823	0	0	$10,102
Board exams	0	$130	0	$165	$295
Health insurance	$2,289	$2,426	$2,572	$2,726	$10,013
Electronic library	$1,446	$1,032	$988	0	$3,466
Laptop/accessories	$2,307	0	0	0	$2,307
Living expenses	$19,025	$19,539	$19,929	$18,439	$77,063
TOTAL	$77,510	$77,180	$74,659	$74,467	$286,473

HARVARD SCHOOL OF DENTAL MEDICINE

Dr. R. Bruce Donoff, Dean

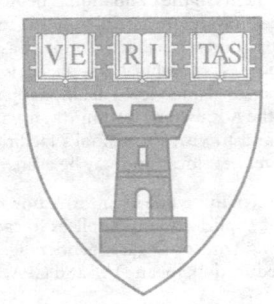

GENERAL INFORMATION

The Harvard School of Dental Medicine (HSDM) was established in 1867 as the first university-based dental school in the United States. This relationship with a great university and its associated world-renowned medical center and teaching hospitals shapes the education of dental students. The Harvard School of Dental Medicine has achieved success in its mission of producing leaders in the field of dental medicine in clinical care, teaching, and research by being educationally innovative and by providing a professional school education that presents multiple opportunities for enrichment. The education of a Harvard dental student prepares women and men for a career of lifelong learning whether that be in clinical practice, teaching, research, oral health care delivery, or a combination of these. The school is proud of its tradition of producing graduates who have excelled in each of these career paths.

In an environment of excellence, shared with medical school classmates during the early years of education, dental students gain an appreciation of the human mind, body, and spirit that gets at the heart of patient care, their main reason for being students of dentistry. The school's philosophy is that dentistry is a specialty of medicine and therefore a certain body of knowledge must be part of every doctor's information repository. Students learn in the tutorial style of education that is emphasized in the New Pathway curriculum at Harvard Medical School. This type of learning is fostered as, at the end of their second year, students enter the clinical phases of their education in the dental school.

The clinical phases of dental education are provided with the same degree of individualized instruction, attention to understanding, and respect for the difficulty of learning. The third year of dental education in the school and its clinics provides the basics of all phases of dentistry. A problem-based program organized through unique treatment teams maximizes this learning experience. This is followed by rotations in the affiliated institutions, allowing students to gain experience and confidence in providing dental care in varying settings to patients with differing needs and levels of general health.

The educational programs at HSDM call upon the wealth of teaching and learning experiences that exist within the dental school, the medical school, the affiliated teaching hospitals, and the entire university. The school believes that the profession needs broadly educated dentists who are outstanding clinicians, who are prepared to develop and teach the new biomedical and biotechnical knowledge needed in dentistry, who can interact effectively with colleagues in the health care professions in hospitals and other health care delivery systems, and who can represent dentistry in health care policy debates and decisions.

The school's new Research and Education Building, opened in fall 2004, is a major catalyst in bringing together the science and practice of dental medicine. The six-story, 68,000 square foot, $30 million, state-of-the-art facility contains educational space, research facilities, faculty and departmental offices, laboratories, seminar/meeting rooms, and common areas. It creates an interdisciplinary environment in which bioengineers, orthodontists, geneticists, restorative dentists, and allied professionals share physical space fostering the concept of putting science into practice, looking for biologic solutions to mechanical problems.

ADMISSION REQUIREMENTS

NUMBER OF YEARS OF PREDENTAL EDUCATION: Formal minimum of three; usual minimum of four.

LIMITATIONS ON COMMUNITY COLLEGE WORK: Maximum of 60 semester hours, all earned before a student enters the third year of study toward a baccalaureate degree.

REQUIRED COURSES:

With lab required	(semester hrs)
Biology	8 or 1 year
Inorganic chemistry	8 or 1 year
Organic chemistry	8 or 1 year
Physics	8 or 1 year

Other courses
Calculus	8 or 1 year
English (preferably composition)	8 or 1 year

SUGGESTED ADDITIONAL PREPARATION: Advanced science courses such as biochemistry, physiology, molecular biology, cell biology, or genetics.

DAT: Mandatory; 19 or above recommended.

GPA: 3.0 or above recommended.

INTERVIEW: Mandatory; scheduled at the discretion of the Admissions Committee.

RESIDENCY: No specific requirements.

ADVANCED STANDING: There is currently no formal advanced standing program.

MASSACHUSETTS

Timetable for the Class Entering Fall 2008

	Earliest Date	Latest Date	School Fee
Regular Admission	6/1/07	12/15/07	$75
Acceptance Notification	12/1/08	9/1/08	

Required Response and Deposit:
Signed letter accepting offer of admission is required to hold acceptance.

45 days after notification if received between 12/1 and 12/31
30 days after notification if received between 1/1 and 1/31
15 days after notification if received after 2/1

No deposit required to hold place.

FOR FURTHER INFORMATION
Anne L. Berg
Director of Admissions & Student Affairs
617-432-1443

Financial Aid
Ann Doherty
Financial Aid Officer
617-432-1527

Minority Affairs
Nadeem Karimbux
Director of Predoctoral Education
617-432-4247

Office of Dental Education
T. Howard Howell
Dean for Dental Education
617-432-1447

Harvard School of Dental Medicine
188 Longwood Avenue
Boston, MA 02115

www.hsdm.harvard.edu

THE DENTAL PROGRAM

The philosophy of education at HSDM is that dentistry is a specialty of medicine. In keeping with this belief, medical and dental students study together in the New Pathway curriculum at Harvard Medical School during the first two years. Dental clinical instruction occurs in treatment teams that utilize a comprehensive approach to patient care. Both didactic and clinical courses are taught by problem-based method of study and discussion in small tutorial groups. In this approach, cases based on actual clinical records or investigative problems are utilized to set the learning objectives. Students learn critical thinking and problem-solving techniques that will equip them for lifelong learning in the field of dental medicine.

YEAR 1. Basic sciences, patient/doctor relationships, preclinical dental sciences, and introduction to research.

YEAR 2. Pathophysiology of human organ systems, psychiatry, introduction to clinical medicine, preclinical dental coursework, and laboratory.

YEAR 3. Clinical dental courses and delivery of comprehensive clinical dental care at HSDM under conditions that approximate small group practices.

YEAR 4. Advanced clinical dentistry at HSDM and at Harvard-affiliated teaching hospitals and community health centers; oral surgery externship; and elective rotations at HSDM affiliates and at other dental schools and hospitals in the United States as well as worldwide.

In addition, students take courses in research and complete a research project, thesis, and formal presentation over the course of the four-year training period.

■ Degrees Offered

DENTAL DEGREE: D.M.D.

ALTERNATE DEGREES: The school offers an M.M.Sc. or D.M.Sc. through its Advanced Graduate division.

■ Other Programs

- Optional Five-Year D.M.D. for students interested in research, international health, etc.
- Health Sciences and Technology (HST) Track
- Oral and Maxillofacial Surgery Research Fellowships
- Other fellowships available through Harvard Medical School
- Employment opportunities available, including dental assisting

COSTS AND FINANCIAL AID

Financial aid is awarded on the basis of need. The school utilizes the Free Application for Federal Student Assistance (FAFSA) to assess eligibility for federal Title IV aid. Students wishing to apply for institutional loans and scholarships must also complete a College Scholarship Service (CSS) Profile application, which must be submitted for each year in which a student requests financial aid, and includes parental information regardless of the student's dependency status. Health Professions Student Loans and school-administered loans and scholarship funds are also available.

Financial Aid Awards to First-Year Students in 2006-07
■ TOTAL NUMBER OF RECIPIENTS: 26   ■ 74% OF CLASS

	Average Award	Range of Awards
Residents	N/A	
Nonresidents	$40,723	$8,500-$57,001

Estimated Total Expenses for Academic Year 2006-07

	YEAR 1	YEAR 2	YEAR 3	YEAR 4	TOTAL
Tuition	$37,200	$37,200	$37,200	$37,200	$148,800
Other expenses charged by school	$3,061	$13,686	$11,611	$11,011	$39,369
Estimated living expenses	$14,890	$14,890	$17,688	$15,128	$62,596
TOTAL EXPENSES*	$55,151	$65,776	$66,499	$63,339	$250,765

*Same resident/nonresident

SELECTION FACTORS

The selection of students is based on a total appraisal of the suitability of the candidates for the program at Harvard. Admission factors include academic achievement in high school and college, performance on the DAT, letters of recommendation (preferably from the Prehealth Professions Advisory Committee or science professors), research experience, leadership potential, and motivation toward a career in dentistry. The school encourages minority and female applicants; selection is made without reference to race, gender, religion, or residence. Recent classes have come from a wide range of colleges and regions of the country.

See chapter 3 of this guide for information regarding numbers of applicants and enrollees to each dental school, along with their race, gender, age, type of predental education, mean DAT and GPA, and state of origin.

ACADEMIC AND OTHER ASSISTANCE

Hispanic, African-American, and Native American students who have been accepted to HSDM are invited to participate in a three-day Multicultural Weekend along with Medical School minority applicants in the spring. Students attend a variety of academic and social events and receive financial aid counseling as part of the recruiting program sponsored by HSDM and Harvard Medical School.

MASSACHUSETTS

TUFTS UNIVERSITY
SCHOOL OF DENTAL MEDICINE

Dr. Lonnie H. Norris, Dean

GENERAL INFORMATION

Tufts University School of Dental Medicine, a private institution, originated in 1868 as the Boston Dental College. It was incorporated in 1899 as a component of Tufts College. The School of Dental Medicine is located in downtown Boston adjacent to the Tufts-New England Medical Center. In addition to the School of Dental Medicine, the Boston Health Sciences Campus is home to the School of Medicine, the Sackler School of Graduate Biomedical Sciences, the Gerald J. and Dorothy R. Friedman School of Nutrition Science and Policy, the Jaharis Family Center for Graduate Biomedical and Nutrition Research, the Jean Mayer Human Nutrition Research Center on Aging, and five hospitals. The School of Dental Medicine, in addition to the D.M.D. program, offers accredited advanced education programs in six dental specialties that lead to a certificate or Master of Science degree. Tufts currently has a seven-year combined degree contractual arrangement with Tufts University and eight-year early assurance programs with Adelphi University (NY), Marist College (NY) and Tougaloo College (MS).

ADMISSION REQUIREMENTS

NUMBER OF YEARS OF PREDENTAL EDUCATION: The Admissions Committee gives preference to applicants who have completed *at* least a baccalaureate degree program. Ninety-nine percent of the class of 2010 has received at least a bachelor's degree, and the remaining students are enrolled in joint-degree programs that award bachelor's degrees after successful completion of the first year of dental school. All coursework must be completed at colleges/universities with accreditation in the United States or Canada.

LIMITATIONS ON COMMUNITY COLLEGE WORK: The Admissions Committee requires all prerequisite coursework to be completed at a four-year accredited college or university.

REQUIRED COURSES: *(semester hrs/semesters)*

Biology	8/2
Inorganic chemistry	8/2
Organic chemistry	4/1
Humanities	4/1
Physics	8/2
Biochemistry	3/1

All requirements must be completed at a four-year college or university (the institution must be accredited). Lab required for all courses except biochemistry.

REQUIRED ADDITIONAL PREPARATION: Applicants must complete a minimum of 30 hours observing or assisting in a dental clinic before matriculation. Proof of experience must be in the form of a formal letter from the supervising dentist.

SUGGESTED ADDITIONAL PREPARATION: The remainder of the candidate's predental program should be designed to achieve a broad educational background. The following subjects are recommended for consideration: microbiology, anatomy, physiology, histology, pathology, pharmacology, general psychology, mathematics, economics, statistics, and humanities courses specifically designed to develop writing technique, vocabulary, and public speaking ability. In addition, a studio art course that stresses manual dexterity, such as sculpture or crafts, is recommended.

DAT: Minimum scores of 16 Academic/15 Perceptual Ability/16 Total Science required for consideration. Preference is given to candidates with scores of 19 or above on all sections. Exam results must be obtained no earlier than June 1, 2005. Scores obtained before June 1, 2005, are no longer valid.

GPA: Preference given to those with cumulative GPA and science GPA of 3.3 or above.

RESIDENCY: No specific requirements.

ADVANCED STANDING: Foreign dental graduates may be admitted with advanced standing. The entry level for foreign dental graduates is at the second-year level. Length of the international program is two years and three months.

Timetable for the Class Entering Fall 2008

	Earliest Date	Latest Date	School Fee
Application Submission	7/1/07	3/1/08	$60
Acceptance Notification	12/1/07	8/15/08	

Required Response and Deposit:
30 days after notification if received between 12/1 and 1/31
15 days after notification if received after 2/1

$1,500 initial deposit to hold place. 2nd deposit of $500 required on 4/15/08.

FOR FURTHER INFORMATION

Admissions
Melissa Bradbury
Assistant Director of Admissions
617-636-6639

Financial Aid
Sandra Pearson
Director of Financial Aid
617-636-6640

Tufts University School of Dental Medicine
One Kneeland Street, DHS-7
Boston, MA 02111

www.tufts.edu/dental

THE DENTAL PROGRAM

The curriculum of the School of Dental Medicine has been designed and modified over the years to reflect the changing needs of the dental profession and the public. The school's primary goal is to develop dental practitioners who are able to utilize their knowledge of the basic principles of human biology and human behavior in conjunction with their technical skills in diagnosing, treating, and preventing oral disease. The D.M.D. program, which extends over a four-year period, consists of a series of didactic, laboratory, and clinical experiences, resulting in the logical development of concepts and skills. Upon completion of the curriculum, the graduate will be both intellectually and technically prepared to practice the profession of dentistry as it exists today, to adapt to future changes, and to initiate and contribute to those changes, all of which will enhance the delivery of dental care.

YEAR 1. The first year consists of basic science and preclinical technique courses. Normal human anatomy and physiology are the main theme of the basic science courses, which include biochemistry, histology, gross anatomy, physiology, embryology, nutrition, and microbiology. The preclinical technique courses focus on dental anatomy, occlusion, and operative dentistry. No formal programs are scheduled during the summer following the first year.

YEAR 2. During the second year, students formally begin their clinical experience. At the outset they treat patients under close supervision of faculty members. Second-year courses are concerned with the pathology of the bodily systems, with special emphasis on the oral cavity. Dental didactic and technique courses, including oral diagnosis, oral radiology, complete dentures, endodontics, oral surgery, periodontology, pediatric dentistry, and orthodontics, begin in the second year and continue into the third year.

YEARS 3 AND 4. The third and fourth years of the program are primarily clinical years devoted to the comprehensive care of patients. Programs related to the treatment of geriatric patients, disabled patients, patients with craniomandibular pain and dysfunction, oral tumors and implantology patients, and related lectures and seminars are included at this time. All of these activities are aimed at the development of increased knowledge and skills in the area of patient care. In the Hospital Clerkship Program, each student practices techniques that will be used in the dental office by participating in a series of workshops and hospital rotations. These experiences demonstrate the integral role of dentistry in total patient care and prepare students to take their rightful position as members of the health care team.

During the third and fourth years, efforts to reinforce the relevance of material presented during the first and second years are carried out in seminars as well as on the clinic floors.

An integral part of the fourth year is the Externship Program. In this program each student is assigned to a clinical facility outside of the dental school for a five-week period. These facilities include sites located throughout the United States. Students are thus able to develop their clinical skills, as well as confidence in their abilities, by treating patients in an environment that more closely resembles dental practice, under the guidance of a preceptor.

■ Degrees Offered
DENTAL DEGREE: D.M.D.

ALTERNATE DEGREES: B.S./D.M.D. with Tufts University College of Arts and Sciences.

■ Other Programs
EARLY ASSURANCE: Programs with Adelphi University, Marist College, and Tougaloo College.

RESEARCH FELLOWSHIPS: Available for academically outstanding students.

COSTS AND FINANCIAL AID

Tufts provides both need- and merit-based funds. Scholarship awards from the school are available in all four years, as is need-based financial aid from school and federal programs.

SELECTION FACTORS

Admission is based on the following considerations: 1) information submitted on the AADSAS application form; 2) recommendations from the predental committee (if the college has no committee, two confidential recommendations, one from a biology professor and one from a biochemistry, chemistry, physics, or mathematics professor) and from the dentist who was observed/assisted. Please note: letters from employers and other faculty members are welcome, but will not replace the required letters; 3) DAT scores; and 4) personal interview at Tufts University (regional interviews are not conducted). The Office of Admissions reserves the right to request additional information at any time to complete an assessment of an applicant's abilities and capabilities. Requested additional information may include, but is not limited to, official TOEFL or TSE scores, additional DAT scores, additional semester grades, and a second interview. Candidates should file and complete their applications as soon as possible after June 1 of any year and should participate in the DAT one year prior to matriculation (scores obtained before June 1, 2005, are no longer valid). Tufts seeks the student who has demonstrated motivation, maturity, compassion, integrity, social awareness, and strong communication skills.

See chapter 3 of this guide for information regarding numbers of applicants and enrollees to each dental school, along with their race, gender, age, type of predental education, mean DAT and GPA, and state of origin.

ACADEMIC AND OTHER ASSISTANCE

Tufts University encourages applications by women and minorities. Currently, the entering class consists of 76 women and 66 minorities. Tutorial programs in the basic sciences and clinical sciences are available to all students.

Financial Aid Awards to First-Year Students in 2006-07
■ TOTAL NUMBER OF RECIPIENTS: 136 ■ 85% OF CLASS

	Average Award	Range of Awards
Residents	$68,016	Up to $75,971
Nonresidents	$68,016	Up to $75,971

Estimated Total Expenses for Academic Year 2006-07

	YEAR 1	YEAR 2	YEAR 3	YEAR 4	TOTAL
Tuition	$45,550	$45,550	$45,550	$45,550	$182,000
Other expenses charged by school	$10,471	$10,601	$7,101	$6,701	$34,874
Estimated living expenses	$20,000	$23,270	$24,420	$17,800	$85,490
TOTAL EXPENSES	**$75,971**	**$79,371**	**$77,021**	**$70,001**	**$302,364**

UNIVERSITY OF DETROIT MERCY
SCHOOL OF DENTISTRY

Dr. H. Robert Steiman, Dean

GENERAL INFORMATION

The University of Detroit Mercy School of Dentistry is an urban-based school located in metropolitan Detroit. The School of Dentistry's goal is to graduate a dentist with the professional competence to assess, diagnose, plan, and treat patients with skill, sensitivity, and cultural awareness. The School of Dentistry is a private, partially state-supported school that was established in 1932. The University of Detroit Mercy is an independent Catholic institution sponsored by the Religious Sisters of Mercy and Society of Jesus.

In January 2008, the School is relocating to a facility located in southwest Detroit. The location of the school provides an opportunity to deliver oral health care to an extensive patient population as well as continue its history of community outreach activities. The relocation allows for a larger clinical facility and an improved environment for learning, research and patient care. The facility houses classrooms, preclinical laboratories, clinics, cafeteria and a library. The location allows for easy access and secure parking for patients and students. A new clinical simulation laboratory containing patient simulator mannequins and clinical workstations is carefully designed to enhance learning. The clinical simulation lab enables students to learn and practice in the laboratory before they provide actual patient care. A 42-chair hospital-based satellite clinic, with additional patient-care opportunities, is located nearby at the University Health Center of Detroit Receiving Hospital. The School of Dentistry is dedicated to educating dentists who are patient-care oriented and skilled in the art of self-evaluation and lifelong learning. The school also offers programs in dental hygiene and graduate and postgraduate studies, as well as continuing education courses for dental professionals.

ADMISSION REQUIREMENTS

NUMBER OF YEARS OF PREDENTAL EDUCATION: Formal minimum of two (60 semester or 90 quarter hours); generally acceptable minimum of three (90 semester or 135 quarter hours).

LIMITATIONS ON COMMUNITY COLLEGE WORK: 60 semester hours.

REQUIRED COURSES:

With lab required	(semester/quarter hrs)*
Inorganic chemistry**	8/12
Organic chemistry	8/12
Physics	8/12
Biology***	8/12

Other courses	
English	6/9

* It is preferred that required courses be taken at a four-year college or university.
** General chemistry is an acceptable alternative.
***Zoology and genetics are acceptable alternatives.

The Office of Admissions reserves the right to modify the prerequisites in exceptional cases when an applicant's background supplants the need for such courses or when additional courses are necessary to improve an applicant's preparation for dental school.

SUGGESTED ADDITIONAL PREPARATION: In addition to the required courses, suggested additional courses are comparative anatomy, histology or embryology, biochemistry (strongly recommended), and courses in the humanities and social sciences. Psychology of human behavior is especially helpful.

It is recommended that high school graduates contemplating a career in dentistry enroll in a four-year degree program at a fully accredited college or university. The student should pursue a full-time program of studies leading to a baccalaureate degree. The choice of a major is not critical as long as the basic course requirements are fulfilled. Prospective applicants are advised to carry a full academic load (15 credits or more per term) and to avoid repetition of courses to improve their grades. Professionally related coursework such as dental hygiene, pharmacy, nursing, as well as engineering, arts, instrumental music, etc., is not counted toward minimum requirements.

DAT: First attempt recommended by October 15, 2008, preferred with a minimum score of 18 in *each category* recommended.

GPA: No official cut-off; 2.95 or above science GPA is recommended.

RESIDENCY: No specific requirement.

ADVANCED STANDING: Appropriately qualified transfer students from U.S. and Canadian dental schools may be admitted with advanced standing into the first, second, or third year. Graduates of foreign dental schools may be admitted with advanced standing into the second year only. Positions are limited by space availability in the designated class.

Timetable for the Class Entering Fall 2008

	Earliest Date	Latest Date	School Fee
Application Submission	6/1/07	2/1/08*	$50**
Acceptance Notification	12/1/07	8/08	$1,500***

(or when class is full)

* Late applications may be considered with special permission. Please contact the school for further information.
** May be waived upon receipt of a letter from financial aid officer at applicant's predental college vouching that applicant merits a waiver or if fee waiver is granted by AADSAS.
***Nonrefundable enrollment fee

Required Response:
45 days if accepted on or after 12/1/07
30 days if accepted on or after 1/1/08
15 days if accepted on or after 2/1/08
Preferred time: immediately.

FOR FURTHER INFORMATION

Office of Admissions
Karin LaRose-Neil
Director
313-494-6611 (A-L); 313-494-6650 (M-Z)
dental@udmercy.edu
University of Detroit Mercy
School of Dentistry, MB 38

Office of Financial Aid
Camellia Taylor, Coordinator
313-494-6617; taylorca2@udmercy.edu
University of Detroit Mercy
School of Dentistry, MB 33

Multicultural Affairs
313-494-6653
University of Detroit Mercy
School of Dentistry, MB 38

Through December 2007:
8200 West Outer Drive
Detroit, MI 48219-3580

Beginning January 2008:
2700 Martin Luther King Jr. Boulevard
Detroit, MI 48208-2576

dental.udmercy.edu

UNIVERSITY OF DETROIT MERCY SCHOOL OF DENTISTRY **MICHIGAN**

THE DENTAL PROGRAM

The objectives of the School of Dentistry are to educate dentists who are patient-centered in their vision of the dental practice, guided by ethics and professional values. Graduates are competent to provide quality, evidence-based oral health care supported by a foundation knowledge in biomedical, dental and behavioral sciences. Graduate dentists are skilled in treating diverse patient populations, sensitive to cultural and ethnic health beliefs and practices.

The basic and preclinical sciences are concentrated in the first two years; however, some of the basic sciences are taught in the third and fourth years to provide for integration with the clinical sciences and to correlate patient care with its rationale. The freshman curriculum is divided between the basic and dental sciences, while in the sophomore year a greater portion of the curriculum is devoted to the dental sciences. Research opportunities are available throughout the curriculum on an elective basis.

Clinical experience on a limited basis begins in the first year and extends through the second year. During the first two years, the students are initially taught to use clinical equipment and to perform various dental procedures on each other. Preclinical courses provide the foundation for patient care in a simulated environment. As part of the second year, students begin treating simple restorative patients. Approximately half of the available time during the third and fourth years is devoted to clinical practice. The student is taught clinical dentistry principally by the method of comprehensive patient care. Individual students are assigned a patient family and are responsible for addressing all the patient's dental needs. This model encourages an important operator-patient relationship that contributes to the professional development of the student. Students provide care to patients in conjunction with dental hygiene students to parallel private practice. Senior dental students are assigned to the southwest clinic, the Detroit Receiving Hospital-University Health Center (UHC) complex and outreach sites located in metropolitan Detroit and Flint, Michigan. The UHC and outreach rotations are designed to enable the student to provide comprehensive patient care in a mode similar to private practice.

Student assessment includes self-evaluation based on established criteria as emphasized in both clinical and didactic courses. Student performance is evaluated by periodic written quizzes or examination: Preclinical practical examinations, discipline-based competency examinations or OSCE (Objective Simulated Clinical Examinations). Students utilize tablet computers as part of the educational and clinical experiences as a resource, evaluation tool and electronic patient chart. The D.D.S. degree is conferred upon students who have completed all requirements and met the minimum grade point average.

■ Degrees Offered
DENTAL DEGREE: D.D.S.

ALTERNATE DEGREES: A six-year program resulting in a joint B.S./D.D.S. degree is available for application by qualified high school seniors.

■ Other Programs
AEGD, Endodontics, Orthodontics, Periodontics, and Program for Graduates of Foreign Dental Schools, Dental Hygiene, Dental Hygiene Degree Completion

COSTS AND FINANCIAL AID

Applicants should consult the Financial Aid Office of the university. Five Dental Merit grants are available for $8,000 for four years. Approximately 91 percent of Michigan residents receive the Michigan Tuition Grant of $2,000, renewable for four years and based on need.

The table below presents minimum estimates of the school expenses an entering student must anticipate. All estimates are based on charges expected for the academic year. Tuition and fees, as well as the types of fees, are subject to change without notice, and all costs are subject to inflation.

Financial Aid Awards to First-Year Students in 2005-06
■ TOTAL NUMBER OF RECIPIENTS: 62   ■ 79% OF CLASS

	Average Award	Range of Awards
Residents	$57,045	N/A
Nonresidents	$57,045	N/A
Noncitizen loans		$34,555-$45,000

Estimated Total Expenses for Academic Year 2006-07

	YEAR 1	YEAR 2	YEAR 3	YEAR 4	TOTAL
Tuition	$39,350	$39,350	$39,350	$39,350	$157,400
Fees	$2,305	$2,029	$579	$579	$5,492
Insurance, equipment usage; ASDA membership; graduation fee					
Equipment rental, books, and supplies	$6,800	$6,500	$5,950	$5,300	$24,550
Registration fee	$570	$570	$570	$570	$2,280
Estimated living expenses	$12,656	$12,656	$12,656	$12,656	$50,624
Rent (11 months), etc.					
TOTAL EXPENSES	$61,681	$61,105	$59,105	$58,455	$240,346

SELECTION FACTORS

Applicants are selected for admission based upon academic performance and difficulty of curriculum in undergraduate studies, DAT scores, and other characteristics as determined by letters of recommendation, personal statement and a personal interview. The Admissions Committee will consider the college attended, course load, and overall and science GPAs. An academic record that progressively increases in quality is a plus factor. Personal characteristics, such as motivation for dentistry and social awareness, are evaluated by letters of recommendation and a personal interview (arranged at the discretion of the Admissions Committee). A composite letter of recommendation is required from the college preprofessional advisory committee or from two science professors (by whom the applicant has been instructed within nonplant or nonenvironmental Biology, Chemistry, or Physics disciplines) if no committee exists, as well as one letter from a practicing dentist attesting to the applicant spending a reasonable amount of time in his or her office observing, shadowing, or investigating the profession. Additional letters are welcome if pertinent.

The University of Detroit Mercy is committed to a policy of nondiscrimination on the basis of race, color, creed, gender, national origin, and age. The School of Dentistry encourages applications from underrepresented groups. Applications from all candidates are evaluated using a single set of standards.

See chapter 3 of this guide for information regarding numbers of applicants and enrollees to each dental school along with their race, gender, age, type of predental education, mean DAT and GPA, and state of origin.

ACADEMIC AND OTHER ASSISTANCE

The UDM School of Dentistry sponsors recruitment and retention programs for all students, including students who are members of underrepresented populations in dentistry. These programs include individual assistance upon request. Upon matriculation, students benefit from a range of academic and personal support services, such as a tutorial program and counseling, as needed.

MICHIGAN

UNIVERSITY OF MICHIGAN
SCHOOL OF DENTISTRY

Dr. Peter J. Polverini, Dean

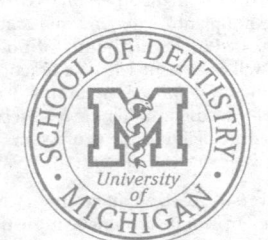

GENERAL INFORMATION

The University of Michigan School of Dentistry, organized in 1875, was the first dental school established as an integral part of a state university and the second to become a part of any university.

The University of Michigan is located in Ann Arbor, a city of 110,000 about 40 miles west of Detroit. The School of Dentistry is housed in a modern complex designed to complement the changing concepts in dental education. Students benefit from the proximity of a large university medical center and the resources of a major public university. Approximately 500 students are enrolled annually in the three basic programs offered by the School of Dentistry: 1) the D.D.S. degree program; 2) advanced programs leading to the degrees of master of science and specialty certification; and 3) a dental hygiene program. In addition to these programs, the school conducts a comprehensive program in continuing dental education and offers a Ph.D. in Oral Health Sciences and a dual D.D.S./Ph.D. program.

Inherent to the mission of the University of Michigan School of Dentistry is a dedication to stimulate the development of the faculty and staff and to inspire students to develop attitudes and skills necessary for continued professional growth. To pursue its mission, the School of Dentistry will foster and exemplify equity, diversity, and multicultural values.

ADMISSION REQUIREMENTS

NUMBER OF YEARS OF PREDENTAL EDUCATION: Formal minimum of three (90 semester or 135 quarter hours) usual and recommended is four.

LIMITATIONS ON COMMUNITY COLLEGE WORK: Maximum of 60 hours. Four-year colleges or universities are strongly preferred.

REQUIRED COURSES: The required course list has been updated for applicants to the Fall 2008 entering class. All science courses must be taken at the premed or predent level to be considered. Laboratory courses are required for Inorganic Chemistry, Organic Chemistry, Physics, and Biological science.

With lab required	(semester/quarter hrs)
Inorganic chemistry	8/12
Organic chemistry	8/12
Physics	8/12
Biological science	8/12

Science courses without lab	
Biochemistry	3/5
Microbiology	3/5

Other courses	
English composition	6/9
Psychology	3/5
Sociology	3/5

SUGGESTED ADDITIONAL PREPARATION: Anatomy, histology, physiology, public speaking (sometimes called speech), and art (drawing, including mechanical drawing; sculpture; photography).

DAT: Should be taken no later than September 1, 2007; no minimum requirements. However, see Selection Factors.

GPA: Typical range 2.7 – 4.0; typical median: 3.50. See Selection Factors.

RESIDENCY: No specific requirements; however, see Selection Factors.

ADVANCED STANDING: Graduates of foreign dental schools may apply for the Internationally Trained Dentist Program (ITDP), which awards a D.D.S. degree after two full years of study. Visit www.dent.umich.edu/prospective/international.html.

Timetable for the Class Entering Fall 2008

	Earliest Date	Latest Date	School Fees
Application Submission	5/15/07	12/1/07	$50
Acceptance Notification	12/1/07	8/25/08	$1,500*

*nonrefundable enrollment fee

Required Response:
45 days if accepted on or after 12/1/07
30 days if accepted on or after 1/1/08
15 days if accepted on or after 2/1/08
Preferred time: immediately

FOR FURTHER INFORMATION
Marilyn W. Woolfolk
Assistant Dean for Student Services
734-763-3313
School of Dentistry

Patricia Katcher
Associate Director, Admissions
734-763-3316
School of Dentistry
www.dent.umich.edu/prospective/dentadmission.html

Kenneth B. May
Interim Director
Office of Multicultural Affairs
734-763-3342
School of Dentistry
www.dent.umich.edu/mac

Internationally Trained Dentist Program
www.dent.umich.edu/prospective/international.html

Housing Information Office
734-763-3164
1500 Student Activities Building
The University of Michigan
Ann Arbor, MI 48109-1316
www.housing.umich.edu

www.dent.umich.edu

THE DENTAL PROGRAM

The general objectives of dental education are to accomplish the following: 1) provide opportunities within a stimulating academic environment for students to develop an appreciation and understanding of philosophical, social, and intellectual problems; 2) emphasize the orientation of the student to the physical and biological sciences upon which the practice of contemporary dentistry is based; 3) provide the opportunities and experiences that enable the student to develop the clinical skills essential to provision of the highest quality oral health service to his or her patients; 4) foster an appreciation within the student of the value, design, and methodology of dental research; 5) attain within all students conformity in letter and spirit to the principles of ethics as an unquestioned part of professional life; 6) encourage students to consider career possibilities in dental research, dental education, and dental public health; 7) develop the potential of the dental graduate for leadership in his or her profession and in the community; and 8) bring conviction to every dental graduate that his or her dental education will serve well only as long as it is refreshed and renewed through lifelong continuing education.

The basic sciences are incorporated into a systems-based course, Integrated Medical Sciences which begins in the first year and continues into the second year. Clinical experiences begin in the first term of the first year; first-year students are part of a clinic team with second-, third-, and fourth-year students. To integrate these areas, dental school faculty teach applied oral science courses in conjunction with the Integrated Medical Science courses that are collectively taught by medical and dental school faculty. An extramural community service-learning program allows students to participate in dental health care delivery in unserved and underserved communities. Beginning at the end of the second year, the clinical program models many aspects of private, group dental practice and is designed with an emphasis on the planning and delivery of comprehensive dental care. Wide-ranging instruction and experience in data retrieval and management systems complement all levels of the curriculum.

Methods used for student evaluation consist of written tests and observations of clinical performance.

YEAR 1. An Integrated Medical Sciences sequence incorporates basic sciences into a course organized by body systems. Clinical and behavioral sciences are introduced in the curriculum and enhanced by weekly observations of clinical experiences.

YEAR 2. Integrated Medical Sciences sequence, clinical, and behavioral science courses continue. Weekly clinical experiences expand to include patient treatment.

YEARS 3 AND 4. Clinical sciences continue with the delivery of comprehensive dental care that approximates private practice, including clinical experiences in extramural programs.

■ Degrees Offered
DENTAL DEGREE: D.D.S.

ALTERNATE DEGREES: A bachelor's degree can be earned only if a liberal arts college awards the degree independently.

■ Other Programs
STUDENT RESEARCH OPPORTUNITIES: Students have the opportunity to participate in research through various programs at the U-M School of Dentistry: the Student Research Program, which requires participation in a competitive application process resulting in stipend support; the Student Research Group, a student membership organization that provides research activities to students; and independent research, in which students seek out faculty willing to mentor them on individual projects.

EXTERNSHIPS: Extramural Clinical Experiences and Service Learning are available to third- and fourth-year students, e.g., Migrant Worker Program, Community-Based Clinics, and other outreach sites.

COSTS AND FINANCIAL AID

A wide variety of loans and scholarships are available to students who might otherwise be unable to continue their education without financial assistance. Applications are evaluated and awards made through the university's Office of Financial Aid. The school tries to assist students who do not have sufficient personal resources. Because of the demands of the curriculum, students are discouraged from holding employment, particularly during the first year. Applications for financial aid and instructions for completion are sent to each student upon payment of enrollment deposit.

Financial Aid Awards to First-Year Students in 2005-06
■ TOTAL NUMBER OF RECIPIENTS: 95   ■ 86% OF CLASS

	Average Award	Range of Awards
Residents	$37,440	$3,911-$49,397
Nonresidents	$56,707	$8,500-$67,483

Estimated Total Expenses for Academic Year 2007-08

	YEAR 1	YEAR 2	YEAR 3	YEAR 4	TOTAL
Tuition, resident	$25,596	$25,596	$25,596	$25,596	$102,384
Tuition, nonresident	$41,244	$41,244	$41,244	$41,244	$164,976
Other expenses					
Fees	$188	$188	$188	$188	$752
Equipment	$3,100	$3,100	$3,100	$3,100	$12,400
Estimated living expenses	$18,554	$20,409	$20,409	$14,843	$74,215
Housing, transportation, personal for 10 months					
TOTAL EXPENSES, RESIDENT	$47,438	$49,293	$49,293	$43,727	$189,751
TOTAL EXPENSES, NONRESIDENT	$63,086	$64,941	$64,941	$59,375	$252,343

SELECTION FACTORS

Because the university is a state-supported institution, preference is given to Michigan residents. Admission to the School of Dentistry is based on evidence of academic training, intellectual capacity adequate to the pursuit of a profession, and other qualifications indicating that the student is fit for the study and practice of dentistry. It is suggested that letters of recommendation include two from instructors in different areas of science and a third from a teacher in a nonscience area or a dentist. Evaluation from a preprofessional committee is also acceptable. Each application is carefully reviewed with special attention to scholastic attainment, character, and personality. To receive serious consideration, applicants should have a GPA of 3.0 (B) or above. Courses should include upper-level courses, with appropriate grades earned and progress made toward a degree. Currently, competitive DAT scores are 20 for Academic Average and 19 for Perceptual Ability. Applicants who appear to meet the necessary academic and scholastic requirements will be invited to the dental school for a campus visit/interview. Noncognitive aspects of a candidate's record such as career or research experiences, student organization activity, volunteer work, missions, other significant life experiences, leadership, social interest, and other characteristics and attributes that might contribute to the diversity of the class are also taken into consideration, as well as potential interest in addressing health disparities and a commitment to or experience in care for underserved communities.

It is the policy of the University of Michigan that no person shall be discriminated against in employment, educational programs and activities, or admission on the basis of race, gender, color, religion, creed, national origin or ancestry, age, marital status, sexual orientation, disability, or Vietnam-era veteran status. Applications from women, veterans, and members of minority groups are encouraged.

See chapter 3 of this guide for information regarding numbers of applicants and enrollees to each dental school, along with their race, gender, age, type of predental education, mean DAT and GPA, and state of origin.

ACADEMIC AND OTHER ASSISTANCE

The University of Michigan has a long-standing commitment to the recruitment, retention, and graduation of a culturally diverse student body. It involves a comprehensive approach targeted toward all levels of preparation for professional school admission, beginning with high school. The approach features enhancement of academic skills, interviewing techniques, preadmissions counseling, DAT preparation courses, and financial aid advising to disadvantaged students. Following admission, disadvantaged students and students from groups underrepresented in the health professions are offered a summer prematriculation orientation and a continuing complementary tutorial program to facilitate their retention in dental school. Please visit the Multicultural Affairs website at www.dent.umich.edu/services/mac. Women, veterans, and members of minority groups are encouraged to apply. Minority students should correspond directly with Dr. Kenneth May (see For Further Information).

UNIVERSITY OF MINNESOTA
SCHOOL OF DENTISTRY

Dr. Patrick M. Lloyd, Dean

GENERAL INFORMATION

The School of Dentistry, established in 1888, is a state institution and part of a great university health center. Since the center is located on the Minneapolis campus of the university, students in dentistry enjoy a variety of academic, cultural, and recreational opportunities. The Minneapolis campus is located in the center of the Minneapolis-St. Paul area, a metropolitan area with a population of over 2.7 million.

The school's teaching and research facilities are in a health sciences building, completed in 1975, which holds shared basic science laboratories and lecture rooms for the health sciences. These quarters, together with other facilities in the center, provide an excellent environment for the study of dentistry. The dental school is an active member of the Academic Health Center, made up of the schools of dentistry, medicine, nursing, pharmacy, public health, and veterinary medicine. A wide range of programs are conducted in the School of Dentistry, including dentistry, dental hygiene, many dental specialties, basic science graduate and other postdoctoral and clinical training programs, and a comprehensive research program. A D.D.S./Ph.D. program and a Program for Advanced Standing Students (UMN PASS) are also available.

ADMISSION REQUIREMENTS

NUMBER OF YEARS OF PREDENTAL EDUCATION: Formal minimum of three (87 semester or 130 quarter hours); generally acceptable minimum of three in liberal arts courses.

LIMITATIONS ON COMMUNITY COLLEGE WORK: A limit of 64 semester hours from community or junior colleges will be applied to the 90 semester hours required, or to the 120 semester credits of a four-year program; 87 semester credits accepted as three years, and 114 semester credits accepted as four.

REQUIRED COURSES:

With lab required	(semester hrs)
General chemistry	8
(complete basic course series)	
Organic chemistry	8
(must include aliphatic and aromatic series)	
Biochemistry	3 (lecture only)
(prerequisite: organic chemistry)	
Physics	8
(complete basic course series)	
Biology	8
(complete basic course series)	

Other courses	
English	8
General Psychology	3
Math	3
(college algebra or precalculus, computer science, statistics)	

SUGGESTED ADDITIONAL PREPARATION: Courses should be selected to give students as broad and liberal an education as possible. However, applicants are also encouraged to take these specific electives: cell biology, histology, physiology, immunology, anatomy, microbiology, and genetics; drawing (3-D preferred) or sculpture; accounting, small business operations, marketing, and management.

DAT: Mandatory; applicants must submit scores no later than December 1, 2007.

GPA: 2.7 required but a substantially higher GPA is necessary to be considered competitive.

EARLY ADMISSION PROGRAM: The School of Dentistry offers an Early Admission Program for qualified applicants. Minnesota residents are given preference in consideration. Eligible candidates must be U.S. citizens and have an overall GPA of ≥3.4 and a science GPA of ≥3.2. Applicants must also have completed their basic science series of biology, general and organic chemistry, have observed in a general dental practice, and meet other *Criteria for DDS Admissions Selection*. If accepted into the Early Admission Program, a provisional acceptance may be granted. For more specific details on the program, please refer to the School of Dentistry website for the *Criteria for Eligibility for Early Admissions Program*.

ADVANCED STANDING: The University of Minnesota School of Dentistry Program for Advanced Standing Students (UMN PASS) is a new two-year program designed for graduates of dental schools outside of the United States and Canada seeking to practice dentistry in the United States. Successful completion of the two-year program leads to a Doctor of Dental Surgery (D.D.S.) degree, allowing a successful graduate to seek a license to practice dentistry in any U.S. state.

Summer Introductory Program: For eight weeks in mid May to mid July, UMN PASS students review lectures, attend seminars, participate in discussion groups on adapting to a new culture, and perform a substantial number of preclinical laboratory exercises. They then complete two weeks of mandatory rotations in University of Minnesota School of Dentistry clinics. The ten-week introductory course is designed to facilitate a smooth transition for UMN PASS student as they merge with the third-year dental students into patient care experiences in September.

For further information on the program, refer to the School of Dentistry web site. The program is directed by Dr. Peter Berthold.

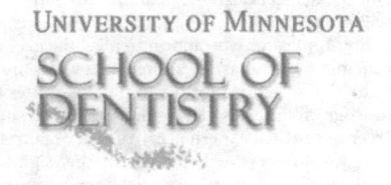

Timetable for the Class Entering Fall 2008

	Earliest Date	Latest Date	School Fee
Application Submission	6/1/07	1/1/08*	$60
Acceptance Notification	12/1/07	approx. 4/1/08	

*In order to receive highest consideration, all application materials should be received by 9/1/2007.

Required Response and Deposit:
45 days after notification if received between 12/1 and 12/31
30 days after notification if received between 1/1 and 2/28
15 days after notification if received after 3/1

A $1,000 nonrefundable, nontransferable tuition deposit is due on the applicant's response date. The deposit will be applied to dental school first year tuition.

FOR FURTHER INFORMATION
Office of Admissions
612-625-7477 (collect)
University of Minnesota
School of Dentistry
15-106 Malcolm Moos Health Sciences Tower
515 Delaware Street S.E.
Minneapolis, MN 55455
Office of Financial Aid
Coordinator of Dental Financial Aid
612-624-4138
Office of Scholarships and Financial Aid
University of Minnesota
210 Fraser Hall
Minneapolis, MN 55455

www.dentistry.umn.edu

UNIVERSITY OF MINNESOTA SCHOOL OF DENTISTRY — MINNESOTA

THE DENTAL PROGRAM

The dental school has a strong reputation for educating fine clinicians and diagnosticians through a curriculum that involves progressive introduction to clinical training, integration of basic and applied clinical skills, and group and problem-based learning situations. During the students' final year, the school offers experiences in outreach clinical practice sites and a comprehensive care clinic setting within the school. The school also encourages students to take elective courses in dental and other disciplines to enhance their clinical, didactic, and research knowledge base.

The goal of the dental curriculum is to educate dental professionals whose scholarly capabilities, scientific acumen, and interpersonal skills are commensurate with their clinical mastery. This is a new and different emphasis for dental education and will provide graduates with the flexibility to adapt to continuing changes in health care and developments in the practice of dentistry.

The curriculum is organized in a vertical fashion; scientific and clinical themes are taught in years one through three. Basic and dental sciences are integrated with clinical topics during these same years. Students begin a clinical curriculum in the first year, and their clinical experiences increase in scope and complexity as they progress.

Clinics are organized into small groups so that students develop close relationships with their peers and with their clinical faculty. During students' fourth year, the school provides a comprehensive care clinical setting, on site, which simulates a group dental practice. Also in the fourth year, students are encouraged to take advanced studies in clinical disciplines or take further coursework in other related disciplines. During the summer preceding and throughout the final year of study, students are offered opportunities in clinical outreach (externships) in the Twin Cities and rural areas of Minnesota and surrounding states.

■ Degrees Offered
DENTAL DEGREE: D.D.S.

ALTERNATE DEGREES: A bachelor's degree can be earned while completing the dental curriculum if the institution where the individual undertook preprofessional coursework offers such a program and awards the degree independently.

■ Other Programs
SUMMER RESEARCH FELLOWSHIPS: The school awards research positions to a selected number of applicants prior to matriculating. In addition, a limited number of research positions are available to students continuing their education.

COMMUNITY OUTREACH: The Minnesota Student District Dental Society (local ASDA chapter) provides a variety of outreach opportunities for interested student members.

FOREIGN EXCHANGE: Available to fourth-year students: Norway, Denmark, Netherlands, and Germany.

EXTERNSHIPS AND ELECTIVES: Available to fourth-year dental students as noted above.

PROFESSIONAL RE-ENTRY PROGRAM: In this program, graduates who have taken time off from dentistry due to illness, disability, or an accident and wish to resume their careers participate in a program tailored to their needs.

D.D.S./PH.D.: The Minnesota Craniofacial Research Training (MinnCReST) Program, funded by a five-year award from the National Institute of Dental & Craniofacial Research (NIDCR), provides generous support for a Dentist-Scientist Training Program (D.D.S. and Ph.D.) degree. MinnCReST trainees can pursue novel research that expands the frontier and scope of dental, craniofacial, and oral health knowledge in their choice of laboratory settings in over 20 research fields and 80 acclaimed, interdisciplinary faculty mentors. The program supports Medical Scientist Training Program (M.D. and Ph.D.); Predoctoral (Ph.D.); Postdoctoral; Post-D.D.S. Postdoctoral/Ph.D.; Post-D.D.S. Postdoctoral/M.S. in Clinical Research; and a short-term research experience for current D.D.S. students. For further information, contact the Office of Admissions at 612-625-7477.

COSTS AND FINANCIAL AID

If students have a demonstrated financial need, every effort is made to offer financial aid during the full length of their dental education on the basis of resources available. The school is able to offer a number of merit scholarships for entering and continuing students. Although students are urged to avoid outside employment during the school year, the Student Employment Bureau assists students in obtaining part-time jobs. Information regarding available aid and methods for application is mailed to the candidate after the School of Dentistry notifies the candidate of acceptance.

Financial Aid Awards to First-Year Students in 2006-07
■ TOTAL NUMBER OF RECIPIENTS: 93   ■ 96% OF CLASS

	Average Award (for Fall, Spring, and Summer Semesters)	Range of Awards
Residents/Reciprocity Students	$48,031	$5,000-$59,308
Nonresidents	$54,588	$2,000-$71,404

Total Expenses for Academic Year 2006-07

	YEAR 1***	YEAR 2	YEAR 3	YEAR 4
Tuition, resident	$19,786	$21,171	$28,709	$30,719
Tuition, nonresident	$34,606	$38,067	$52,144	$57,357
Other expenses				
Equipment fee	$319	$479	$493	$508
University registration fee	$950	$1,500	$1,575	$1,650
Student service fee	$599	$925	$953	$982
Univ. sponsored hospitalization insurance*	$1,646	$1,695	$1,746	$1,799
Miscellaneous fees	$67	$104	$107	$110
Implant materials fee	0	0	$355	0
Microscope rental	$52	0	0	0
Precious metals (costs vary due to market rates)	$155	$500	0	0
Dental partial framework fee	0	$82	0	0
Articulator	$400	0	0	0
Stone study teeth	$22	0	0	0
Oral anatomy manual	$16	0	0	0
Disability insurance	$71	$72	$72	$75
Instrument usage fee	$2,410	$3,615	$3,723	$3,723
Instrument replacement fee**	0	$28	$67	0
Books	$3,142	$1,772	$2,698	$311
Estimated living expenses:				
Room and board	$8,738	$13,500	$13,905	$14,322
Transportation	$750	$773	$1,194	$1,230
Personal miscellaneous	$1,676	$1,726	$2,667	$2,747
TOTAL EXPENSES, RESIDENT	$40,797	$47,942	$58,264	$58,175
TOTAL EXPENSES, NONRESIDENT	$55,617	$64,838	$81,699	$84,813
Int'l. student fee	$124	$155	$159	$164
Int'l. student aid fee	$19	$20	$21	$22
TOTAL EXPENSES, INTERNATIONAL	$55,760	$65,013	$81,879	$84,999

*Insurance coverage, when purchased spring semester, will extend through summer session.
**Students may incur additional charges due to instrument breakage or losses. These charges will be assessed during the students' second and third years.
***Second-, third-, and fourth-year students complete a mandatory summer term.

SELECTION FACTORS

Admission is based on the quality of college study, including such factors as consistency, improvement, quality of coursework, completion of required courses, and limited use of "P" (passing) or "S" (satisfactory) grades and avoidance of withdrawal and incomplete grades, and the quantity of academic work per quarter or semester. It is required that all prerequisite/elective courses be completed by the end of the 2007-08 academic year. Scores on the DAT are also considered. Competitive applicants are invited to visit the School of Dentistry for a tour, formal interview, academic counseling, and transcript evaluation. Recommendations must come from persons closely familiar with the applicant within the last four years. Two should come from science faculty; one must be sent from an employer. Applicants must also demonstrate interest in and knowledge of dentistry through close observation of, or participation in, patient care; interest and experience in personal services requiring empathy for people and social sensitivities; and interest and experience in activities requiring fine manual dexterity.

All applicants who are not native speakers of English must submit written evidence of a Test of English as a Foreign Language (TOEFL).

Admission is granted without regard to race, religion, color, gender, national origin, disability, age, veteran status, sexual orientation, creed, marital status, or public assistance. Since Minnesota is a state-supported institution, preference for admission is given to Minnesota residents. Minnesota has an admissions contract with Montana and reciprocity agreements with North Dakota, South Dakota, and Manitoba. In addition, the School of Dentistry encourages well-qualified applicants from states other than those listed above to apply for admission. Refer to the school website for more detailed information on selection factors.

See chapter 3 of this guide for information regarding numbers of applicants and enrollees to each dental school, along with their race, gender, age, type of predental education, mean DAT and GPA, and state of origin.

UNIVERSITY OF MISSISSIPPI
SCHOOL OF DENTISTRY

Dr. James R. Hupp, Dean

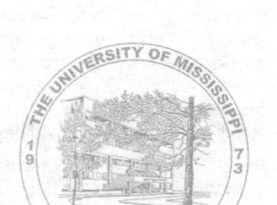

GENERAL INFORMATION

The Mississippi state legislature authorized the establishment of the School of Dentistry at the University of Mississippi Medical Center in the 1973 regular session. The primary goal of the School of Dentistry is to provide an educational experience that will prepare scientifically minded, clinically competent, community-oriented, ethical health professionals to serve the oral and general health needs of their patients and society. In addition, the school is committed to generating a scholarly environment that encourages a lifelong spirit of inquiry and learning, promotes critical attitudes, nurtures compassion, and develops the ability to accept and incorporate beneficial change.

The University of Mississippi Medical Center, a state-supported institution, is the state's only academic health sciences center. The Medical Center includes the Schools of Dentistry, Medicine, Nursing, and Health Related Professions, graduate programs in the medical sciences, and the University Hospital. The interrelated components share a common commitment to education, research, and service to improve the quality of life in the state and region. All contribute to, and benefit from, the total health care environment.

The University of Mississippi's dental education program is structured to meet the state's long-term dental health needs. The curriculum emphasizes extensive training in general dentistry that allows graduates to provide comprehensive care for the greatest possible number of their patients. To develop essential clinical skill and confidence, students' contact with patients begins in the first quarter of the freshman year. As experience and skills increase, so do patient care responsibilities and opportunities for more independent decision-making.

The innovative and stimulating approach to dental education at the University of Mississippi Medical Center has the ultimate goal of graduating mature, clinically proficient, community-oriented health professionals who will serve the dental health needs of Mississippi and the nation.

ADMISSION REQUIREMENTS

NUMBER OF YEARS OF PREDENTAL EDUCATION: Required minimum of three (90 semester hours); preferred minimum of four (128 semester hours)

LIMITATIONS ON COMMUNITY COLLEGE WORK: 65 semester hours.

REQUIRED COURSES:

With lab required	(number of semesters)
Inorganic chemistry	2
Organic chemistry	2
Physics	2
Biology	2
Advanced biology or chemistry	2

Other courses	
Statistics	1
English*	1
Mathematics	2
(college algebra, trigonometry, or calculus)	

*Must be in composition

SUGGESTED ADDITIONAL PREPARATION: Biochemistry, computer science, comparative anatomy, quantitative analysis, embryology, cell biology, immunology, psychology, and courses in the humanities are highly recommended.

DAT: No test date or minimum score is required; however, test results must not be older than three years.

GPA: No official cut-off; average GPAs for recent entering classes have been in the 3.5 range.

RESIDENCY: Preference is given to legal residents of Mississippi, and all applicants must be U.S. citizens.

ADVANCED STANDING: Under exceptional circumstances, students attending another U.S. school who are residents of Mississippi may be considered for advanced standing. Graduates of foreign dental schools are not eligible for advanced standing.

Timetable for the Class Entering Fall 2008

	Earliest Date	Latest Date	School Fee
Application Submission	7/1/07	11/1/07	$50
Acceptance Notification	12/1/07	6/1/08	

Required Response:
15 days after notification

FOR FURTHER INFORMATION
J. David Duncan
Assistant Dean, Student Affairs
601-984-6009
University of Mississippi School of Dentistry
2500 North State Street
Jackson, MS 39216

Office of Student Financial Aid
601-984-1117

Office of Multicultural Affairs
Wilhelmina O'Reilly
Special Assistant to the Dean
601-984-1340

University of Mississippi Medical Center
2500 North State Street
Jackson, MS 39216

dentistry.umc.edu

THE DENTAL PROGRAM

The major emphasis of the dental curriculum is to train practitioners of general dentistry to provide total health care. This is accomplished by employing a systems approach to a problem-oriented curriculum. Clinical experience begins in the second year, and a team approach to patient care is used on a limited basis through all four years. A team is comprised of one student from each class. Basic science and clinical science courses are integrated. Off-campus clinical experiences begin in the first year with a one-week community project somewhere in the state. These continue throughout the four years. A written evaluation of all courses and instructors is completed by each student at the end of each quarter. Audiovisual facilities and student learning laboratories are provided where applicable.

■ Degrees Offered

DENTAL DEGREE: D.M.D., Ph.D.

ALTERNATE DEGREES: By prior arrangement, students entering without a degree may earn their bachelor's degree while completing the dental program.

COSTS AND FINANCIAL AID

The University of Mississippi School of Dentistry provides both need- and merit-based funds. For more information contact the Financial Aid Office.

Financial Aid Awards to First-Year Students in 2005-06
■ TOTAL NUMBER OF RECIPIENTS: 28   ■ 90% OF CLASS

	Average Award/Range of Awards
Residents	$10,733-$27,343

Estimated School-Related Expenses for Academic Year 2007-08

The table below presents minimum estimates of the school expenses an entering student can anticipate. All estimates are based on charges expected for the academic year. Tuition and fees, as well as the types of fees, are subject to change without notice, and all costs are subject to inflation.

	YEAR 1	YEAR 2	YEAR 3	YEAR 4	TOTAL
Tuition (including fees)					
Resident	9,030	9,030	9,030	9,030	36,120
Approximate additional expenses					
Computer	2,200	0	0	0	2,200
Health Insurance	1,782	1,782	1,782	1,782	7,128
Books	1,042	1,042	1,172	1,042	4,298
Lab Coats	84	54	54	54	246
Supplies	370	450	436	0	1,256
Articulator	934	0	0	0	934
State Exam Fees	0	0	2,175	0	2,175
National Board Exam Fees	0	215	0	290	505
Total Additional Expenses	6,412	3,543	5,619	3,168	18,742
TOTAL EXPENSES, RESIDENT	**15,442**	**12,573**	**14,649**	**12,198**	**54,862**

* Summer tuition is charged after the spring quarter of the fourth year.

SELECTION FACTORS

Selection of applicants is very competitive and is made without regard to sex, race, color, creed, religion, or national origin. Decisions are based on objective and subjective components. Major consideration is given to objective components such as college academic records and DAT scores. Subjective components include: knowledge of the profession, communication skills, integrity, motivation, leadership, maturity, overcoming adversity, and social awareness. Also included are recommendations of preprofessional advisors and faculty and a personal interview with members of the Admissions Committee. Preference is given to legal residents of Mississippi, and all applicants must be U.S. citizens.

See chapter 3 of this guide for information regarding numbers of applicants and enrollees to each dental school, along with their race, gender, age, type of predental education, mean DAT and GPA, and state of origin.

ACADEMIC AND OTHER ASSISTANCE

The University of Mississippi School of Dentistry sponsors recruitment and retention programs for all students, including students who are members of underrepresented populations in dentistry. These programs include summer enrichment and preparation programs and individual assistance upon request. Upon matriculation, students also benefit from a range of academic and personal support services.

MISSOURI

UNIVERSITY OF MISSOURI-KANSAS CITY
SCHOOL OF DENTISTRY

Dr. Michael J. Reed, Dean

GENERAL INFORMATION

The University of Missouri-Kansas City (UMKC) School of Dentistry is a publicly supported institution located on "Hospital Hill" in midtown Kansas City, a city of half a million located in a metropolitan area of one and three-quarters million people. The Kansas City Dental College (founded in 1881) and the Western Dental College (founded in 1890) merged in 1919 to form the Kansas City-Western Dental College. In 1941 this school joined the University of Kansas City, a private institution. In 1963 the University of Kansas City became part of the University of Missouri. It has the largest and most active alumni association of all dental schools (its annual alumni meeting typically attracts 1,500 D.D.S. registrants). The UMKC School of Dentistry is the only dental school in the University of Missouri system; 100 predoctoral, 30 dental hygiene, and 25 graduate students enter each year. Teaching relationships exist with six hospitals in the Kansas City and adjacent areas, in addition to the UMKC School of Medicine.

ADMISSION REQUIREMENTS

NUMBER OF YEARS OF PREDENTAL EDUCATION: All applicants must have completed the equivalent of a minimum of 90 semester hours at the time of application. Preference is given to candidates who have completed a baccalaureate degree before entry.

LIMITATIONS ON COMMUNITY COLLEGE WORK: No more than 60 hours of college credit can be earned at a community college. Candidates are expected to complete the science prerequisites of a four-year institution.

REQUIRED COURSES: Although no specific college major is required, students must successfully complete all of the following college coursework by the end of the winter/spring semester of the year they wish to begin the dental program:

- Four semesters of biology (general biology 1, anatomy, physiology, and cell biology); other courses that have counterparts in the dental curriculum (such as histology, neuroscience, microbiology) are strongly recommended
- Two semesters (8-10 semester hours) of general chemistry
- Two semesters (8-10 semester hours) of organic chemistry
- Two semesters (8-10 semester hours) of physics
- Two semesters (six semester hours) of English composition

SUGGESTED ADDITIONAL PREPARATION: It is advantageous to have course credit in mathematics, formal logic, biochemistry, business, social/behavioral sciences (such as psychology), communication skills, computer science, the humanities, and applied arts (such as sculpting, jewelry, etc.).

DAT: Required. Must be taken prior to submitting the AADSAS application. A DAT academic average score of at least 17 is preferred to be considered for admission.

GPA: Preference is given to candidates with 90 or more hours of college credit at the time of application with a science GPA of 3.40 or higher and/or a DAT academic average of 17 or higher; the overall GPA will be considered although it will not receive the same weight as the science GPA. A candidate with 90 or more hours of college credit and a science GPA of 3.0 and a DAT academic average of 16 or higher can be considered for interview; the overall GPA will be considered although it will not receive the same weight as the science GPA.

SUBJECTIVE CRITERIA:

1. Investigation of the profession of dentistry: it is strongly suggested that you observe in a minimum of five different dental offices and acquire a minimum of 80-100 hours of observation.
2. Social conscience and compassion evidenced by active and ongoing participation in volunteer activities.
3. Fundamental personal character such as integrity, maturity, self-reliance, and leadership skills.
4. Critical thinking/problem solving ability exhibited in courses involving formal logic or research experiences.
5. Interpersonal communication skills, including speaking, listening, and writing skills.
6. Effective/efficient time management: your ability to balance full academic schedules with extracurricular involvement or employment.

RESIDENCY: The School of Dentistry is state-supported and has a primary responsibility to candidates who are U.S. citizens and permanent residents of Missouri and Kansas. The school has reciprocal or contractual agreements to accept defined numbers of qualified applicants from Arkansas, New Mexico, and Hawaii.

ADVANCED STANDING: An advanced standing program is not available for graduates of foreign dental schools. Transfer applicants from U.S. or Canadian dental schools who are Missouri residents in good standing can be considered only when vacancies occur. Normally, transfer applicants will be placed in the first or second year of study. After recommendation for admission, level of entry will be determined on a space available basis.

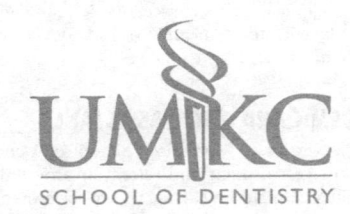

Timetable for the Class Entering Fall 2008

	Earliest Date	Latest Date	School Fee
Application Submission	6/1/07	2/1/08*	$35
Acceptance Notification	12/1/07	2/1/08	

*Preference given to applications received at the school before 11/01/07.

Required Response and Deposit:
30 days after notification if received between 12/1 and 1/31
15 days after notification if received on or after 2/1

$200 to hold position in entering class.

FOR FURTHER INFORMATION

Office of Student Programs
816-235-2080/800-776-8652
UMKC School of Dentistry
650 East 25th Street
Kansas City, MO 64108

Student Financial Aid Office
816-235-1154
University of Missouri-Kansas City
5115 Oak Street
Kansas City, MO 64110

Minority Recruitment Program
816-235-2085/800-776-8652
UMKC School of Dentistry
650 East 25th Street
Kansas City, MO 64108

Off-Campus Housing Association
816-235-1428
University of Missouri-Kansas City
4825 Troost Avenue
Kansas City, MO 64110

www.umkc.edu/dentistry

THE DENTAL PROGRAM

The curriculum (eight semesters, two summer terms) offers an education leading to an effective and enriching career of public service, professional growth, and contribution. The program provides a sound background in the biomedical, behavioral, and clinical sciences with an emphasis on comprehensive oral health care delivered through a "generalist based team" system of clinical education. The early exposure to clinical dentistry and the multidisciplinary, integrated preclinical curriculum are hallmarks of the program.

YEAR 1. The first year focuses on topics in the biomedical sciences that provide a foundation for clinical studies. The first-year student also studies dental behavioral science and introductory courses in oral diagnosis and in dental restorative techniques with associated preclinical laboratories; assists third- and fourth-year students in the dental clinic; and begins the study of preventive dentistry. Early clinical exposure is emphasized with an additional clinic-based course in the first semester (clinical assisting) and another in the second semester (oral diagnosis).

YEAR 2. Biomedical science courses continue, but emphasize preclinical coursework of increasing complexity, including laboratory work. Students continue learning the fundamental procedures in operative dentistry, prosthodontics (fixed and removable), and endodontic therapy. Classroom lecture sessions are conducted in these areas of dentistry along with periodontics, oral diagnosis, oral radiology, and oral surgery. Clinically, second-year students provide oral prophylaxis and disease prevention treatment to patients and begin to perform simple restorative procedures.

YEAR 3. The primary emphasis is clinical practice. The general clinic is organized into three subunits called teams. Each generalist-based team is comprised of faculty with extensive general dentistry experience as well as faculty who represent the clinical disciplines of dentistry. Patients are assigned to students for comprehensive care, from initial oral diagnosis and treatment planning through procedures for successful case completion. Clinical students are assigned operatories for treating their patients. Students also attend advanced classes in periodontics, prosthodontics, oral surgery, orthodontics and dentofacial orthopedics, pediatric dentistry, operative dentistry, and oral diagnosis/oral medicine.

YEAR 4. The fourth year involves extensive clinical practice. There are a few seminars and courses (e.g., practice management), but the students' major responsibility is to perfect diagnostic, patient management, and technical patient treatment skills.

■ Degrees Offered

DENTAL DEGREE: D.D.S.

ADDITIONAL DEGREES: B.S. in Dental Hygiene; M.S. in Dental Hygiene Education; M.S. in Oral Biology; interdisciplinary Ph.D. program; graduate professional certificates in advanced education in general dentistry, oral and maxillofacial radiology, oral and maxillofacial surgery, orthodontics and dentofacial orthopedics, pediatric dentistry, periodontics, and endodontics; and a variety of continuing education courses.

COSTS AND FINANCIAL AID

Estimated Total Expenses for Academic Year 2006-07

	YEAR 1	YEAR 2	YEAR 3	YEAR 4	TOTAL
Tuition, resident	$25,993	$25,993	$32,282	$32,282	$116,550
Tuition, nonresident	$47,766	$47,766	$60,949	$60,949	$217,430
Other expenses					
Fees: student activity, building, etc.	$937	$937	$1,130	$1,130	$4,134
Equipment/books and supplies	$700	$700	$700	$700	$2,800
Estimated living expenses	$18,840	$18,840	$18,840	$18,840	$75,360
TOTAL EXPENSES, RESIDENT	$46,370	$46,370	$52,952	$52,952	$198,644
TOTAL EXPENSES, NONRESIDENT	$68,233	$68,233	$73,622	$75,292	$285,380

Financial Aid Awards to First-Year Students in 2006-07

■ TOTAL NUMBER OF RECIPIENTS: 94   ■ 94% OF CLASS

	Average Award	Range of Awards
Residents	$36,031	$13,100-$59,677
Nonresidents	$46,702	$8,500-$64,522

SELECTION FACTORS

Candidates are chosen after thorough consideration of their college academic record (including the amount, nature, and quality of completed coursework and overall, science GPAs), DAT scores, and the Dental Student Admission Committee's (DSAC) evaluation of the promise of the candidate as a future dentist. In addition, the DSAC considers the general knowledge, maturity, motivation to dentistry, integrity, social awareness, and ability of the applicant to communicate and interact with others. The applicant's concern for the oral health care of others, evidence of time management skills, previous career competence and involvement, and leadership in student or community activities will be included in the evaluation.

Three letters of recommendation are required, with at least one from a faculty member of the academic department in which the applicant has had a major area of study. If there is a prehealth advisory committee at the applicant's school, a letter of recommendation from this committee is required. Personal interviews are granted to those who meet the minimum academic criteria. In addition to the above GPA screening criteria for personal interview, applicants will be evaluated as to whether or not the prerequisite courses have been or can easily be completed during the academic year the application is being considered. For those candidates who meet the minimum criteria, the DSAC will consider the cases individually.

A qualified applicant with experience or training in any of the health care specialties (dental hygiene, dental assisting, dental lab technician, pharmacy, nursing, physical therapy, medicine, etc.) will be given special consideration. The school does not discriminate on the basis of race, gender, creed, or national origin; applications from members of racial/ethnic minority groups (i.e., those underrepresented in the dental profession) and women are strongly encouraged.

See chapter 3 of this guide for information regarding numbers of applicants and enrollees to each dental school, along with their race, gender, age, type of predental education, mean DAT and GPA, and state of origin.

ACADEMIC AND OTHER ASSISTANCE

Academic support systems include continuous academic monitoring, study/test-taking skills, relaxation training, and an Instructional Resources Library. Nonacademic support systems include housing referrals, financial aid assistance/referral, counseling assistance/referral, and verification services. Certain academic assistance, such as tutoring and counseling, are available as needed at the school. Specific programs for women, racial/ethnic minorities, or other special students are available.

CREIGHTON UNIVERSITY
SCHOOL OF DENTISTRY

Dr. Steven W. Friedrichsen, Dean

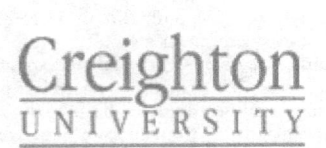

GENERAL INFORMATION

Creighton University, a private Jesuit school with a total enrollment of approximately 6,700 students, is one of the most diverse educational institutions of its size in the nation. In addition to the College of Arts and Sciences, Creighton conducts a College of Business Administration and Schools of Law, Dentistry, Medicine, Pharmacy, Nursing, Allied Health, and Graduate Studies. It is located in Omaha, Nebraska, a city of 400,000 and a metropolitan area of 700,000.

Creighton University was founded in 1878, and the School of Dentistry was established in 1905. Completed in 1973, the dental facility is a modern, three-level, 150,000-square foot structure containing classrooms, teaching and research laboratories, and clinics with over 175 patient treatment stations. The School of Dentistry completed a five-year renovation program of classrooms, laboratories, and clinical operatories in the summer of 1998. The teaching hospital offers additional clinical facilities. The award-winning Bio-Information Center, which serves all the health science schools and the hospital, is directly connected to the School of Dentistry. It is comprised of a Bio-Medical Communications Center, the Health Sciences Learning Resources Center, and the Health Sciences Library. Described as the most "user-oriented" facility of its kind in the country, it offers a variety of services and is open 105 hours each week. In addition, the School of Dentistry is affiliated with a number of area hospitals and maintains a close working relationship with the other health science schools by participating in a Health Sciences Management Team and sharing health sciences faculty.

The major effort of the School of Dentistry is directed toward its education program leading to the D.D.S. degree. Creighton does, however, offer continuing dental education courses and cooperates with several local junior colleges in the training of dental auxiliaries. In addition, Creighton conducts research, provides dental health and dental health education services to the local community, and participates in an outreach program to the Dominican Republic.

Creighton School of Dentistry is a regional resource. Creighton students come from all parts of the United States, its territories, and some foreign countries. Creighton has traditionally served the dental health education needs of a number of states that do not have schools of dentistry and is currently engaged in compacts with the states of Idaho, New Mexico, North Dakota, Utah, and Wyoming. Idaho residents enrolled in IDEP can enroll in either Creighton University or Idaho State University for their freshman year. Utah residents who are eligible for consideration in RDEP can enroll in either Creighton University or the University of Utah for their freshman year. Students from compact states receive a substantial tuition remission.

ADMISSION REQUIREMENTS

NUMBER OF YEARS OF PREDENTAL EDUCATION: Formal minimum of two (64 semester hours); generally acceptable minimum of four (120 semester hours).

LIMITATIONS ON COMMUNITY COLLEGE WORK: None.

REQUIRED COURSES:

With lab required	(semester/quarter hrs)
Inorganic chemistry	8/12
Organic chemistry	6/9
Biology*	6/9

Other courses	
English	6/9
Physics	6/9

*Zoology is an acceptable alternative.

SUGGESTED ADDITIONAL PREPARATION: Courses in psychology, modern languages, history, speech, economics, biochemistry and comparative anatomy are recommended. Programs that contribute to the applicant's total development are encouraged.

DAT: No test date or minimum score requirement.

GPA: No specific requirements.

RESIDENCY: No specific requirements.

ADVANCED STANDING: Students transferring from U.S. and Canadian schools may be admitted with advanced standing. Foreign dental graduates may be considered for advanced standing, the maximum level of entry being the third year.

Timetable for the Class Entering Fall 2008

	Earliest Date	Latest Date	School Fee
Application Submission	7/1/07	4/1/08	$45
Acceptance Notification	12/1/07	8/20/08	

Required Response and Deposit:
45 days after notification if received between 12/1 and 12/31
30 days after notification if received between 1/1 and 1/31
15 days after notification if received after 2/1

$500 initial deposit to hold place and $300 final deposit when all coursework is completed and final acceptance has been received; both deposits credited toward tuition and nonrefundable.

FOR FURTHER INFORMATION

Admissions
402-280-2695; 800-544-5072
denschadm@creighton.edu
Creighton University School of Dentistry
Creighton Dental Admissions Office
2500 California Plaza
Omaha, NE 68178

Financial Aid
Director of Financial Aid
402-280-2731; 800-282-5835

Minority Affairs
Director of Multicultural and Community Affairs
402-280-2981

Housing
Director of Student Housing
402-280-3016

cudental.creighton.edu

THE DENTAL PROGRAM

The basic goal of the School of Dentistry is to provide primary care practitioners to address the oral health needs of society, particularly the segment of society that experiences inadequate dental health perpetuated by isolation and the absence or unavailability of dental health education facilities. In the fulfillment of this basic goal, the institution addresses its efforts to the following primary objective: to educate dental practitioners who are biologically oriented, clinically competent, socially sensitive, and ethically and morally responsible. As part of a Jesuit institution, adhering to the fundamental principles set forth by the Society of Jesus during its almost five centuries of existence, the school promotes a value orientation that is Judeo-Christian in philosophy. Incidental to the education program, the school attempts to provide an environment complementary to the development of the whole person.

The four-year program is designed to provide maximum opportunity for clinical application of basic concepts. Essentially, the curriculum is a progression of experiences from basic and preclinical sciences to mastery of clinical skills. Basic sciences are cooperatively taught by both dental and medical school faculty under the aegis of the Department of Oral Biology. Clinical sciences are taught by full-time clinical faculty with the assistance of part-time faculty. The full-time faculty, representing both basic and clinical science disciplines by training and experience, ensure integration of basic and clinical sciences. The part-time faculty bring extensive and varied experience, based on their own private practices, to add another dimension to the program and to reinforce the concepts being taught.

YEAR 1. Basic and preclinical sciences with introduction to clinical situations.

YEAR 2. Continuation of basic and preclinical sciences with more emphasis on preclinical technique courses and introduction of definitive patient care.

YEAR 3. Continuation of clinical courses, initiation of practice management curriculum, and comprehensive clinical care.

YEAR 4. Continuation of clinical and practice management coursework and delivery of comprehensive dental care that attempts to approximate private practice; senior elective courses also available.

■ Degree Offered
DENTAL DEGREE: D.D.S.

■ Other Programs
RESEARCH: Opportunities to participate in research conducted by the School of Dentistry are available through the Associate Dean for Research Office.

FELLOWSHIPS: A limited number are available for academically outstanding students.

EXTERNSHIPS: Available to third- and fourth-year students only.

COSTS AND FINANCIAL AID

The Financial Aid Office is committed to employing every available means in aiding prospective students to meet the expenses of dental education. In addition to federal loan programs, smaller university-based loans and scholarships are available. Student employment is permitted, provided it does not impede academic performance or interfere with clinical activity. Entering students may request financial assistance information and application material any time after confirmation of acceptance by writing to the director of financial aid.

Financial Aid Awards to First-Year Students in 2006-07
■ TOTAL NUMBER OF RECIPIENTS: 79   ■ 94% OF CLASS

	Average Award	Range of Awards
Residents	$50,250	$1,000-$70,050
Nonresidents	$50,250	$1,000-$70,050

Estimated Total Expenses for Academic Year 2006-07

	YEAR 1	YEAR 2	YEAR 3	YEAR 4	TOTAL
Tuition, resident and nonresident	$39,090	$39,090	$39,090	$39,090	$156,360
Other expenses					
Student health insurance*	$1,732	$1,732	$1,732	$1,732	$6,928
University fee	$760	$760	$760	$760	$3,040
HEP vaccination	$230	0	0	0	$230
Instruments	$4,700	$5,400	$3,104	$3,104	$16,308
Books and manual	$1,200	$1,200	$1,000	$540	$3,940
Estimated living expenses					
Room/board	$13,500	$16,500	$16,500	$13,500	$60,000
	(9 mos.)	(11 mos.)	(11 mos.)	(9 mos.)	
TOTAL EXPENSES, RESIDENT AND NONRESIDENT	$61,212	$64,682	$61,186	$58,726	$245,806

*Mandatory if not covered by another plan.

SELECTION FACTORS

It is the policy of Creighton University to accept all qualified students whom its facilities and resources will accommodate, regardless of race, color, national origin, gender, or religion and to administer its education policies, scholarship and loan programs, and other programs without any such discrimination. All applicants are considered for admission on the basis of their potential to successfully complete the predoctoral program without compromise of the established standards of academic and clinical performance expected of all graduates of the School of Dentistry and their potential to best serve the needs of society.

Selection of all students is based upon both objective and subjective evaluation. Objective criteria include GPA, DAT scores, and science grades. Applicants with higher scores and satisfactory subjective evaluation are given primary consideration. However, applicants with lesser objective qualifications are considered on the basis of more subjective factors, such as: 1) evidence of predisposition to provide dental health care in underserved areas; 2) evidence of participation in worthwhile community activities; 3) recommendation from teachers, known alumni, and other members of the profession; 4) quality of preprofessional educational program; 5) residence in states having educational compact agreements with the school; and 6) evidence of good moral character, motivation, and emotional and intellectual maturity.

See chapter 3 of this guide for information regarding numbers of applicants and enrollees to each dental school, along with their race, gender, age, type of predental education, mean DAT and GPA, and state of origin.

ACADEMIC AND OTHER ASSISTANCE

Creighton University sponsors recruitment and retention programs for all students including those who are members of underrepresented populations in dentistry. These programs include summer enrichment and preparation programs, a postbaccalaureate program for disadvantaged students, and individual assistance upon request.

NEBRASKA

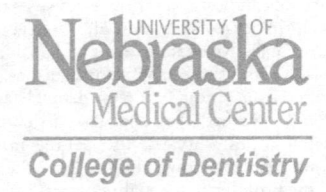

UNIVERSITY OF NEBRASKA MEDICAL CENTER
COLLEGE OF DENTISTRY

Dr. John W. Reinhardt, Dean

GENERAL INFORMATION

The College of Dentistry, University of Nebraska Medical Center (UNMC) is a public institution. The Lincoln Dental College was founded in 1899 and was operated as a private school until 1917, when it became affiliated with the University of Nebraska. The college became part of the university's Medical Center on July 1, 1979. The college is located in Lincoln, Nebraska (population 200,000). The total number of students enrolled is 270, including 48 students enrolled in a two-year dental hygiene program and 50 postgraduate and graduate students. Postgraduate dental programs are offered in endodontics, general practice residency, prosthodontics, advanced education in general dentistry, orthodontics, pediatric dentistry, and periodontics. A graduate program in dentistry leads to a clinically oriented M.S. degree. A graduate program in the oral biology department leads to a more traditional M.S. or Ph.D. degree. The postgraduate programs in general practice and pediatric dentistry are located primarily at the UNMC University Hospital in Omaha. The residency program in periodontics is associated with the Veterans Administration Hospital in Lincoln. The college currently has dental education contracts with the states of Wyoming and North Dakota.

ADMISSION REQUIREMENTS

NUMBER OF YEARS OF PREDENTAL EDUCATION: Three years (90 semester or 134 quarter hours).

LIMITATIONS ON COMMUNITY COLLEGE WORK: None.

REQUIRED COURSES:*

With lab required	(semester/quarter hrs)
Inorganic chemistry	8/12
Organic chemistry	8/12
Biology or zoology	8/12
Physics	8-10/12-15

Other courses	
English composition	6/9

*No pass/fail courses accepted.

SUGGESTED ADDITIONAL PREPARATION: Completion of a three-year postsecondary program of 90 semester hours of credit represents the minimum requirement for matriculation. The required courses can generally be completed in the first two years of college. Therefore, while completing the three years of college, students are encouraged to work toward a baccalaureate degree in their chosen field of interest, since admission cannot be assured. The average number of postsecondary hours (130 semester hours) completed by the entering class is high. Sixty percent of these students have earned a baccalaureate degree. All students will be considered for acceptance to only the class for which they have applied.

DAT: Recommended to be taken no later than October 2007; see Selection Factors.

GPA: See Selection Factors.

RESIDENCY: See Selection Factors.

ADVANCED STANDING: Applicants will be required to have completed a 24-month minimum postgraduate program in a clinically related dental discipline at an ADA-accredited institute in the United States or Canada before being eligible to matriculate at the College of Dentistry.

Timetable for the Class Entering Fall 2008

	Earliest Date	Latest Date	School Fee
Application Submission	5/15/07	1/1/08	$50
Acceptance Notification	12/1/07	5/1/08	$200

Required Response:
45 days after notification if received between 12/1 and 12/31
30 days after notification if received between 1/1 and 1/31
15 days after notification if received after 2/1

FOR FURTHER INFORMATION

Office of Admissions
402-472-1363
University of Nebraska Medical Center
College of Dentistry
40th & Holdrege
Lincoln, NE 68583-0740

Office of Financial Aid
Judith Walker
402-559-4199
984265 Nebraska Medical Center
Omaha, NE 68198-4265

Minority Student Affairs Office
402-559-4437
University of Nebraska Medical Center
Student Life Center
42nd & Dewey
Omaha, NE 68105-4275

unmc.edu/dentistry

THE DENTAL PROGRAM

The dental program is 44.5 months in duration, with 36.5 months in actual attendance. There are eight semesters of 16 weeks each. In addition, attendance is required at three summer sessions (eight weeks each), one between each academic year until graduation.

Objectives of the college are to: 1) select applicants who have the personal and moral qualifications, technical potential, and scholastic ability for a professional career in dentistry; 2) provide, within a flexible curriculum, a solid foundation of fundamental scientific knowledge and the basic technical skills necessary for using this education; 3) motivate students to recognize and fulfill their social and moral responsibilities to their patients, their civic responsibility to the community, and their ethical obligation to the profession of dentistry; and 4) inspire students to see the need for continuing education and for personal and professional evaluation throughout their dental careers.

The basic sciences are taught during the first two years of the dental curriculum. Students are introduced to clinical observation and personal participation during the first year. Patients are assigned and clinical activity is amplified in the sophomore year. Integration of basic and clinical sciences is achieved each day as the faculty evaluates and teaches the student's clinical activity. Off-campus clinical experiences are scheduled via institutional assignments and a rural rotation program. Research projects may be undertaken while students are in school. Several courses have the self-pacing feature, and electives may be assigned during the senior year. The clinical program is designed to familiarize the students with all aspects of total patient care. A learning center is available where the computer facilities and development programs are located.

■ Degree Offered
DENTAL DEGREE: D.D.S.

■ Other Programs
The opportunity exists for concurrent studies leading to an M.S. or Ph.D.

COSTS AND FINANCIAL AID

Estimated Total Expenses for Academic Year 2006-07

	YEAR 1	YEAR 2	YEAR 3	YEAR 4	TOTAL
Tuition, resident	$18,205	$18,205	$18,205	$14,561	$69,179
Tuition, nonresident	$49,182	$49,182	$49,182	$39,346	$186,892
Other expenses					
Student fees	$1,120	$1,070	$1,070	$813	$4,073
Equipment: books and instruments	$8,030	$8,030	$8,030	$8,030	$32,120
Estimated living expenses	$18,000	$18,000	$18,000	$13,500	$67,500
TOTAL EXPENSES, RESIDENT	$45,355	$45,305	$45,305	$41,404	$77,369
TOTAL EXPENSES, NONRESIDENT	$76,332	$76,282	$76,282	$66,189	$295,085

Financial Aid Awards to First-Year Students in 2006-07

■ NUMBER OF RECIPIENTS: Residents: 33; Nonresidents: 13

	Average Award	Range of Awards
Residents	$42,468	$398-$50,855
Nonresidents	$75,303	$62,976-$77,671

SELECTION FACTORS

The college has no specific requirements regarding the absolute minimal scholastic average or DAT scores. In some cases, applicants who have a low scholastic average will be evaluated on their performance over the last three or four semesters of college. Applicants in this situation should have included some science courses in their schedule, with a suggested load of 14-16 hours per semester, and shown significant scholastic improvement.

Students must possess the intellectual capability, emotional adaptability and stability, and social and perceptual skills, along with the physical capability to observe, communicate, and perform the motor skills, to satisfactorily complete the full curriculum.

International students may be considered for admission who are academically prepared. Nonimmigrant foreign students who want to be issued Form 1-20 (certificate of eligibility for a student visa) must meet the following requirements before they can be considered for admission: 1) supply official or certified transcripts, mark sheets, and degree statements from all institutions they have attended; 2) furnish evidence of adequate financial resources for self-support required of each foreign student; 3) demonstrate English proficiency for students whose first language is not English by a TOEFL score of at least 575 or an appropriate equivalent; and 4) complete at least one academic year at an accredited college or university in the United States prior to application for admission.

Students under serious consideration will be contacted to arrange a personal interview with the Admissions Committee. Personal interviews are required for those applicants chosen for admission or the position of alternate to the entering class. The UNMC College of Dentistry is an equal opportunity institution and does not discriminate on the basis of gender, disability, race, color, religion, marital or veteran status, or national or ethnic origin. The University of Nebraska supports Affirmative Action programs. The scholastic quality over the last ten years shows the average GPA of accepted students was 3.6. The College of Dentistry does not require letters of recommendation; however, evaluation of a student's progress and potential by a predental adviser or committee is appreciated.

See chapter 3 of this guide for information regarding numbers of applicants and enrollees to each dental school, along with their race, gender, age, type of predental education, mean DAT and GPA, and state of origin.

ACADEMIC AND OTHER ASSISTANCE

Counseling is available for underrepresented minority applicants. Tutoring is available for students who need it.

UNIVERSITY OF NEVADA, LAS VEGAS
SCHOOL OF DENTAL MEDICINE

Dr. Karen P. West, Dean

GENERAL INFORMATION

The University of Nevada, Las Vegas School of Dental Medicine is located on the new UNLV Shadow Lane Campus. This 18.2 acre campus is shared with the university's Biotechnology Center, with the dental school occupying over 110,000 square feet of space and equipped with more than 165 patient treatment areas. This campus is just several miles from the main UNLV campus, which is located on a beautifully landscaped 335 acres of land. Since its founding in 1957, UNLV has seen dramatic growth in its student population and its academic programs. UNLV consists of 12 colleges offering over 22,000 students more than 148 undergraduate, master's, and doctoral degree programs.

Las Vegas is one of the country's fastest growing metropolitan areas. Averaging 310 days of sunshine per year, Las Vegas lies in a desert valley surrounded by mountains and offers abundant recreational opportunities. The surrounding area is one of the Southwest's most picturesque, offering outdoor recreation year-round at such areas as Lake Mead, Red Rock Canyon, Brian Head Ski Resort, and the Grand Canyon. The area also offers cultural events including concerts, plays, art exhibits, and a Shakespearean Festival.

The UNLV School of Dental Medicine's first class started in September 2002.

ADMISSION REQUIREMENTS

NUMBER OF YEARS OF PREDENTAL EDUCATION: Formal minimum of three years (90 semester units); bachelor's degree preferred.

LIMITATIONS ON COMMUNITY COLLEGE WORK: Maximum of 60 semester hours.

REQUIRED COURSES:

With lab required	(semester hrs)
Biology	8
General chemistry	8
Organic chemistry	8
Physics	8
Other courses	
English	6
Biochemistry	3

SUGGESTED ADDITIONAL PREPARATION: It is strongly suggested that students take additional science courses in human or comparative anatomy, physiology, microbiology, histology, and genetics. Communication, art, sculpture, and business courses are also recommended. Computer skills are highly desirable.

DAT: Mandatory; recommended to be taken no later than October 2007. Test scores must not be older than three years.

GPA: No specific requirements.

RESIDENCY: No specific requirements.

ADVANCED STANDING: None.

Timetable for the Class Entering Fall 2008

	Earliest Date	Latest Date	School Fee
Application Submission	6/1/07	2/1/08	$50
Acceptance Notification	12/1/07		

Required Response and Deposit:
45 days after notification if received between 12/1 and 12/31
30 days if received between 1/1 and 1/31
15 days after 2/1

$500 due with acceptance letter is applied toward tuition and is nonrefundable. A second nonrefundable deposit of $500 is due on June 1.

FOR FURTHER INFORMATION

Office of Admissions
Christine C. Ancajas
Director
702-774-2520

Office of Financial Aid
Jodi L. Gerber
Senior Coordinator of Student Enrollment,
Client Services
702-774-2526

Office of Student Services
Marshall P. Brownstein
Associate Dean for Student Affairs
702-774-2520

UNLV School of Dental Medicine
1001 Shadow Lane, MS7410
Las Vegas, NV 89106-4124

dentalschool.unlv.edu

THE DENTAL PROGRAM

MISSION. The UNLV School of Dental Medicine will be a driving force toward improving the health of the citizens of Nevada through unique programs of oral health care services to the community, integrated biomedical, professional, and clinical curricula, and biomedical discovery. The school's vision statement is "Toward Perfect Health Through Oral Health."

The goals of the school will be achieved in the following areas:

- **Patient Care and Service**
  Provide excellence in patient-centered clinical care, patient education, and statewide community outreach programs.
- **Education**
  Implement a vertical and horizontal curriculum that integrates biomedical sciences, professional studies, and clinical sciences to ensure competent and contemporary oral health care providers.
- **Scholarship**
  Provide an environment productive of collaborative research and other scholarly activities.
- **Faculty Development**
  Cultivate a faculty of excellence through a unique program of professional academic opportunities, internal development, recruitment, and retention.

■ Degrees Offered

DENTAL DEGREE: D.M.D.

ALTERNATE DEGREE: D.M.D./M.B.A.

COSTS AND FINANCIAL AID

Note that the expenses below are for students living off campus. For students living on campus or with parents, the estimated living expenses will be lower. The costs of tuition and fees may increase in future years.

Estimated Total Expenses for Academic Year 2006-07

	YEAR 1	YEAR 2	YEAR 3	YEAR 4	TOTAL
Tuition, resident	$30,825	$30,825	$30,825	$30,825	$123,300
Tuition, nonresident	$53,325	$53,325	$53,325	$53,325	$213,300
Books and supplies	$6,400	$6,400	$6,400	$6,400	$25,600
Estimated living expenses (room, board, transportation, and personal)*	$16,359	$16,359	$16,359	$16,359	$65,436
Loan fees	$680	$680	$680	$680	$2,720
Laptop computer**	$2,500	0	0	0	$2,500
TOTAL EXPENSES, RESIDENT	$56,764	$54,264	$54,264	$54,264	$219,556
TOTAL EXPENSES, NONRESIDENT*	$79,964	$77,464	$77,464	$77,464	$312,356

*An additional $700 is allocated for living expenses for nonresident students.
**Required of new students.

SELECTION FACTORS

Applicants to the School of Dental Medicine will be evaluated by an admissions committee composed of faculty members. Selection factors will include academic achievement, DAT scores, letters of recommendation from a preprofessional committee or individual professors, interview, commitment and motivation, interpersonal skills, work experience, community service, and the number of semester units in college. Additionally, applicants will be required to obtain a letter of recommendation from a dentist whom they have observed or worked for.

As a public institution, UNLV gives preference to Nevada residents. Out-of-state residents are strongly encouraged to apply. However, preference will be given to those applicants from states without dental schools.

The University of Nevada, Las Vegas is committed to ensuring that all programs and activities are readily accessible to all eligible persons without regard to race, color, religion, gender, national origin, ancestry, disability, Vietnam-era and/or disabled veteran status, protected class under relevant state and federal laws, and, in accordance with university policy, sexual orientation.

See chapter 3 of this guide for information regarding numbers of applicants and enrollees to each dental school, along with their race, gender, age, type of predental education, mean DAT and GPA, and state of origin.

NEW JERSEY

UNIVERSITY OF MEDICINE AND DENTISTRY OF NEW JERSEY
THE NEW JERSEY DENTAL SCHOOL

Dr. Cecile A. Feldman, Dean

GENERAL INFORMATION

Created by the state legislature in 1970, the University of Medicine and Dentistry of New Jersey (UMDNJ) is now a statewide network of academic health centers that includes eight schools on five campuses, enrolling more than 4,500 students. With a network of more than 100 affiliates, teaching hospitals, and educational partners spanning the state, UMDNJ touches the lives of almost every New Jerseyan every day. It is dedicated to the pursuit of excellence in the education of health professionals and scientists, the conduct of research, the delivery of health care, and service to the people of New Jersey.

The New Jersey Dental School (NJDS), one of the eight health professional schools of UMDNJ, graduated its first class of students over four decades ago. The school was established as part of the Seton Hall College of Medicine and Dentistry, admitting its first students in 1956. The school has since grown into the state's major resource for dental education, research, and community service.

The first class for the D.D.S. degree was admitted in 1956 and graduated in 1960. The class of 1965 was the first to receive the D.M.D. degree. The dental school moved to new facilities in Newark in 1976. The dental school offers graduate dental educational specialty training in six areas: Endodontics, Orthodontics, Pediatric Dentistry, Periodontics, Prosthodontics, and Advanced Education in General Dentistry. Hospital residencies are offered in General Practice and in Oral and Maxillofacial Surgery (which leads to a Doctor of Medicine degree). A fellowship in Oral Medicine is also available. The dental school serves as a clinical training site for programs of the UMDNJ-School of Health Related Professions in dental assisting and dental hygiene.

New Jersey Dental School maintains an impressive 6-to-1 ratio of students to faculty. The internationally recognized faculty has been recruited from throughout the country and abroad. In addition to the unique e-curriculum—a schoolwide wireless network of educational resources designed to provide students with instant access to course materials, computer-aided instruction, clinical information, email, and the World Wide Web—the basic, clinical, and behavioral sciences curriculum includes extramural programs, hospital dentistry, selective/elective programs, and instruction in the utilization of dental auxiliaries in the treatment of patients.

ADMISSION REQUIREMENTS

NUMBER OF YEARS OF PREDENTAL EDUCATION: Formal minimum of three; usual minimum of four.

REQUIRED COURSES:

With lab required (semester/quarter hrs)
Inorganic chemistry	8/16
Organic chemistry	8/16
Biology	8/16
Physics	8/16

Other courses
English	6/12

Electives sufficient to complete three full years of study.

SUGGESTED ADDITIONAL PREPARATION: A strong background in the natural sciences is essential both as a criterion for admission and as a basis for successful performance in dental school.

DAT: Mandatory. For the class that entered in 2006, the average of the Academic Average section was 19.28. For the class that entered in 2005, the average of the Academic Average section was 19.31.

GPA: For the class that entered in 2006, the average GPA was 3.47. For the class that entered in 2005, the average GPA was 3.53.

RESIDENCY: Applicants must be citizens of the United States or possess a green card as a permanent resident of the United States.

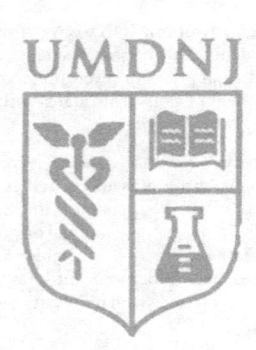

Timetable for the Class Entering Fall 2008

	Earliest Date	Latest Date	School Fee
Application Submission	6/1/07	2/1/08	$75
Acceptance Notification	12/1/07	First day of orientation	

Required Response and Deposit:
45 days after notification if received between 12/1 and 12/31
30 days after notification if received between 1/1 and 1/31

$1,000 initial deposit; $1,000 subsequent deposit due 5/1/08.

FOR FURTHER INFORMATION
Office of Admissions
Jeffrey Linfante
Director of Admissions and Recruitment
973-972-1614; linfante@umdnj.edu

Kathleen Wood
Admissions Coordinator
973-972-5362; kathy.wood@umdnj.edu

UMDNJ-New Jersey Dental School
110 Bergen Street, Room B-830
Newark, NJ 07103-2400

Office of Student Financial Aid
Cheryl White
Associate Director
973-972-4376
UMDNJ-New Jersey Dental School
30 Bergen Street, ADMC #1208
Newark, NJ 07107-3000

Office of Multicultural Affairs
Rosa Chaviano-Moran
Director
973-972-1103
UMDNJ-New Jersey Dental School
110 Bergen Street, Room B-829
Newark, NJ 07103-2400

Housing
973-972-8796
UMDNJ-New Jersey Dental School
110 Bergen Street, Room B-829
Newark, NJ 07103-2400

dentalschool.umdnj.edu

THE DENTAL PROGRAM

UMDNJ-New Jersey Dental School is a publicly supported institution. Its mission is to promote professional standards of excellence among its students, faculty, and staff in meeting the health needs of New Jersey citizens through the coordination of education, research, and service.

The goal of the dental curriculum is to prepare competent general practitioners who are able to manage the oral health care of the public. The curriculum will also provide a foundation for graduates who seek advanced training in the dental specialties, biomedical research, and/or dental education. To accomplish this, graduates must understand the interrelationship of the biological, physical, clinical, and behavioral sciences to effectively practice three overlapping areas of professional responsibility: 1) comprehensive patient care; 2) participation in community dental health programs; and 3) continuation of professional development.

YEAR 1. Basic sciences with introduction to clinical dentistry.

YEAR 2. Additional basic sciences and patient treatment.

YEAR 3. Continued didactic education paired with clinical rotations.

YEAR 4. Comprehensive dental care with a family of patients.

■ Degrees Offered

DENTAL DEGREE: D.M.D.

ALTERNATE DEGREES: B.S./D.M.D. with the following schools:

- Caldwell College
- Fairleigh Dickinson University
- New Jersey City University
- Montclair State University
- New Jersey Institute of Technology
- Ramapo College
- Richard Stockton College
- Rowan University
- Rutgers University
- St. Peters College
- Stevens Institute of Technology

Combined (with UMDNJ-Graduate School of Biomedical Sciences) D.M.D./Ph.D. program in biomedical sciences: anatomy, cell biology, and injury science; biochemistry and molecular biology; neurosciences; microbiology and molecular genetics; laboratory medicine and pathology; pharmacology and toxicology; physiology.

Combined (with UMDNJ-School of Public Health) D.M.D./M.P.H.

■ Other Programs

SUMMER RESEARCH FELLOWSHIPS: Available to all students.

EXTERNSHIPS: Available to fourth-year students only.

COSTS AND FINANCIAL AID

Because of frequent and major changes in the eligibility guidelines for financial aid, the information given here is general. More specific information is given to applicants at the time of their interviews. Financial aid packets with current requirements and forms are sent to all accepted applicants and distributed to all continuing students. For more information, contact the Financial Aid Office.

SELECTION FACTORS

Applicants are interviewed only at the discretion of the Admissions Committee. No candidate will be accepted without an interview. An interview is granted based on undergraduate science and overall grade point averages, DAT scores, and recommendations. There are no restrictions placed on prospective applicants because of their color, creed, race, gender, age, marital status, or national origin. Admission of disabled students is governed by the University Policy on the Americans with Disabilities Act.

See chapter 3 of this guide for information regarding numbers of applicants and enrollees to each dental school, along with their race, gender, age, type of predental education, mean DAT and GPA, and state of origin.

ACADEMIC AND OTHER ASSISTANCE

The school sponsors recruitment and retention programs for all students, including students who are members of underrepresented minorities. The Students for Medicine and Dentistry Program is for incoming first-year students and is a comprehensive introduction to basic and clinical sciences and study skills. It is held during the summer prior to first-year matriculation. Upon matriculation, students will find various academic and personal support services available. For example, the Foundation of UMDNJ offers more than one million dollars in scholarships for disadvantaged students.

Financial Aid Awards to First-Year Students in 2006-07
■ TOTAL NUMBER OF RECIPIENTS: 87   ■ 96% OF CLASS

Estimated Total Expenses for Academic Year 2006-07

	YEAR 1	YEAR 2	YEAR 3	YEAR 4	TOTAL
Tuition, resident	$22,246	$22,246	$22,246	$22,246	$88,984
Tuition, nonresident	$34,811	$34,811	$34,811	$34,811	$139,244
Other expenses					
UHP health insurance *	$1,917	$1,917	$1,917	$1,917	$7,668
Parking**	$150	$150	$150	$150	$600
Activity fee	$300	$300	$300	$300	$1,200
Student health service fee	$300	$300	$300	$300	$1,200
Criminal background check	$85	0	0	0	$85
DVD $700	$700	$700	$1,500		$3,600
Debit card	$500	$100	$100	$100	$800
Equipment use fee	$2,400	$2,100	$1,800	$1,800	$8,100
Expendable supply fee	$1,859	$1,540	$295	0	$3,694
Gold usage fee	0	$250	0	0	$250
Graduation fee	0	0	0	$80	$80
Handpiece	$2,150	0	$2,150	0	$4,250
Handpiece cassette	$45	0	$45	0	$90
Implant kit	0	$360	0	0	$360
Laptop computer	$1,700	0	0	0	$1,700
Manuals	$232	$174	$185	$84	$675
Surgical scrubs***	$230	0	$161	0	$391
Tooth atlas CD	$115				$115
Technology fee	$325	$325	$325	$325	$1,300
TOTAL EXPENSES, RESIDENT	**$35,254**	**$30,463**	**$30,674**	**$28,802**	**$125,463**
TOTAL EXPENSES, NONRESIDENT	**$47,819**	**$43,028**	**$43,238**	**$41,367**	**$175,452**

*May be waived with proof of alternate insurance.
**Optional.
***Purchased directly from supplier.

The amount of tuition and fees as well as the type of fees are subject to change without notice. A deferred payment plan may be arranged with the Office of Administration and Finance. Although the New Jersey Dental School is on an academic trimester calendar, tuition and fees are assessed on a semester (twice a year) basis. The University's policy on Student Residence and In-State Tuition is at http://www.umdnj.edu/oppmweb/Policies/HTML/StudentServices/00-01-25-15_05.html.

NEW YORK

COLUMBIA UNIVERSITY
COLLEGE OF DENTAL MEDICINE

Dr. Ira B. Lamster, Dean

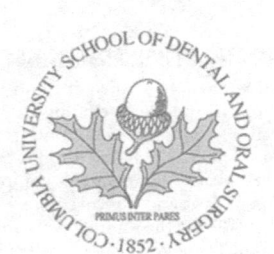

GENERAL INFORMATION

The College of Dental Medicine of Columbia University is a private dental school in the city of New York. The College is an integral part of the world-famous Columbia University Medical Center. It traces its origin to the year 1852, when the New York State legislature chartered the College. The college became the School of Dental and Oral Surgery of Columbia University in 1916, when dentistry was recognized as an integral part of the health sciences and dental education as a true university discipline. Many departments of the university contribute to, and collaborate in, the education of dental and postdoctoral students, and students are thus assured a broad foundation for sound professional development. The educational philosophy of Columbia University is the constant pursuit of excellence. In keeping with this ideal, the primary goal of the College of Dental Medicine is the preparation of graduates equipped to fulfill their obligation to the individual, to society, and to the profession. A special mission of the school is the creation of dental educators, researchers, and policy consultants through several dual degree programs including the M.B.A., M.P.H., Ph.D. in Informatics, and the M.A. in Education with Columbia Teachers College.

The dental/clinical teaching center occupies three floors in the Medical Center and houses the clinics, research facilities, faculty offices, and student facilities for all programs—D.D.S., postdoctoral, and continuing education. Most basic science courses are taken jointly with medical students. The library facilities and lecture, conference, and seminar rooms are shared by all health science programs.

ADMISSION REQUIREMENTS

NUMBER OF YEARS OF PREDENTAL EDUCATION: Preferred minimum of four years; formal minimum of 90 credits, or the equivalent of three years. It is expected that applicants with only 90 credits will have exceptional GPA, DAT scores, and experience.

LIMITATIONS ON COMMUNITY COLLEGE WORK: None.

REQUIRED COURSES:

With lab required	(semester hrs/years)
Organic chemistry	8/1
Biology	8/1
Physics	8/1
Inorganic chemistry	8/1

Other courses	
English composition/literature	6/1

SUGGESTED ADDITIONAL PREPARATION: Coursework in biochemistry is strongly recommended. Courses in chemistry, anatomy, physiology, mathematics, foreign languages, sociology, history, and the fine and industrial arts are also recommended. It is not necessary to complete the academic requirements before applying, but all requirements must be completed before registration.

DAT: Mandatory. Applications are not considered without DAT scores; thus it is advised that applicants take the earliest possible DAT exam.

GPA: 3.3 or above recommended.

RESIDENCY: No requirements.

ADVANCED STANDING: Qualified graduates of non-U.S. dental schools are considered in July for January entrance. Program runs 30 months. Applicants must have official report of scores from National Board, Part I, prior to applying. Call 212-305-3478 for program information.

Timetable for the Class Entering Fall 2008

	Earliest Date	Latest Date	School Fee
Application Submission	7/1/07	1/19/08	$75
Acceptance Notification	12/1/07	8/25/08	

Required Response and Deposit:
45 days after notification if received on or after 12/1
30 days after notification if received on or after 1/1
14 days after notification if received on or after 2/1

$2,000 deposit, nonrefundable, applied toward tuition at time of registration; $1,000 secondary deposit, nonrefundable, due May 1, 2008.

FOR FURTHER INFORMATION
Office of Admissions
Joseph McManus
Assistant Dean for Admissions
212-305-3478
Columbia University
College of Dental Medicine

Office of Student Financial Planning
Sandra Garcia
Assistant Director
212-305-4100

Office of Diversity and Multicultural Affairs
Dennis Mitchell
Associate Dean
212-342-3716

630 West 168th St.
New York, NY 10032

www.dental.columbia.edu

COLUMBIA UNIVERSITY COLLEGE OF DENTAL MEDICINE **NEW YORK**

THE DENTAL PROGRAM

The curriculum at the College of Dental Medicine is unique in both content and approach and is particularly medically oriented. Case-based and problem-based learning is central to the educational approach, as well as small group teaching. Students begin with two years of study in the challenging biomedical-based curriculum; they take courses in dentistry, human anatomy, cell biology, biochemistry, pharmacology, pathophysiology, and physical diagnosis. This provides the knowledge and skills necessary to become a competent 21st-century health care provider. Two three-week duration different hospital rotations include physical evaluation and pathophysiology. In the third year students focus intensively on clinical skills through our mentor model of comprehensive care clinical education, as students work side-by-side with a faculty member who serves as a preceptor.

YEAR 1. Biomedical science classes, concentration on normal human biology; preclinical lab.

YEAR 2. Biomedical science classes, concentration on abnormal human biology; clinical dentistry courses; preclinical lab continues.

YEAR 3. Primarily clinical; area of concentration begins.

YEAR 4. Clinical; independent intramural comprehensive care group practices.

■ Degrees Offered

DENTAL DEGREE: D.D.S.

ADDITIONAL DEGREES: D.D.S/M.A. and D.D.S./Ph.D in Bioinformatics is available. The D.D.S./M.B.A and the D.D.S./M.P.H. programs require joint admission and one additional year to complete the course requirements.

COSTS AND FINANCIAL AID

Estimated Total Expenses for Academic Year 2006-07

	YEAR 1	YEAR 2	YEAR 3	YEAR 4	TOTAL
	10 mos.	10 mos.	12 mos.	10.5 mos.	
Tuition*	$41,609	$41,609	$41,609	$41,609	$166,436
Fees*					
Student health and hospitalization insurance	$3,006	$3,006	$3,006	$3,006	$12,024
Disability insurance	$68	$68	$68	$68	$272
Student activity fee	$210	$210	$210	$210	$840
Dental kit	$3,427	$3,427	$3,427	$3,427	$13,708
Computer access fee	$80	$80	$80	$80	$320
Transcript fee	$75	0	0	0	$75
Educational expenses					
Books and supplies	$1,410	$1,380	$600	$625	$4,015
Dissection kit	$50	0	0	0	$50
Exams*	0	$545	0	$2,080	$2,625
Estimated living expenses					
Housing	$7,255	$8,518	$9,796	$8,944	$34,513
Food	$5,433	$4,799	$5,519	$5,309	$20,790
Clothing, laundry	$818	$820	$941	$860	$3,439
Miscellaneous	$1,782	$1,777	$2,044	$1,871	$7,474
TOTAL EXPENSES	**$65,233**	**$66,238**	**$67,300**	**$67,819**	**$266,580**

*Projected figures, subject to change without notice.

Financial Aid Awards to First-Year Students in 2006-07

■ TOTAL NUMBER OF RECIPIENTS: 67	■ 90% OF CLASS
Average Award (7.8% grant; 92.2% loan)	Range of Awards
$49,280	$14,500-$65,240

SELECTION FACTORS

The College of Dental Medicine seeks a diverse student body that is diverse in gender, geography, ethnicity, and culture, reflecting New York City and our patients. We welcome applications from students of all ethnic and national origins and do not discriminate on the basis of physical disability. Preference is given to applicants with bachelor's degrees from accredited American colleges of arts and sciences. We do not employ any rigid cut-off for grades, DAT scores, etc. Academic and scholastic standing is most important in evaluating an application. Letters of recommendation from predental advisory committees play an important part in elaborating on personal qualities, such as intellectual capacity, social awareness, and motives. The DAT scores help us select from highly recommended applicants with excellent scholastic standing.

Interviews are by invitation only and are mandatory. The Committee on Admissions invites candidates with the above qualifications for an interview. Personality, maturity of expression, English language skills, presentation, and evidence of potential professional growth are ascertained in the interview. We interview approximately 10 percent of all applicants. No telephone interviews will be granted.

The College of Dental Medicine encourages applications from underrepresented and disadvantaged groups. The school has a nationally active program of recruitment and retention aimed at qualified applicants interested in the pursuit of a dental career. More than 20% of enrollees in recent classes have been from student groups underrepresented in dentistry. For further information contact the associate dean for diversity and multicultural affairs.

See chapter 3 of this guide for information regarding numbers of applicants and enrollees to each dental school, along with their race, gender, age, type of predental education, mean DAT and GPA, and state of origin. Columbia University is an international university and we accept applications from qualified students without regard to their country or state of origin.

NEW YORK

NEW YORK UNIVERSITY
COLLEGE OF DENTISTRY

Dr. Richard I. Vogel, Interim Dean

GENERAL INFORMATION

New York University College of Dentistry (NYUCD) is a private institution that offers students the advantage of a metropolitan setting. Founded in 1865, the college is the largest and the third oldest dental school in the United States. The college offers professional training leading to the D.D.S. degree, as well as postgraduate and specialty training.

The College of Dentistry is administered by the David B. Kriser Dental Center, New York University, which is comprised of two buildings located on First Avenue from East 24th Street to East 25th Street in New York City. The Kriser Dental Center houses all of the basic and clinical science departments, research facilities, and 580 clinical operatories in the 11-story Arnold and Marie Schwartz Hall of Dental Sciences and the adjoining K.B. Weissman Clinical Science Building. Additional programs offered include a bachelor's degree and associate degree in dental hygiene, continuing dental education programs, Program for Advanced Study in Dentistry for International Graduates, M.S. program in Oral Biology in collaboration with the New York University Graduate School of Arts & Science, an M.S. in Clinical Research, and an M.S. in Biomaterials.

ADMISSION REQUIREMENTS

NUMBER OF YEARS OF PREDENTAL EDUCATION: A bachelor's degree from an accredited U.S. or Canadian college or university, including all prerequisite courses, DAT, and GPA of 3.1 or higher, or a GPA of 3.5 at an accredited college or university from the U.S. or Canada, with 90 credits including all prerequisite courses.

REQUIRED COURSES:

With lab required	(year/semester hrs)
Inorganic chemistry*	1/6-8
Organic chemistry*	1/6-8
Physics*	1/6-8
Biology**	1/6-8

Other courses	
English*	1/6-8

* Required courses included in the minimum of 90 credits.
** May include a half year of genetics and a half year of botany.

SUGGESTED ADDITIONAL PREPARATION: While a broad undergraduate education with a major in a chosen field is the background of choice, certain courses beyond the minimum requirements are recommended. Courses such as comparative anatomy, histology, embryology, genetics, physics, physiology, and mathematics are strongly recommended.

DAT: Mandatory.

GPA: 3.2 or above.

RESIDENCY: No specific requirement (except for New York state beginning 2007).

ADVANCED PLACEMENT: Consideration is given to students transferring from U.S. and Canadian dental schools for advanced placement in the first or second year of the program only. International dental graduates may be accepted for a three-year program, beginning at the sophomore level.

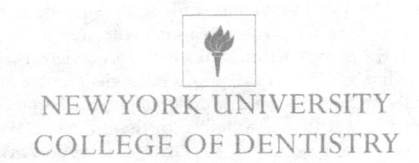

NEW YORK UNIVERSITY
COLLEGE OF DENTISTRY

Timetable for the Class Entering Fall 2008

	Earliest Date	Latest Date	School Fee
Application Submission	7/15/07	3/15/08	$75
Acceptance Notification	12/1/07	8/1/08	

Required Response and Deposit:
*Deposit due in 45 days if accepted on or after 12/1/07
*Deposit due in 30 days if accepted on or after 1/1/08
*Deposit due in 15 days if accepted on or after 2/1/08

*$1,500 initial deposit to hold place. A second deposit of $1,000 is also required.

FOR FURTHER INFORMATION

Office of Student Affairs & Admissions
Eugenia E. Mejia
Director of Admissions
212-998-9818; dental.admissions@nyu.edu

Office of Financial Aid
Tanya Cunningham
212-998-9825; tac2@nyu.edu

Minority Affairs Office
Eugenia E. Mejia
eem1@nyu.edu

New York University
College of Dentistry
345 East 24th Street
New York, NY 10010-4086

nyu.edu/dental

THE DENTAL PROGRAM

NYUCD's educational philosophy is based upon the conviction that "real life" is not the rote of repetition of information; rather, it is the application of knowledge to solve problems associated with disease. Thus, NYUCD has initiated a hands-on approach early in the learning process in combination with a rigorous program that requires critical thinking and problem-solving.

NYU implemented a new curriculum in September 2001. The four-year curriculum is fully integrated and does not teach along traditional departmental structure. The biomedical sciences are taught in three segments over the first three years. The clinical sciences emphasize general dentistry and are also fully integrated. Education is broad in scope, yet focused and applied to real-world problems and issues. Patient contact begins in the first year, and students earn patient care privileges through achievement.

YEAR 1. The D1 year is balanced between the study of Sciences Basic to the Practice of Dentistry and General Dentistry Simulation—an integrated sequence of courses that build foundation skills in dentistry and therapy. Students take an immersion course in the Application of Technology to Health Professions to enable them to use an extensive array of digital resources for inquiry. By the end of the D1 year, students have an excellent understanding of the basic elements of human form and function in health. They will understand health in the United States, major health issues, and problems. They will be based in dentistry as a profession and how dentists maintain the patient's oral health. In addition, the student will have an excellent background in factors relevant to the practice of dentistry, such as clinical records.

YEAR 2. In the D2 year, the biological sciences are directed toward pathology and pathogenesis. The student will gain an excellent background in systemic and oral disease. The D2 curriculum provides an intensive background in the process of data collection, evaluation assessment of risk, and determining the state of a patient's oral health. Esthetics and the management of oral diseases are a major focus. In the General Dentistry Simulation program, students are challenged to do more complex procedures and apply principles to design approaches to unique situations. The role of the dental specialist is explored in the D2 curriculum. The D2 curriculum completes the major components of the skills and knowledge to be utilized by students in the management of their patients.

YEAR 3. In the D3 year, the student devotes the majority of time to the treatment of patients. The entire patient care program is integrated. D3 and D4 students work in Group Practices with a group faculty. This two-year program not only provides an excellent environment for learning and productivity, but D3 students will gain new skills as well as perfecting skills from earlier experiences. A series of courses called Advanced Dental Specialties provides the connections with the dental specialties, the value-added experiences from faculty who are specialists, and the synergy that comes from a collegial group. This patient care setting is productive and enriching, and students can establish a clinical practice in an area where they will remain for two years.

YEAR 4. The capstone of the curriculum is the D4 year. Students' effort is directed toward patient care in a general practice setting. The continuity that is afforded from a two-year contact in the same clinical practice provides important experiences in such areas as health promotion and having opportunities to see the results of treatment. During the D4 year, each student will serve as a Group Practice Coordinator and have the opportunity to provide leadership in the clinical practice. Each student will be given the opportunity to prepare and present the results of a major treatment plan. This case presentation experience will provide valuable insights in patient assessment, therapy, and health promotion. In addition, the curriculum gives coursework for the background necessary and practice in preparation for examination for licensure.

■ Degrees Offered

DENTAL DEGREE: D.D.S.. D.D.S./M.P.H.

ALTERNATE DEGREES: Institutes participating in the B.A./D.D.S. program (seven-year combined degree program) include:

- New Jersey Institute of Technology
- Alfred University
- Caldwell College
- Fairleigh Dickinson University
- University of Hartford
- Manhattanville College
- NYU College of Arts and Sciences
- Mt. Saint Vincent
- Stern College for Women (Yeshiva University)
- Wagner College
- Ramapo College
- Staten Island University
- Saint Francis College
- Tuskegee University (eight-year program)

■ Honors Program

Available to fourth-year students only, this program provides academically outstanding students with the opportunity to receive instruction on an advanced level for one day each week in the following disciplines: implant dentistry, orthodontics, oral and maxillofacial surgery, endodontics, periodontics, and prosthodontics. Students are selected from among the upper 10 percent of the junior class by the appropriate department chairpersons.

COSTS AND FINANCIAL AID

NYUCD offers a limited number of Dean's Academic Enrichment scholarships to applicants who demonstrate academic excellence. Financial aid and awards are based solely on demonstrated financial need and availability of funds. For more information, contact the Financial Aid Office.

SELECTION FACTORS

Selection criteria include the quality of quantity of the undergraduate credits completed. Special emphasis is placed on the grades achieved in the prerequisite courses. Accepted applicants generally have cumulative and science GPAs of 3.2 or higher (A=4.0). Letters of recommendation are required. A pre-health advisors committee letter is preferred, or you may submit three letters from faculty (two must be from the sciences). Ongoing commitment to community service and leadership initiatives is considered in addition to academic performance.

NYUCD does not discriminate on the basis of race, gender, creed, national origin, or financial situation. It is expected that an applicant will be able to offer service to the community for a reasonable period of time; will be healthy enough to withstand the rigorous schedule and study demands of the curriculum; and will be physically able to perform technical dental procedures.

See chapter 3 of this guide for information regarding numbers of applicants and enrollees to each dental school, along with their race, gender, age, type of predental education, mean DAT and GPA, and state of origin.

ACADEMIC AND OTHER ASSISTANCE

NYUCD sponsors recruitment and retention programs for all students, including students who are members of underrepresented populations in dentistry. These programs include individual assistance upon request. Upon matriculation, students also benefit from a range of academic and personal support services.

Financial Aid Awards to First-Year Students in 2006-07
■ TOTAL NUMBER OF RECIPIENTS: 230   ■ 100% OF CLASS

	Average Award (15% grants, 85% loans)	Range of Awards
Residents	$45,500	$7,000-$55,000

Total Expenses for Academic Year 2006-07*

	YEAR 1	YEAR 2	YEAR 3	YEAR 4	TOTAL
Tuition and fees	$49,347	$49,347	$49,347	$49,347	$197,388
Books and Instrument rental	$6,083	$6,083	$6,083	$6,083	$24,332
Estimated living expenses, university housing/meals, personal expenses, transportation, health insurance	$25,779	$30,525	$30,525	$23,406	$110,235
TOTAL EXPENSES	**$81,209**	**$85,955**	**$85,955**	**$78,836**	**$331,955**

*Estimated at time of printing.

STONY BROOK UNIVERSITY
SCHOOL OF DENTAL MEDICINE

Dr. Barry R. Rifkin, Dean

GENERAL INFORMATION

The primary mission of the School of Dental Medicine at Stony Brook University is to graduate dentists who are highly skilled general practitioners, able to integrate clinical, biomedical, and behavioral knowledge to advance the health and well-being of their patients and their communities. They learn to provide compassionate patient-centered care while consistently demonstrating the highest level of professionalism and sensitivity to the diverse personal and cultural contexts in which dental care is delivered. Furthermore, the educational experience encourages students to pursue postdoctoral training in general dentistry, the various clinical specialties, and/or research.

The School of Dental Medicine was established in 1968 and admitted its first class in 1973. It is a component of the Health Sciences Center, which also includes the schools of health, technology and management, medicine, nursing, and social welfare. Stony Brook is a public institution situated about 60 miles east of New York City in Suffolk County, on the wooded north shore of Long Island. From its location at the geographical center of Long Island in the historic village of Stony Brook, both the cultural life of New York City and the tranquil, recreational countryside and seashore of Suffolk County are readily accessible.

The School of Dental Medicine is fully accredited by the Commission on Dental Education and the State Education Department. Admission to the School of Dental Medicine is highly competitive. The grade point averages and Dental Aptitude Test scores of incoming freshmen typically place Stony Brook in the top tier among dental schools in the nation. Dental students take courses in anatomy, biochemistry, microbiology, pathology, pharmacology, and physiology at the medical school along with medical students. In the clinical component of the dental curriculum, students take courses in behavioral sciences, dental anesthesiology, dental materials, dental medicine, endodontics, practice development, operative dentistry, oral biology, oral pathology, oral and maxillofacial surgery, orthodontics, pediatric dentistry, periodontics, and prosthodontics.

The School of Dental Medicine offers postdoctoral education in orthodontics, endodontics, pediatric dentistry, periodontics, and care for the developmentally disabled. A general practice dental residency is offered in conjunction with Stony Brook University Hospital. In addition, the School of Dental Medicine is affiliated with the oral and maxillofacial surgery residency program at Long Island Jewish Medical Center. The Master of Science and Doctor of Philosophy degrees are offered through the Graduate School of Stony Brook University and the School of Dental Medicine's Department of Oral Biology and Pathology.

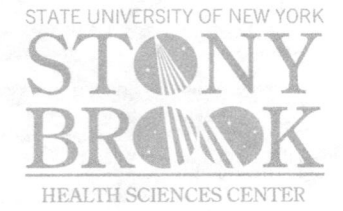

ADMISSION REQUIREMENTS

NUMBER OF YEARS OF PREDENTAL EDUCATION: Minimum of three generally required; bachelor's degree strongly preferred.

LIMITATIONS ON COMMUNITY COLLEGE WORK: Maximum of 60 semester hours, preferably earned prior to the third year of study toward a baccalaureate degree.

REQUIRED COURSES:

With lab required (Full Year)
Biology
Inorganic (general) chemistry
Organic chemistry
Physics

Other courses
Mathematics (calculus or statistics)   6 credits

SUGGESTED ADDITIONAL PREPARATION: Success in dental school is highly correlated with a student's competence in science. Applicants should gain familiarity with the fundamentals of the natural and social sciences that are relevant to the delivery of health care. Virtually all candidates accepted into dental school possess a baccalaureate degree in the arts and sciences. Although preference for admission is not based on a particular field of academic concentration, all candidates are required to demonstrate competence in biology, inorganic and organic chemistry, physics, mathematics, and social and behavioral sciences. It is strongly suggested that applicants also take courses in biochemistry or physiology, the social sciences, and English composition.

DAT: Mandatory.

GPA: 3.0 or above preferred.

ADVANCED STANDING: There is currently no formal advanced standing program.

Timetable for the Class Entering Fall 2008

	Earliest Date	Latest Date	School Fee
Application Submission	7/1/07	1/15/08	$75
Acceptance Notification	12/1/07	8/26/08	$350

Required Response:
30 days if accepted between 12/1 and 12/31
20 days if accepted between 1/1 and 1/31
10 days if accepted on or after 2/1
Applicants accepted after 5/1 may be required to respond within seven days or sooner, depending on proximity to the start of the academic year.

FOR FURTHER INFORMATION

Office of Admissions
Debra Cinotti
Associate Dean for Admissions & Student Affairs
631-632-8871

Office of Financial Aid
Deborah Schade
631-632-3027
Director of Financial Aid

School of Dental Medicine
Stony Brook University
Stony Brook, NY 11794-8709

www.hsc.stonybrook.edu

THE DENTAL PROGRAM

The basic science disciplines are presented primarily in year one and conclude in year two. The dental students take these courses together with the medical students at the medical school. Preclinical training in dentistry also begins in year one. Dental students begin patient care in year two, with extensive clinical training continuing during the third and fourth years. Students are responsible for the complete care of their patients, following a comprehensive care model. The clinical component of the educational program is provided by the departments of children's dentistry, general dentistry, dental medicine, oral biology and pathology, oral and maxillofacial surgery and periodontics. The professional staff closely supervises all phases of patient care.

During the fourth year, students enter the General Practice Program (GPP). The goal of the GPP program is to duplicate as closely as possible the manner in which a general dental practice is conducted. Students conduct their practices in operatories equipped and maintained as private general dental offices. Students are supervised by faculty who are general dentists. When the services of a specialist are required, the student participates in the treatment as provided by the appropriate dental consultant.

The newly renovated clinical facility includes state-of-the-art computerization. Each student operatory is equipped with computerization and functions as a paperless office.

■ Degrees Offered

DENTAL DEGREE: D.D.S.

ALTERNATE DEGREES: Combined D.D.S./M.P.H. program administered through the graduate program in public health at the health sciences center.

M.S. and Ph.D. degrees from the department of Oral Biology and Pathology through the Stony Brook University Graduate School.

Some undergraduate schools may credit certain School of Dental Medicine courses toward a bachelor's degree in cases where students have been accepted to the school with less than the four years of study usually required. Such arrangements must be made by the student directly with the undergraduate school.

COSTS AND FINANCIAL AID

All estimates below are based on charges expected for the current academic year, are subject to change without notice, and are subject to inflation.

Financial Aid Awards to First-Year Students in 2006-07
■ TOTAL NUMBER OF RECIPIENTS: 38   ■ 97% OF CLASS

Estimated Total Expenses for Academic Year 2006-07

	YEAR 1	YEAR 2	YEAR 3	YEAR 4	TOTAL
Tuition, resident	$14,800	$14,800	$14,800	$14,800	$59,200
Tuition, nonresident	$29,600	$29,600	$29,600	$29,600	$118,400
University Fees	$1,058	$840	$1,140	$805	$3,843
Books/computers*	$1,896	$1,283	$810	$1,892	$5,881
Supplies/instruments	$7,007	$7,170	$5,639	$4,166	$23,982
Transportation	$4,700	$4,700	$4,850	$4,650	$18,900
Rent/utilities	$8,250	$8,250	$8,250	$7,500	$32,250
Food/household	$3,850	$3,850	$3,850	$3,500	$15,050
Clothing/laundry	$750	$750	$750	$750	$3,000
Healthcare	$500	$500	$500	$450	$1,950
Personal	$1,000	$1,000	$1,000	$1,000	$4,000
TOTAL EXPENSES, RESIDENT	**$43,811**	**$43,143**	**$41,589**	**$39,513**	**$168,056**
TOTAL EXPENSES, NONRESIDENT	**$58,611**	**$57,943**	**$56,389**	**$54,313**	**$227,256**

*Students entering Year 1 without the required laptop computer can purchase one for up to $2,500 and receive budget and loan increases to accommodate this purchase.

Budgets represent an eleven-month period from September to July for years one through three and a ten-month period from September to June for year four students. All financial aid awarded will be based on the net difference between the standard student budgets as specified and available student/family resources as determined by the Federal Methodology Need Analysis System. The above budget does not include medical insurance costs. University approved medical insurance is mandatory. A required Student Health Insurance fee of $3,036 per year is charged if a student does not have approved private health insurance coverage. A corresponding budget increase and additional financial aid are offered to those charged for health insurance. Student health insurance is nondeferrable

SELECTION FACTORS

The School of Dental Medicine strives to select highly qualified students who are representative of a variety of backgrounds, experiences, and interests. As such, the school is committed to the selection of a student body that is representative of society at large. Selection is based on an overall appraisal of the applicant's suitability for dentistry. Factors such as academic achievement, letters of recommendation, performance on the DAT, and the personal interview are considered in the admission process. As a component of the State University of New York, the School of Dental Medicine gives preference to well-qualified residents from all areas of New York State.

See chapter 3 of this guide for information regarding numbers of applicants and enrollees to each dental school, along with their race, gender, age, type of predental education, mean DAT and GPA, and state of origin.

ACADEMIC AND OTHER ASSISTANCE

The School of Dental Medicine encourages applications from individuals from those groups that have been, in the past, underrepresented in the dental profession or that have been socioeconomically deprived. Because of the small class size, students attending the school are trained in a supportive environment. Tutoring, faculty and peer counseling, and remedial clinic sessions are available to students under special circumstances as determined by the faculty.

NEW YORK

UNIVERSITY AT BUFFALO
SCHOOL OF DENTAL MEDICINE
Dr. Richard N. Buchanan, Dean

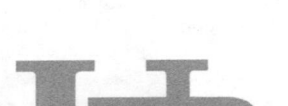

GENERAL INFORMATION

Founded in 1892 by a group of Buffalo physicians and dentists as the fourth unit of the private University of Buffalo, the School of Dental Medicine is now in its second century of serving the dental health care needs of New York State. In 1962, the University of Buffalo was incorporated into the State University of New York, and the School of Dental Medicine, along with the rest of the university, underwent a period of sustained growth. A new North Campus was constructed in suburban Amherst, and the undergraduate program, many of the graduate programs, and the law school were moved to that site. The South Campus, the former main campus of the university, was transformed into a Health Science Center to house the schools of dental medicine, medicine and biomedical sciences, nursing, public health and health professions and, in the near future, pharmacy. In the fall of 1986, the School of Dental Medicine moved to Squire Hall, the fourth location in its history. With over 400 operatories for patient care, Squire Hall is among the most modern facilities for dental education in the country. The School of Dental Medicine is also affiliated with six area hospitals to provide extramural training in oncology, oral and maxillofacial surgery, pediatric dentistry, oral medicine, and restorative dentistry.

Metropolitan Buffalo has a population in excess of 1,250,000. The city has undergone a period of revitalization and now boasts a developing waterfront, a new downtown baseball stadium, a subway system, and a 20,000-seat sports arena. The University at Buffalo is the largest of the four University Centers in the State University System and has an enrollment of nearly 28,000. In addition to dentistry, the university offers professional degree programs in medicine, law, and social work.

ADMISSION REQUIREMENTS

NUMBER OF YEARS OF PREDENTAL EDUCATION: Formal minimum of three; usual minimum of four with a minimum of 60 credit hours (two years of study) at a U.S. or Canadian college or university.

LIMITATIONS ON COMMUNITY COLLEGE WORK: Maximum of 60 semester hours, earned in lower level courses leading to a baccalaureate degree.

REQUIRED COURSES:

With lab required (full-year)
General chemistry
Organic chemistry
General biology
General physics

Other courses (full-year)
English, including composition

SUGGESTED ADDITIONAL PREPARATION: Biochemistry, quantitative chemistry, physical chemistry, developmental biology, genetics, calculus, statistics, social sciences (advanced), and humanities (advanced).

DAT: Mandatory; minimum score of 14 required for the academic average and perceptual ability test scores.

GPA: 3.0 or better.

RESIDENCY: No requirements.

ADVANCED STANDING: Applications for advanced standing are accepted on a space-available basis for the second-year program. To be considered, an applicant must be in good academic standing and have no outstanding "F" grades. The deadline for applications is April 1. Graduates of foreign dental schools who hold citizenship or permanent resident status may be considered for the International Dentist Program. The deadline for application is February 1. Interested individuals should contact Student Admissions at the School of Dental Medicine or visit the school's website at www.sdm.buffalo.edu. Additional information and an online application can be found under Programs of Study.

Timetable for the Class Entering Fall 2008

	Earliest Date	Latest Date	School Fee
Application Submission	5/15/07	2/1/08	$50
Acceptance Notification	12/1/07	8/6/08	

Required Response and Deposit:
30 days after notification if received between 12/1 and 12/31
14 days after notification if received after 1/1

$350 deposit to hold a position in the incoming class (refundable until 4/1)

FOR FURTHER INFORMATION
Office of Student Admissions
Robert B. Joynt
Director of Student Admissions
716-829-2839 or 716-829-2862
joynt@buffalo.edu

Barbara D. Weinberg
Admissions Coordinator
716-829-2839; bdw3@buffalo.edu

Office of Financial Aid
Karen Miller
Director, Student Services
716-829-2839; klmiller@buffalo.edu

University at Buffalo School of Dental Medicine
315 Squire Hall, South Campus
Buffalo, NY 14214

Housing Office
General Housing Information
716-645-2181
University at Buffalo, Richmond Building 4
Elicott Complex, North Campus
Buffalo, NY 14216

www.sdm.buffalo.edu

UNIVERSITY AT BUFFALO SCHOOL OF DENTAL MEDICINE **NEW YORK**

THE DENTAL PROGRAM

The dental curriculum is designed to prepare a student for a career as a practicing dentist. The strong clinical program introduces students to patient care early in their dental school experience. However, with a strong program in the basic sciences and the opportunity to become involved in research while in dental school, a graduate is prepared for a number of career options including specialty training, academics, and research.

YEAR 1. Primary focus on the basic sciences with an introduction to the preclinical courses.

YEAR 2. Continuation of the basic science curriculum with a primary focus on the preclinical courses; first semester (one day/week) and second semester (two days/week) devoted to patient treatment in restorative dentistry and periodontics.

YEAR 3. Completion of the basic science curriculum; three days a week devoted to comprehensive patient treatment in one of four group practices comprised of third- and fourth-year students; each student assigned operatory for his or her exclusive use; rotation to area hospitals and medical center for additional clinical experience in oncology, pediatric dentistry, restorative dentistry, and oral maxillofacial surgery; completion of preclinical courses.

YEAR 4. Increase in time devoted to patient care with students assigned to clinics or rotations five days a week; clinical experience in comprehensive patient treatment gained as part of a group practice experience; students assigned to operatories for their exclusive use; additional clinical experience in oncology, pediatric dentistry, restorative dentistry, and oral maxillofacial surgery gained in rotation to area hospitals and medical centers.

■ Degrees Offered
DENTAL DEGREE: D.D.S.

ALTERNATE DEGREES: B.S./D.D.S. with the following schools:

- Canisius College (Buffalo, NY)
- LeMoyne College (Syracuse, NY)
- Niagara University (Niagara University, NY)
- St. Bonaventure University (St. Bonaventure, NY)
- St. Lawrence University (Canton, NY)
- SUNY Fredonia (Fredonia, NY)
- SUNY Geneseo (Geneseo, NY)
- University at Buffalo (Buffalo, NY)
- Utica College (Utica, NY)

Combined D.D.S./Ph.D. program administered through the Department of Oral Biology with major areas of study in the basic sciences.

■ Other Programs
RESEARCH FELLOWSHIPS: Available to those students interested in participating in summer research programs in the basic and clinical sciences.

MINORS PROGRAM: A limited number of senior students have the opportunity to participate in additional didactic and clinical experiences in a clinical discipline of their choice. Students may select from programs in prosthetics, pediatric dentistry, oral medicine, periodontics, and oral and maxillofacial prosthetics.

COSTS AND FINANCIAL AID

The university and the School of Dental Medicine provide both need- and merit-based funds to assist students in financing their dental education. Scholarship funds are awarded to second-, third-, and fourth-year students on the basis of academic achievement at the school.

Financial Aid Awards to First-Year Students in 2006-07
■ TOTAL NUMBER OF RECIPIENTS: NA   ■ NA% OF CLASS

	Average Award	Range of Awards
Residents	$31,858*	NA
Nonresidents	$34,848*	NA

*Subsidized and unsubsidized.

Estimated Total Expenses for Academic Year 2006-07

	YEAR 1	YEAR 2	YEAR 3	YEAR 4	TOTAL
Tuition, resident	$14,800	$14,800	$14,800	$14,800	$59,200
Tuition, nonresident	$29,600	$29,600	$29,600	$29,600	$118,400
Educational expenses					
Comprehensive fee	$1,223	$1,223	$1,223	$1,223	$4,890
Activity fee	$200	$200	$200	$200	$800
Student medical insurance	$1,299	$1,299	$1,299	$1,299	$5,196
Microscope fee	$150	$150	0	0	$300
Clinic mgmt. system fee	$2,500	$2,500	$2,500	$2,500	$10,000
Gross anatomy fee	$255	0	0	0	$255
Articulator, magnification	$1,200	0	0	0	$1,200
Supply purchase	$6,635	$4,503	$2,150	$890	$14,178
Fees and licensing	$1,500	$1,720	$1,500	$1,795	$6,515
Living expenses					
Housing and board	$9,581	$9,581	$9,581	$9,581	$38,324
Personal allowance	$1,600	$1,600	$1,600	$1,600	$6,400
Transportation allowance	$2,500	$2,500	$2,500	$2,500	$10,000
TOTAL EXPENSES, RESIDENT	**$43,443**	**$40,076**	**$37,353**	**$36,388**	**$157,258**
TOTAL EXPENSES, NONRESIDENT	**$58,243**	**$54,876**	**$52,153**	**$51,188**	**$216,458**

SELECTION FACTORS

Consideration is extended to those applicants whose scholastic progress has placed them in the upper portion of their class. Prime consideration is given to students with cumulative grade point averages of 3.0 (on a 4.0 scale) or better, BCP (biology, chemistry, physics) GPAs of 3.0 or better, and DAT scores of 16 academic average and 16 PAT or better. In cases where students have had a relatively low GPA in the first year of college but have recovered with two years at a much higher GPA, consideration may be extended if DAT scores are high. Preference will be given to those who will have completed a bachelor's or higher degree prior to enrolling.

The Student Admissions Committee prefers a composite letter generated through a health sciences preprofessional committee. Applicants are encouraged to become familiar with the process for generating a composite letter of recommendation at their undergraduate school, so they can complete their applications in a timely fashion.

Applicants who have demonstrated the academic potential necessary to complete the program will be asked to visit the school to meet with faculty and students. It is the purpose of this visit, along with letters of recommendation, to ascertain a sense of the applicant's motivation for dentistry, integrity, maturity, social awareness, and intellectual ability. Preference is extended to residents of New York, but applications from out of state and foreign students are encouraged.

See chapter 3 of this guide for information regarding numbers of applicants and enrollees to each dental school, along with their race, gender, age, type of predental education, mean DAT and GPA, and state of origin.

ACADEMIC AND OTHER ASSISTANCE

All students experiencing academic difficulty may receive assistance through retention programs at the department level. The university and School of Dental Medicine student support services are available to all dental students. An active Minority Student Affairs Committee provides support to all minority students.

UNIVERSITY OF NORTH CAROLINA AT CHAPEL HILL
SCHOOL OF DENTISTRY

Dr. John N. Williams, Dean

GENERAL INFORMATION

The University of North Carolina (UNC) at Chapel Hill has the honor of being the first state university in America. Chapel Hill is a small college community of 52,400 located near the center of the state in close proximity to the Research Triangle Park. The campus is widely regarded as one of the most beautiful and historic of the major universities, and the mild climate permits virtually year-round enjoyment of the surroundings.

The School of Dentistry accepted its first class in 1950. It currently occupies its original building plus a dental research building, a five-story 110,000-square foot addition to the teaching and clinical facilities, and a 15,000-square foot office building. A new five-story patient-care facility opened in January 1998. A new basic science building and the Division of Health Sciences Library provide direct support to programs in the School of Dentistry-School of Medicine-UNC Hospitals, which are interconnecting and serve as a functional unit. In addition, the schools of nursing, pharmacy, and public health surround the dental school and are closely associated with its programs.

The school offers graduate specialty training in 13 dental disciplines and training programs for dental hygienists and dental assistants, as well as a master's level course of study that prepares dental hygienists for teaching careers.

ADMISSION REQUIREMENTS

NUMBER OF YEARS OF PREDENTAL EDUCATION: Formal minimum of three (96 semester or 144 quarter hours); usual minimum of four.

LIMITATIONS ON COMMUNITY COLLEGE WORK: Maximum of 64 semester hours.

REQUIRED COURSES:

With lab required (semester/quarter hrs)
Inorganic chemistry 8/12
Biology 8/12
 (includes human anatomy or vertebrate zoology)

Other courses
Organic chemistry*
Physics**
English 6/9

* Two sequenced lecture courses with minimum of 4 semester hours.
** Sequenced course(s) covering mechanics, wave motion, optics, electricity, energy, and nuclear physics.

SUGGESTED ADDITIONAL PREPARATION: Choose from among molecular biology, genetics, biochemistry, statistics, business, writing skills, and computer science.

DAT: Mandatory; April or May test date preferred.

GPA: 3.0 or above recommended.

RESIDENCY: Priority is given to North Carolina residents; approximately 20 percent of the class is selected from nonresident applicants. To qualify as a resident, a student must have maintained a domicile in North Carolina for at least 12 months immediately prior to the date of matriculation. Out-of-state students may request a change of residency status after enrollment; however, the student must establish that his or her presence in the state was for purposes of maintaining a bona fide domicile rather than for temporary residence incident to enrollment in the school.

ADVANCED STANDING: Transfer requests for advanced standing from candidates from other ADA-accredited dental schools will be considered on an individual basis. Factors considered will be prior academic record and background, available space in the class, consistency between the curriculum of the two schools, and residency status. Transfers may be made no later than into the second-year class.

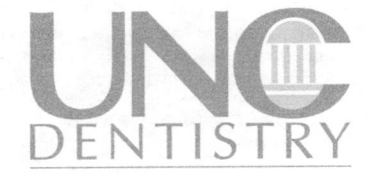

Timetable for the Class Entering Fall 2008

	Earliest Date	Latest Date	School Fee
Application Submission	6/1/07	11/1/07	$74*
Acceptance Notification	12/07 and 2/08	6/08	

*Nonrefundable

Required Response and Deposit:
A signed acceptance letter and provisions letter
A $500 nonrefundable deposit
30 days after notification if received between 12/1 and 12/31
30 days after notification if received between 1/1 and 2/28
15 days after notification if received after 3/1

UNC Supplementary Application also required. Supplemental application deadline is December 1.

FOR FURTHER INFORMATION

Admissions
Albert D. Guckes
Assistant Dean
919-966-4451

Minority Affairs and Financial Aid
Tom Luten
Director of Student Services
919-966-4451

University of North Carolina School of Dentistry
CB #7450, Brauer Hall
Chapel Hill, NC 27599-7450

www.dent.unc.edu

THE DENTAL PROGRAM

The program consists of eight semesters of 16 weeks each, plus three required nine-week summer sessions. Although the majority of students require four years to meet the degree requirements, circumstances may necessitate an extended period of study.

The Health Sciences Library, located next to the dental school, has a fully equipped learning laboratory available for student use. Students have full membership on all standing committees and assume responsibility for several other functions within the institution. During the entire four years, an active career counseling service is available for students. Features include third-year seminars to help students apply to postgraduate programs; fourth-year seminars in practice management; and an ongoing practice placement service.

YEAR 1. The first year includes courses in the core basic sciences, introductory dental sciences, and Introduction to Patient Care, which focuses on the special relationship between a health care provider and the patient. Students begin patient care in the summer.

YEAR 2. Students continue taking biological science and dental science courses, as well as the physical diagnosis course, which consists of lecture and laboratory experiences. After introduction to patient care in the fall, students assume full patient-care privileges in the spring.

YEAR 3. Students spend a significant amount of time caring for their patients in the comprehensive care service, as well as the several specialty services. A series of intermediate dental science and elective courses are offered. During the summer, students are encouraged to participate in research projects or elective patient-care externships.

YEAR 4. Students assume responsibility for patients who require more advanced dental care. The fall is free of any core didactic coursework so that students may participate in elective courses, research, and required extramural rotations. The spring is highlighted by advanced dental science courses, updates, and practice-related courses.

■ Degrees Offered

DENTAL DEGREE: D.D.S.

ALTERNATE DEGREES: D.D.S./Ph.D. program: Although programs pursued have been with basic science departments only, a joint program with a Ph.D. in a behavioral science is also possible.

Master's level programs and a joint D.D.S./M.P.H. program are also available. Master's degree programs will require one or one and a half additional years of study. The doctoral degree programs will require at least two additional years of study.

■ Other Programs

Student research is encouraged throughout the dental curriculum, and funding is available for elective credit research projects. The Student Research Group sponsors speakers and assists students in their research activities. Several students are selected each year to present their findings at national/international research meetings.

COSTS AND FINANCIAL AID

Our Admissions Committee does not consider the financial status of a student during the application and admission process. Once a student is accepted, the school will strive to assist in funding his or her documented need within set allowable living expenses for single and married students. Most awards are in the form of loans. The school does not have private funds to meet the needs of students. Therefore, we are dependent upon the availability of federal and state resources. Applications for financial aid are due in March or following acceptance to the school. Tuition and fees, as well as the types of fees listed below, are subject to change without notice, and are subject to inflation.

Financial Aid Awards to First-Year Students in 2006-07
■ TOTAL NUMBER OF RECIPIENTS: 70   ■ 86% OF CLASS

	Average Award	Range of Awards
Residents	$26,619	$5,000-$38,776
Nonresidents	$49,700	$40,228-$52,799

Estimated Total Expenses for Academic Year 2006-07

	YEAR 1	YEAR 2	YEAR 3	YEAR 4	TOTAL
Tuition, resident*	$14,390	$14,390	$14,390	$7,835	$51,005
Tuition, nonresident*	$41,131	$41,131	$41,131	$41,131	$164,524
Other expenses	$8,795	$5,442	$4,124	$4,436	$22,797
Photocopying, educational materials, basic science expenses, textbooks, state board fees, laptop computer, insurance					
Equipment rental	$1,500	$1,500	$1,500	$1,500	$6,000
Estimated living expenses	$15,765	$15,765	$15,765	$15,765	$63,061
Transportation, housing, meals. Does not include medical insurance					
TOTAL EXPENSES, RESIDENT	$40,450	$37,097	$35,779	$29,536	$137,463
TOTAL EXPENSES, NONRESIDENT	$67,191	$63,838	$62,520	$62,832	$250,982

*Includes tuition for mandatory summer session.

SELECTION FACTORS

The school seeks applicants who will benefit from and contribute to the educational environment and the dental profession and who will, upon graduation, have a wide range of career opportunities. Therefore, the dental school expects students to demonstrate the following: First, an applicant must possess satisfactory academic abilities and have completed the required predental courses and DAT at an acceptable level of performance. Second, an applicant should possess psychomotor skills sufficient to perform the technical tasks necessary in dentistry evidenced by performance on the perceptual ability exam of the DAT and participation in relevant hobbies and experiences. Third, an applicant must demonstrate a commitment to service and desire to help others as evidenced by extracurricular and volunteer activities that require interactions with others and courses in social science, history, literature, economics, philosophy, and psychology. Fourth, an applicant should possess the potential to be a self-directed, life-long learner by evidencing a high level of independent thinking and intellectual curiosity. Fifth, an applicant must demonstrate a knowledge of the dental profession and some important issues facing the profession.

Admission criteria are applied equally to all applicants, regardless of race, age, gender, color, national origin, or religion. Applicants are encouraged to contact the Admissions Office as early as possible to discuss dentistry as a career. Following a review of applications, candidates may be invited for a personal interview. Applicants may also contact the Admissions Office to arrange a tour of the school. Typically 50 percent of the class will be filled at the December acceptance. The size of the 2006-07 entering class was 81.

See chapter 3 of this guide for information regarding numbers of applicants and enrollees to each dental school, along with their race, gender, age, type of predental education, mean DAT and GPA, and state of origin.

ACADEMIC AND OTHER ASSISTANCE

The Schools of Dentistry and Medicine sponsor the Medical Education Development Program for students from disadvantaged backgrounds. This program involves a nine-week period for which all expenses of the dental participants are met by the School of Dentistry. The program is designed to review and reinforce areas in the basic sciences; develop and strengthen reading, study, and test-taking skills; allow the participant to become familiar with a professional environment; and introduce the participant to certain dental techniques.

OHIO

CASE SCHOOL OF DENTAL MEDICINE

Dr. Jerold S. Goldberg, Dean

GENERAL INFORMATION

The School of Dental Medicine was organized in 1892 as the Dental Department of Western Reserve University. Since 1969 the facilities of the school of dentistry have been located in the Health Science Center of Case Western Reserve University adjacent to the schools of medicine and nursing and University Hospitals of Cleveland, Ohio. Since its organization, the School of Dental Medicine has conferred degrees on more than 4,200 graduates.

Education in the basic sciences and technique, as well as preclinical laboratory work, is carried out by each student in an individually assigned area in the multidisciplinary laboratories. The 50,000-square foot dental clinic floor consists of two major clinics and five specialty clinics. The major clinics are made up of individual cubicles, fully equipped as private operatories. Drawing from a population of more than one million people, the clinics provide a broad spectrum of care to the population, affording the student substantial clinical experience.

The School of Dental Medicine also has working relationships with many hospitals and health clinics in the Greater Cleveland community. Third- and fourth-year students have the opportunity to function as dentists and observe hospital routine and operating room technique in these hospitals.

ADMISSION REQUIREMENTS

NUMBER OF YEARS OF PREDENTAL EDUCATION: Formal minimum of two; desired minimum of four.

LIMITATIONS ON COMMUNITY COLLEGE WORK: Maximum of 60 semester hours, all earned before student enters the third year of study toward a baccalaureate degree.

REQUIRED COURSES:

With lab required	(semester/quarter hrs)
Inorganic chemistry	6/10
Organic chemistry	6/10
Physics	6/10
Biology	6/10

Other courses
English   6/10

SUGGESTED ADDITIONAL PREPARATION: Choose from among biochemistry, comparative anatomy, cell biology, microbiology, and physiology.

DAT: 18 or above recommended.

GPA: 3.2 or above recommended.

RESIDENCY: No requirements.

ADVANCED STANDING: A graduate of a foreign dental school may be considered for advanced standing on a space-available basis.

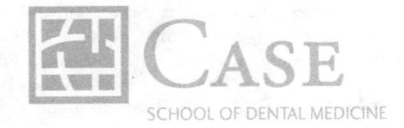

Timetable for the Class Entering Fall 2008

	Earliest Date	Latest Date	School Fee
Application Submission	5/15/07	1/1/08	$45
Acceptance Notification	12/1/07	6/1/08	

Required Response and Deposit:
45 days after notification if received between 12/1 and 12/31
30 days after notification if received after 12/31

$1,000 to hold place.

FOR FURTHER INFORMATION

Office of Admissions
David A. Dalsky
Director
216-368-2460

Financial Aid Office
Barbara A. Sciulli
Advisor
216-368-3256

Student Services Office
Philip C. Aftoora
Director
216-368-3201

Housing
Donald J. Kamalsky
Director
216-368-3780

Case Western Reserve University
Yost Hall, Room 115
Cleveland, OH 44106

dental.case.edu2

THE DENTAL SCHOOL

The Case School of Dental Medicine provides contemporary programs that educate and train students to become competent dentists and offers programs of postgraduate and continuing education that improve the knowledge and skills of members of the dental profession.

YEAR 1. Basic sciences, problem-based learning, technical courses, and limited patient treatment.

YEAR 2. Continue basic science and preclinical courses with increased clinical patient treatment.

YEAR 3. Clinical science courses with comprehensive patient care in preceptor groups.

YEAR 4. Practice management and clinical problem-solving courses with continuation of comprehensive patient care in preceptor groups.

■ Degrees Offered

DENTAL DEGREE: D.M.D.

COMBINED DEGREE: D.M.D./M.D.

ALTERNATE DEGREES: Combined degree programs by arrangement, a privilege accorded undergraduates in their senior year whereby the first year of professional study may be substituted for the last year of liberal arts education.

PREPROFESSIONAL SCHOLARS PROGRAM: Six-year D.M.D. program; two years in the College of Arts and Sciences, four years in the School of Dental Medicine. Eight-year program: four years in the College of Arts and Sciences, and four years in the School of Dental Medicine.

■ Other Programs

EXPANDED FUNCTION: Nondegree certificate course in expanded dental functions to dental auxiliaries with requisite training and experience.

DENTAL EXTERNSHIPS: Available to third- and fourth-year students only.

SELECTION FACTORS

The Admissions Committee considers undergraduate academic records, DAT scores, and letters of recommendation in its selection process. A personal interview at the School of Dental Medicine, by invitation of the Admissions Committee, is necessary prior to acceptance. The interviewee will tour the school, receive information about financial aid, and have an opportunity to talk with faculty and students. During the interview the committee looks for evidence of such personal qualities as integrity, motivation, and maturity.

See chapter 3 of this guide for information regarding numbers of applicants and enrollees to each dental school, along with their race, gender, age, type of predental education, mean DAT and GPA, and state of origin.

ACADEMIC AND OTHER ASSISTANCE

The School of Dental Medicine has a minority coordinator who assists in the recruitment of minority students and monitors their progress through the dental program. The Office of Student Affairs assists students in identifying special needs and providing resources.

COSTS AND FINANCIAL AID

The primary sources of financial aid are federally supported loan and scholarship programs. For more information, contact the Financial Aid Office.

Financial Aid Awards to First-Year Students in 2006-07

■ TOTAL NUMBER OF RECIPIENTS: 70   ■ 93% OF CLASS

	Average Award	Range of Awards
Residents	$40,500	$8,500-$62,705
Nonresidents	$40,500	$8,500-$62,705

Estimated Total Expenses for Academic Year 2006-07

	YEAR 1	YEAR 2	YEAR 3	YEAR 4	TOTAL
Tuition, resident	$42,500	$42,500	$44,225	$44,225	$173,450
Tuition, nonresident	$42,500	$42,500	$44,225	$44,225	$173,450
Other expenses					
Activity fees	$200	$200	$200	$200	$800
Lab fees	$390	$390	$390	$390	$1,560
Equipment	$10,688	$4,998	0	0	$15,686
Estimated living expenses	$14,474	$14,474	$17,374	$17,374	$63,696
TOTAL EXPENSES, RESIDENT	**$68,252**	**$62,562**	**$62,189**	**$62,189**	**$255,192**
TOTAL EXPENSES, NONRESIDENT	**$68,252**	**$62,562**	**$62,189**	**$62,189**	**$255,192**

THE OHIO STATE UNIVERSITY
COLLEGE OF DENTISTRY

Dr. Carole A. Anderson, Interim Dean and Vice Provost

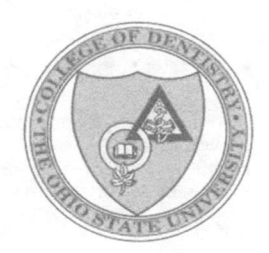

GENERAL INFORMATION

The Ohio State University is a state supported university located in the state's capital, Columbus. The College of Dentistry is located in the Health Sciences Center on the main campus in Columbus (2005 city population 693,983, Franklin County population 1,068,080, U.S. Census Bureau). The dental school was originally organized in 1890 as a department of the Ohio Medical University and was merged with Starling Medical College in 1906. In 1914, the Dental Department of Starling Ohio Medical College became the College of Dentistry of The Ohio State University and in 1925 was moved to the main campus. The College of Dentistry has been located in the University Health Sciences Center since 1951. The Division of Dental Hygiene was established in 1944 and is now the largest university-affiliated dental hygiene program in the United States. The College of Dentistry also conducts programs of continuing education and offers 11 graduate education programs.

The College of Dentistry building is a five-floor structure housing all administrative offices, classrooms, clinics, laboratories, and research facilities for dentistry and dental hygiene. The main clinics were renovated in 1992. Renovations throughout the college continue, including the recently renovated Oral Surgery wing. Classrooms and laboratories are equipped with computer-controlled movie and slide projectors. A student computer lab is available for online instruction. Additionally, dental clinics are located at the University and Children's Hospitals and in the Nisonger Center. A close relationship is maintained with the Colleges of Medicine & Public Health, Biological Sciences, and the Schools of Nursing and Allied Medical Professions.

ADMISSION REQUIREMENTS

NUMBER OF YEARS OF PREDENTAL EDUCATION: Formal minimum of two years (60 semester or 90 quarter hours); usual acceptable minimum prior to applying is a minimum of three years (90 semester hours or 135 quarter hours). Most students matriculate after four years and earning their undergraduate degree (120 semester hours or 180 quarter hours). The completion of your undergraduate degree is strongly desired. **Two thirds of the prerequisites (9 of 13 semester courses or 10 of 14 quarter courses) must be complete with grades prior to submitting the AADSAS application.**

COMMUNITY COLLEGE COURSEWORK: Not suggested.

REQUIRED COURSES: Courses must be at premed, predent, or Bachelor of Science levels to be considered.

With lab required	(semesters/quarters)
Biological science	2/2
General chemistry	2/3
Physics	2/2

With lab recommended	(semesters/quarters)
Human anatomy	1/1
Organic chemistry	2/2
Microbiology	1/1
Biochemistry	1/1

Other courses	(semesters/quarters)
Freshman English	1/1
Advanced writing course	1/1
Total Courses	13/14

REQUIRED ADDITIONAL PREPARATION: Office Observation Report. Each applicant must spend a minimum of 20 hours observing a general dentist in a private practice in the United States. This general dentist may NOT be a family member and cannot work in a teaching facility. Additional time spent with specialists is strongly encouraged. Applicants must submit all hours completed on the required form.

Community Service Report. Applicants must report their top five community service activities on the required online form.

The required documents and guidelines for both the office observation and community service are located on our website at www.dent.osu.edu/admissions/before_you_apply.php.

DAT: It is strongly suggested that applicants take the DAT no later than the end of August 2007 for admission into the entering class of 2008. You do not need to take the DAT prior to submitting your AADSAS application.

GPA: 3.4 or above recommended.

SUPPLEMENTAL APPLICATION: Required of all applicants. The applicant is notified by email when the AADSAS application is received and provided with the link to the online supplemental application. The application fee can be submitted only online by credit or debit card ($60 U.S. applicants/$70 international applicants).

INTERVIEW: By invitation ONLY. Interviews for the 2007-2008 cycle are scheduled for Saturday 9/29/07, Saturday 10/06/07, Saturday 12/01/07, and Saturday 1/26/08. The admissions calendar is located at www.dent.osu.edu/admissions/admissions_calendar.php.

SUGGESTED ADDITIONAL PREPARATION: It is strongly recommended that students have a well-rounded liberal arts education, including courses in drawing, three-dimensional art, psychology, and interpersonal communication.

RESIDENCY: Preference is given to residents of Ohio.

TRANSFER APPLICANTS: Applications for transfer with advanced standing are limited to students currently enrolled in another dental school in the United States. Students must be in good standing at their current

---

Timetable for the Class Entering Fall 2008

	Earliest Date	Latest Date	School Fee
AADSAS Application Submission	5/15/07	9/15/07	see below
First Round Acceptance Notification	12/1/07		
Second Round Acceptance Notification	12/3/07		
Third Round Acceptance Notification	1/28/08		

Required Response and Deposit:
45 days if accepted on or after 12/3
30 days if accepted on or after 1/28

A total acceptance fee of $750 (subject to change) is due on receipt of acceptance notification. $725 of this fee applies toward tuition. The remaining $25 is used as the acceptance fee and does not apply towards tuition. The total deposit of $750 is nonrefundable. The submission of this acceptance fee signifies the applicant's understanding of all college policies and requirements provided at the time of acceptance, including immunizations and health requirements. More information is located at www.dent.osu.edu/admissions/immunization.php.

FOR FURTHER INFORMATION
Recruitment and Admissions
The Ohio State University College of Dentistry
305 W. 12th Avenue, Box 195
P.O. Box 182357
Columbus, OH 43218-2357
Phone 614-292-3361; fax 614-292-0813
dentadmit@osu.edu
www.dent.osu.edu/admissions

Recruitment & Admissions Personnel
Joen M. Iannucci
Director of Admissions & Professor of Clinical Dentistry
Donald F. Bowers
Emeritus Director of Admissions & Professor Emeritus
Amy Mason, Admissions Counselor
Norman Burns, Recruitment Officer

Additional Information
Tammy Lewis
Registrar & Financial Aid
Postle Hall Room 1159
614-292-7768/lewis.36@osu.edu

www.dent.osu.edu

institution to enroll at Ohio State. Students seeking admission are considered on the strength of their previous academic performance and recommendations. More information is located at www.dent.osu.edu/admissions/transferstudents.htm.

INTERNATIONAL APPLICANTS: Ohio State does not offer an advanced standing program for foreign-trained dentists. Applicants with a foreign degree of any kind must follow the requirements located at www.dent.osu.edu/admissions/applicants_international_students.php.

THE DENTAL PROGRAM

YEAR 1. The major basic sciences are taught by lecture, self-instruction, visual aid, and laboratory experience; introduction to clinical dentistry experience.

YEAR 2. Continuation of basic sciences and laboratory experience; introduction to clinical dentistry.

YEAR 3. Clinic experience is provided under faculty supervision in the college, hospital, and remote-site clinics. Clinical sciences are integrated with the basic sciences by faculty members during clinical practice and basic sciences courses.

YEAR 4. Delivery of comprehensive dental care under conditions that approximate private practice, with extramural programs in locations nationwide, including the OHIO Project.

■ Degrees Offered

DENTAL DEGREE: D.D.S. (Doctor of Dental Surgery)

ALTERNATE DEGREES: M.S. and certificate programs in all eleven specialties. More information can be found at www.dent.osu.edu/AdvancedEducation/Admissions.php.

D.D.S./Ph.D.: Available for predoctoral students. More information can be found at www.dent.ohio-state.edu/oralbio/combined.htm.

■ Other Programs

RESEARCH: Opportunities are available to students on an elective basis in both basic and dental sciences. Information is located at www.dent.osu.edu/Research.php.

EXTERNSHIPS: Programs available are special general practice, care for homebound patients, and training at remote-site clinics. Off-campus clinical experiences are available in remote-site clinics, such as the Children's Hospital, Veterans Administration hospitals, and other Ohio hospitals with active dental programs.

SERVICE: The OHIO Project: The Oral Health Improvement through Outreach Project is a program for students to provide dental care to the underserved in community clinics. More information can be located at www.dent.osu.edu/ohioproject.

SELECTION FACTORS

The Admissions Committee considers the following factors: overall GPA, science GPA, DAT scores, knowledge of dentistry, contribution to diversity, personal qualities and attributes, community service activities, and activities or hobbies indicative of manual skills. Interviews are held on campus and are by invitation only. More information can be located at www.dent.osu.edu/admissions/our_selection_process.php.

The policy of The Ohio State University is that discrimination against any individual for reasons of race, color, creed, religion, national origin, gender, age, disability, or Vietnam-era veteran status is specifically prohibited. Accordingly, equal access to employment opportunities, educational programs, and all other university activities is extended to all persons, and the university promotes equal opportunities through a positive and continuing Affirmative Action Program. Preference will be shown to applicants who are residents of the state of Ohio, as defined by the university.

ACADEMIC AND OTHER ASSISTANCE

The Ohio State University College of Dentistry sponsors recruitment and retention programs for all students, including students who are members of underrepresented populations in dentistry. The Ohio State University provides both need- and merit-based funds. For more information, please contact Tammy Lewis.

COSTS AND FINANCIAL AID

Estimated Total Expenses for Academic Year 2006-07

	YEAR 1	YEAR 2	YEAR 3	YEAR 4	TOTAL
Tuition, resident	$22,674	$22,674	$30,232	$30,232	$105,812
	(3 quarters)	(3 quarters)	(4 quarters)	(4 quarters)	
Tuition, nonresident	$50,091	$22,674	$30,232	$30,232	$133,229
Other expenses (books and supplies—original fee)	$5,109	$5,391	$5,596	$5,864	$21,960
Health insurance	$1,350	$1,365	$1,820	$1,820	$6,370
Equipment	$2,952	$2,952	$3,936	$3,936	$13,776
Estimated living expenses	$13,463	$14,960	$17,952	$17,952	$64,328
Rent, utilities, telephone, groceries, laundry, clothing, and transportation					
TOTAL EXPENSES, RESIDENT	$41,526	$43,304	$54,420	$54,152	$193,402
TOTAL EXPENSES, NONRESIDENT	$68,943	$43,304	$54,420	$54,152	$220,819

UNIVERSITY OF OKLAHOMA
COLLEGE OF DENTISTRY
Dr. Stephen K. Young, Dean

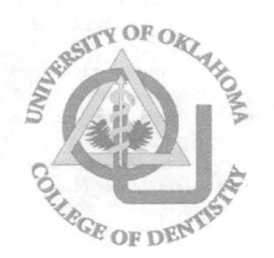

GENERAL INFORMATION

The University of Oklahoma (OU) College of Dentistry is a state-supported institution located at the Health Science Center in Oklahoma City, which includes the colleges of Allied Health, Public Health, Medicine, Nursing, Pharmacy, and a Graduate College. The College of Dentistry graduated its first class in 1976.

The college is located in the Dental Clinical Sciences Building, a modern, attractive facility with five general practice clinics, and additional operatories for oral diagnosis, radiography, oral surgery, pedodontics, periodontics, graduate programs, and residencies. There are a total of 228 dental operatories for student use. The building also includes a preclinical laboratory, lecture halls, seminar rooms, full-service dental laboratory, research space, faculty offices, and student activity areas.

The college conducts a baccalaureate dental hygiene program. The Dental Clinical Sciences Building houses graduate programs in Orthodontics, Periodontics and an AEGD residency. There is an oral and maxillofacial residency at University Hospital and a GPR residency at Children's Hospital in the OU Medical Center.

ADMISSION REQUIREMENTS

NUMBER OF YEARS OF PREDENTAL EDUCATION: Minimum of three (90 semester hours); majority have four or more years. Applicants who have or are completing a baccalaureate degree will be the most competitive.

LIMITATIONS ON COMMUNITY COLLEGE WORK: None, but applicants should have a minimum of 30 hours of upper-division coursework.

REQUIRED COURSES:

With lab required	(semester/quarter hrs)
Biology	8/12
Inorganic chemistry	8/12
Organic chemistry	8/12
Physics	8/12

With or without lab	(semester/quarter hrs)
Biochemistry	3 or 4/4 or 6

Other courses	
English*	6/9
General psychology	3/4.5

Grade of "C" or above required.

*Composition and literature are acceptable alternatives.

SUGGESTED ADDITIONAL PREPARATION: Applicants should observe in one or more dental offices, seeking as much knowledge as possible regarding the profession (100 hours minimum). Additional courses in biology are also recommended (e.g., physiology, microbiology, cell biology, comparative anatomy, genetics).

INTERVIEW: Mandatory, by invitation of the Admissions Committee.

DAT: Mandatory. *Nonresident*—must be taken no later than September 1 (Canadian DAT may be substituted). *Resident*—must be taken before interview can be scheduled. Interviews begin October 1. Academic average should be at or above the national average. For multiple scores, the DAT report showing the highest academic average will be used in evaluating the applicant.

GPA: A minimum of 2.5 (A=4.0) required.

RESIDENCY: No specific requirements.

ADVANCED STANDING: None.

Timetable for the Class Entering Fall 2008

	Earliest Date	Latest Date	School Fee
Application Submission	6/1/07	9/1/07	$65 U.S. citizen
			$90 non-U.S. citizen
Acceptance Notification	12/1/07	2/15/08	

Oklahoma residents missing the 9/1/07 deadline may apply directly to the dental school with a 12/1/07 deadline.

Required Response and Deposit:
45 days after notification if received between 12/1 and 12/14
30 days after notification if received between 1/15 and 2/1
15 days after notification if received after 2/1

$500 nonrefundable deposit should accompany student's letter of acceptance of offer and applies toward first semester tuition.

FOR FURTHER INFORMATION

Office of Admissions
Randy Jones
Director of Admissions and Student Affairs
Judy Peterson
Admissions Coordinator
405-271-3530
College of Dentistry, Rm 512

Office of Financial Aid
Pam Jordan
Director
405-271-2118
Student Union, Rm 301

HSC Student Affairs
Kate Stanton
Executive Director
405-271-2416
Student Union, Rm 300

University of Oklahoma
P.O. Box 26901
Oklahoma City, OK 73190

Housing**
405-325-2511
University of Oklahoma
1406 Asp Avenue, Rm 126
Norman, OK 73019-6091

dentistry.ouhsc.edu

**Located on the University of Oklahoma Health Sciences Center campus, the University Village Apartments is the ideal living environment for HSC students. For more information visit www.ou.edu/universityvillage.

THE DENTAL PROGRAM

The first year starts the last week of June. The length of the program is 45 months; students are in actual attendance for 40 months including an eight-week clinic session at the end of the third year.

The dental curriculum is designed to produce a competent general practitioner. The objectives of the professional education program are to produce graduates who will 1) be competent in the diagnosis and treatment of oral disease; 2) practice preventive dentistry in relation to total health; 3) assume positions of responsibility within the community; 4) be sensitive to the needs, aspirations, and apprehensions of patients and others; 5) competently manage dental practice and dental auxiliary personnel; and 6) have developed an initiative for continuing education and adaptation to progress within the profession. These objectives are the foundation of the instructional format.

YEAR 1. Basic sciences, preclinical sciences, introduction to clinics and patient treatment.

YEAR 2. Continuation of basic and preclinical sciences with clinical patient treatment.

YEAR 3. Pharmacology and clinical patient treatment.

YEAR 4. Clinical patient treatment.

■ Degrees Offered

DENTAL DEGREE: D.D.S.

ALTERNATE DEGREES: B.S. following first year of dental school; arrangements with undergraduate institution are the responsibility of the student involved.

ADVANCED DEGREES: The College of Dentistry offers postdoctoral programs leading to a M. S. degree in orthodontics or periodontics. A three-year residency program leading to a certificate in oral and maxillofacial surgery and a one-year residency for Advanced Education in General Dentistry are also available at the postdoctoral level.

■ Other Programs

EXTERNSHIPS: Required during both third and fourth years.

SELECTION FACTORS

The Committee on Admissions places substantial importance on: 1) quality and adequacy of academic background; 2) performance on the DAT; 3) letter of recommendation from a predental advisory committee or letters from two science instructors; 4) letters from general practitioners supporting your exposure to or employment in the dental field; and 5) a personal interview. Preference is given to Oklahoma residents. Admissions criteria are applied equally to all applicants, regardless of race, color, creed, gender, national origin, or disability.

The latest date for filing a completed AADSAS application is September 1. First offers will be made on December 1; additional offers will be made through February. Applicants are therefore encouraged to apply early.

A limited number of Arkansas residents are eligible to qualify for resident tuition rates under an agreement administered by the Southern Regional Education Board.

See chapter 3 of this guide for information regarding numbers of applicants and enrollees to each dental school, along with their race, gender, age, type of predental education, mean DAT and GPA, and state of origin.

COSTS AND FINANCIAL AID

Assistance is available to those students who demonstrate financial need. Dental students are eligible to apply for the following aid programs: Health Professions Loan, Federal Perkins Loan, Lew Wentz Loan, Baker Loan, and ADEAL loans. Oklahoma residents can apply for the Oklahoma Tuition Aid Grant and Tuition Waiver Scholarships. Also, a number of scholarships are awarded to students based on academic performance. Requests for financial aid application packets should be directed to the Office of Financial Aid.

The recommended filing date for fall/spring semesters is March 1. Many of the need-based programs have a May 1 deadline. Although applications cannot be processed until the student has been admitted, students are encouraged to submit applications before admission to the college.

Financial Aid Awards to First-Year Students in 2006-07

■ TOTAL NUMBER OF RECIPIENTS: 58 ■ 96% OF CLASS

	Average Award	Range of Awards
Residents—48	$50,822	$38,500-$58,222
Nonresidents—10	$71,242	$38,500-$71,242

Estimated Total Expenses for Academic Year 2006-07

	YEAR 1	YEAR 2	YEAR 3	YEAR 4	TOTAL
Tuition, resident	$13,512	$13,512	$13,512	$13,512	$54,048
Tuition, nonresident	$33,389	$33,932	$33,932	$33,389	$134,636
Other expenses and fees					
Activity	$182	$152	$158	$113	$605.00
Connectivity	$395	$520	$520	$442	$1877
Equipment	$200	$200	$200	$200	$800
Facility	$409	$340	$355	$252	$1356
Health service	$160	$128	$128	$160	$576
Instruments	$6,100	$6,300	$6,100	$950	$1,945
Lab utilization	$150	$150	$150	$150	$600
Library resource	$350	$291	$304	$200	$1145
Microscope	0	$75	0	0	$75
Parking	$200	$200	$200	$200	$800
Professional liability	$30	$30	$30	$30	$120
Registration	$45	$30	$30	$45	$150
Student ID card	$10	0	0	0	$10
Books	$945	$1,340	$705	$160	$3,150
Computer	$2,500	0	0	0	$2,500
Graduation expenses	0	0	0	$150	$150
Inoculation/vaccination	$150	0	0	0	$150
Magnification loupes (optional)	$900	0	0	0	$900
Travel (clinical training/residency	0	0	$700	$2,200	$2,900
Uniforms/shoes	$300	$50	$50	$50	$450
National boards	0	$220	0	$295	$515
Western regional board	0	0	0	$1,900	$1,900
OK state licensure (optional)	0	0	0	$200	$200
Estimated living expenses	$23,221	$17,415	$17,416	$23,221	$81,274
TOTAL EXPENSES, RESIDENT	**$49,834**	**$40,879**	**$40,558**	**$44,505**	**$175,776**
TOTAL EXPENSES, NONRESIDENT	**$69,711**	**$60,756**	**$60,435**	**$64,382**	**$255,284**

OREGON

OREGON HEALTH & SCIENCE UNIVERSITY
SCHOOL OF DENTISTRY

Dr. Jack W. Clinton, Dean

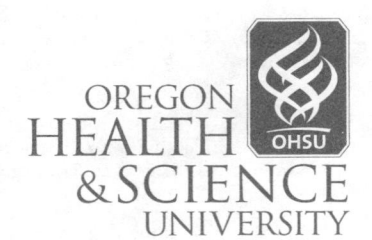

GENERAL INFORMATION

The Oregon Health & Science University (OHSU) School of Dentistry is a nonprofit public corporation with a public mission located in Portland, a city of 556,370 residents in a greater metropolitan area of approximately 2 million. The School of Dentistry is located in the wooded hills of southwest Portland on a 116-acre campus. Paths for joggers, bicyclists, and pedestrians connect the University with the heart of the city just two miles away. The dental school was established in 1898, and the School of Dentistry became incorporated into the Oregon State System of Higher Education in 1945. Since 1974, the School of Dentistry has been part of the Oregon Health & Science University, an institution devoted solely to educating health professionals and biomedical researchers. A dental school is more than just an institution, courses, classrooms, and clinics—it's people. OHSU dental students find friendly people who work together as a team toward one goal: providing each student with the best dental education available.

ADMISSION REQUIREMENTS

NUMBER OF YEARS OF PREDENTAL EDUCATION: Formal minimum of three years (90 semester or 135 quarter hours) from an accredited U.S. or Canadian college or university.

LIMITATIONS ON COMMUNITY COLLEGE WORK: A student who begins a predental program at a community college should plan to attend no more than one year and then transfer to an accredited four-year institution.

REQUIRED COURSES:

Inorganic chemistry, with lab	1 yr. sequence
Organic chemistry, with lab	2 qtrs./2 semesters
General biology, with lab	1 yr. sequence
Physics, with lab	1 yr. sequence
Anatomy	1 semester
Physiology	1 semester
Biochemistry*	1 semester
English composition	1 yr. or equivalent

Courses must be at predent, premed, or baccalaureate levels to be considered.

*Laboratory recommended but is optional if taught separately from lecture course.

SUGGESTED ADDITIONAL PREPARATION: Additional science courses such as microbiology, cell biology, molecular biology, histology, and neuroscience are highly recommended. Study of the social and behavioral sciences, as well as the fine arts and humanities, will enhance the student's ability to practice dentistry.

INTERVIEW: Mandatory; by invitation from Admissions Committee.

DAT: Official scores must be received by November 1. It is recommended that the DAT be taken far enough in advance to retake the exam if needed. Scores from the most recent exam will be considered during the review process. Both American and Canadian DAT scores are accepted. DAT scores should be at or above the national average. See characteristics of the entering class for average DAT scores.

GPA: A 3.0 GPA or above in required predental courses is recommended.

DENTAL EXPLORATION: Minimum of 50 hours prior to the time of application, of which 25 should be in a general practitioner's office.

RESIDENCY: The School of Dentistry recognizes that its primary obligation is to provide an opportunity in dental education for residents of Oregon. Selection, as far as residency is concerned, is based on the following order of priorities: Oregon residency; residency in the Western Interstate Commission for Higher Education (WICHE)—Alaska, Arizona, Hawaii, Montana, New Mexico, North Dakota, and Wyoming; residency in the remaining states; and Canadians. With the exception of Canadian course work, international students applying with foreign courses are not eligible for admission.

ADVANCED STANDING: There is no advanced standing program for foreign-trained dentists. The School of Dentistry does not accept transfer students.

Timetable for the Class Entering Fall 2008

	Earliest Date	Latest Date	School Fee
Application Submission	6/1/07	11/1/07	$75
Acceptance Notification	12/1/07-2/15/08		

Alternates may be notified of acceptance until classes begin (third week of August).

Allow six weeks for AADSAS processing. It is highly recommended that applicants submit the AADSAS application by Labor Day. Applicants reduce the possibility of acceptance if their application is received by OHSU after November 1.

Required Response and Deposit:
$500 deposit due with applicant's letter accepting offer; deposit is applied toward tuition and is nonrefundable.

FOR FURTHER INFORMATION

Office of Admissions and Student Affairs
Mark D. Mitchell
Associate Dean, Admissions and Student Affairs
503-494-5274; sodadmit@ohsu.edu
School of Dentistry
Oregon Health & Science University
611 SW Campus Drive, Room 214
Portland, OR 97239-3097

Financial Aid Office
503-494-7800; finaid@ohsu.edu
Oregon Health & Science University
3181 SW Sam Jackson Park Road
Portland, OR 97239-3098

www.ohsu.edu/sod

THE DENTAL PROGRAM

The dental curriculum is designed to prepare graduates for the practice of general dentistry. Emphasis is placed on the prevention of dental diseases as well as on technical, diagnostic, and treatment planning skills essential to treating patients.

Students see their first patient during the fall quarter of their freshman year as part of a course dealing with the prevention of dental diseases. During the first two years, there is additional clinical experience, although most emphasis is placed on the biological sciences and preclinical techniques. The summer session between the second and third years focuses on clinical experience and oral pathology. The third and fourth years deal mostly, but not entirely, with clinical practice and include courses in practice planning and management. Honors clinical electives are offered in advanced restorative techniques, implantology, and specialty areas (e.g., endodontology, behavioral science). Development of ethical standards of practice, opportunities for community service, and elective courses augment the development of clinical skills.

■ Degrees Offered

DENTAL DEGREE: D.M.D.

ALTERNATE DEGREES: On rare occasions, students entering without a degree may earn a bachelor's degree in cooperation with the predental undergraduate college or university. Students who intend to transfer School of Dentistry courses for their baccalaureate degree should consult with predental faculty advisors and the college or university degree progress office to ensure that all courses from the school will articulate to fulfill undergraduate degree requirements. The Office of Admissions must approve arrangements for concurrent degree completion. Concurrent degree should be completed by the end of the first term while enrolled at the School of Dentistry.

ADVANCED DEGREES: The School of Dentistry offers programs leading to a M.S. degree in the basic and material sciences and a certificate or M.S. degree in the dental specialty areas.

■ Other Programs

ACADEMIC MERIT AWARDS: Entering dental students with outstanding undergraduate academic achievement may be eligible for an academic merit award. This award may provide financial support for four years, reducing tuition. Selection criteria for the merit awards are based on demonstrated academic excellence (all previous college work) and performance on the Dental Admission Test (DAT).

Applicants will automatically be considered for these awards when all of their regular application materials have been received. Awards are allocated after the entering class has been finalized, during the spring prior to matriculation into the program. For more information concerning these awards, contact the Associate Dean for Admissions and Student Affairs.

SELECTION FACTORS

Students are selected on the basis of demonstrated scholastic ability in both required and elective courses. Quality and quantity of courses taken per quarter are also considered. Performance on the DAT is compared with the science GPA. Letters of evaluation are screened for personal qualities and demonstrated interest in, and knowledge of, the profession of dentistry. Selected applicants will be invited to visit the campus to interview with members of the admissions committee and visit with student representatives. Applicants are evaluated using established criteria without regard to national origin, color, race, religion, disability, veteran status, age, sexual orientation, or gender.

See chapter 3 of this guide for information regarding numbers of applicants and enrollees to each dental school, along with their race, gender, age, type of predental education, mean DAT and GPA, and state of origin.

ACADEMIC AND OTHER ASSISTANCE

OHSU sponsors recruitment and retention programs for all students, including tours for applicants and other interested parties. A tutorial program is available to assist all enrolled dental students. Faculty and peer advisors, psychological counseling, and learning specialists are available to provide assistance with study skills. The School of Dentistry works closely with the Office for Student Access to facilitate and support equal access for students with disabilities. The Center for Diversity and Multicultural Affairs offers a full range of programs during the year to enrich students' experience at OHSU. For further information, please contact the Office of Admissions and Student Affairs, at 503-494-5274.

COSTS AND FINANCIAL AID

The School of Dentistry is committed to making dental education available to admitted students and meeting the demonstrated financial need of students through loans, grants, scholarships, and limited work-study opportunities. The University maintains a financial aid office to assist students in obtaining a variety of aid. Students are encouraged to complete the Free Application for Federal Student Aid (FAFSA) by the March deadline. FAFSA forms are available online at www.fafsa.ed.gov. More information about financial aid at OHSU can be easily accesed at www.ohsu.edu/finaid, or by contacting the OHSU Financial Aid Office at 503-494-7800.

Financial Aid Awards to First-Year Students in 2005-06

■ TOTAL NUMBER OF RECIPIENTS: 74*   ■99% OF CLASS

	Average Award	Range of Awards
Residents	$39,160	$9,500-$52,200
Nonresidents	$53,674	$26,000-$60,438

Every School of Dentistry student who was eligible for assistance received an award.

* Ninety-four percent of all School of Dentistry students receive financial aid. The school awarded $12.5 million in financial aid to dental students in the 2005-06 school year.

Estimated Total Expenses for Academic Year 2006-07

	YEAR 1	YEAR 2	YEAR 3	YEAR 4	TOTAL
Tuition, resident	$18,042	$18,042	$21,049	$21,049	$78,182
Tuition, nonresident	$31,308	$31,308	$36,526	$36,526	$135,668
Other expenses					
Student health fees	$627	$627	$836	$836	$2,926
Major Medical insurance	$2,388	$2,171	$2,605	$2,605	$9,769
Miscellaneous fees	$1,801	$1,801	$2,344	$2,344	$8,290
Equipment purchase	$10,922	$8,139	$2,877	$934	$22,872
Books	$900	$800	$400	$250	$2,350
Supplies	$400	$1,000	$2,300	$2,200	$5,900
Estimated living expenses*	$15,840	$14,400	$17,280	$17,280	$64,800
TOTAL EXPENSES, RESIDENT	**$50,920**	**$46,980**	**$49,691**	**$47,498**	**$195,089**
TOTAL EXPENSES, NONRESIDENT	**$64,186**	**$60,246**	**$65,168**	**$62,975**	**$252,575**

*Estimate includes transportation, room and board, and other personal expenses for single students.

UNIVERSITY OF PENNSYLVANIA
SCHOOL OF DENTAL MEDICINE

Dr. Marjorie K. Jeffcoat, Dean

GENERAL INFORMATION

With a history deeply rooted in forging precedents in dental education, research, and patient care, the University of Pennsylvania School of Dental Medicine is continuously evaluating and adapting its programs to remain at the forefront of dental medicine, preparing its graduates to do the same. Established in 1878, the school is among the oldest university-affiliated institutions in the nation and an integral part of the larger University of Pennsylvania community.

Penn Dental attracts students from throughout the country and around the world, awarding D.M.D. degrees to approximately 135 students each year. Penn Dental is consistently among the top ten American dental schools in federally funded research and one of the few schools with its own basic sciences faculty. The school is also a leading provider of dental care for the Philadelphia community, exposing students to diverse patient populations and a depth of clinical experience.

Penn Dental's academic and clinical resources employ the most recent advances in technology and patient care. Virtual reality-based technology is used to develop students' preclinical skills in basic dentistry beginning the first semester of the freshman year. As the world's first academic testing site of this dental simulation technology, Penn Dental remains at the forefront of its application and research, with the second largest lab of this type in the nation. In addition, Penn Dental integrates options into its program that cross the usual boundaries of the predoctoral program. From unique electives and community outreach programs to diverse externship and research opportunities, students are able to explore all aspects of dentistry and shape a course of study that meets their individual goals.

Penn Dental is located on the western edge of the university campus, within walking distance of the other graduate and professional schools and a multitude of on-campus resources, from libraries, museums, and performing arts centers to athletic and recreational facilities. The three buildings of Penn Dental—the state-of-the-art Robert Schattner Center, the Leon Levy Center for Oral Health Research, and the historic Thomas W. Evans Museum and Dental Institute—are all linked to create their own campus atmosphere, with surrounding courtyards and cafes.

Penn Dental's educational programs include a predoctoral D.M.D. program; postgraduate programs in endodontics, oral medicine, oral and maxillofacial radiology, oral and maxillofacial surgery, orthodontics, orthodontics/periodontics, pedodontics, periodontics, and periodontal prosthetics; an Advanced Education in General Dentistry Program; and an M.S. in Oral Biology, which prepares students for an academic career. As part of the University of Pennsylvania community, the school also offers some unique dual-degree opportunities.

ADMISSION REQUIREMENTS

NUMBER OF YEARS OF PREDENTAL EDUCATION: Formal minimum of three; usual minimum of four.

LIMITATIONS ON COMMUNITY COLLEGE WORK: Maximum of 60 semester hours, all earned before a student enters the third year of study toward a baccalaureate degree.

REQUIRED COURSES:

With lab required (semester/quarter hrs)
Inorganic chemistry	8/12
Organic chemistry	8/12
Biochemistry	1/3
Biology	8/12
Physics	8/12

Other courses
Mathematics	1/3
English	3/6

SUGGESTED ADDITIONAL PREPARATION: Choose from among upper division biology, quantitative analysis, microbiology, genetics, or histology.

DAT: Mandatory; can be taken at any time but no later than December 31 prior to the year of matriculation.

GPA: 3.2 or above recommended.

RESIDENCY: No requirements.

ADVANCED STANDING: Foreign dental graduates are considered for a special advanced standing program. Contact the Office of International Relations at 215-898-0558 for information.

Timetable for the Class Entering Fall 2008

	Earliest Date	Latest Date	School Fee
Application Submission	6/1/07	1/1/08	$50
Acceptance Notification	12/1/07	8/25/08	

Required Response and Deposit:
45 days after notification if received on or after 12/1/07
30 days after notification if received on or after 1/1/08
15 days after notification if received on or after 2/1/08

$1,000 nonrefundable deposit due in two installments; applied to tuition.

FOR FURTHER INFORMATION

Office of Admissions
Corky Cacas
Director of Admissions
215-898-8943;
Dental-admissions@pobox.upenn.edu

Office of Student Affairs
Susan Schwartz
Assistant Dean for Student Affairs
215-898-4550; susanz@pobox.upenn.edu

Office of Minority Affairs
Rose Wadenya
215-573-2650; wadenya@pobox.upenn.edu

University of Pennsylvania
School of Dental Medicine
The Robert Schattner Center
240 South 40th Street
Philadelphia, PA 19104-6030

On-Campus Housing Office
215-898-8271
University of Pennsylvania
Residential Living
3901 Locust Walk
Philadelphia, PA 19104-6180

www.dental.upenn.edu

THE DENTAL PROGRAM

The length of program spans 45 months, with 38 months for which students are in actual attendance. Four-week summer sessions between years two and three and years three and four are mandatory. The freshman year continues through the month of June.

The basic science courses are taught in the first and second years through lectures, seminars, and laboratory experiences. Clinical experience begins with dental health education in the first year. The third and fourth years emphasize the general practice of dentistry. Much effort is made to integrate basic and clinical sciences throughout the four-year program. A highlight of the program is an offering of more than 50 selective courses in a variety of areas. Fourth-year students spend six weeks gaining additional clinical skills in a hospital setting. Opportunities for separate admission to programs in education, biomedical engineering, and business are available. Seniors can also participate in foreign exchange programs for one month at 29 different locations in Europe, Asia, Middle East, Central America, and Africa.

The school takes a leadership role in the incorporation of technology into its curriculum, including the use of virtual reality to teach psychomotor skills. Faculty members are very active in basic and applied research in the life sciences. There are abundant opportunities for students to participate in research programs.

The University of Pennsylvania School of Dental Medicine operates on an "A," "B," "C," "F" evaluation system. Student performance in lecture and basic science labs is measured by written objective examination, usually of the multiple-choice and slide identification variety. Achievement in preclinical dental labs is determined by practical exams. Evaluation of clinical performance is based on a composite of daily grades, faculty comments, and competency evaluations. Students who fail a course(s) are reviewed individually by the school's Committee on Student Advancement, which prescribes the course of action to be followed by the student.

■ Degrees Offered
DENTAL DEGREE: D.M.D.

ALTERNATE DEGREES: B.S./D.M.D. with the following schools:

- University of Pennsylvania
- Lehigh University
- Muhlenberg College
- Villanova University
- Hampton University
- Xavier University of Louisiana

Opportunities to earn other degrees concurrently are possible for a limited number of highly qualified students, and include the following combinations:

- D.M.D./M.S. in education (Graduate School of Education)
- D.M.D./M.S. in bioengineering and basic sciences
- D.M.D./M.S. in public health
- D.M.D./Ph.D. in basic sciences

Opportunities to pursue other degrees are determined on an individual basis.

■ Other Programs
RESEARCH FELLOWSHIPS: A limited number between the first and second year.

EXTERNSHIPS: Available to fourth-year students only.

SELECTION FACTORS

The University of Pennsylvania School of Dental Medicine seeks highly qualified, academically prepared, caring individuals who will contribute to the advancement of high-quality oral health care. The school encourages underrepresented minority and female applicants to apply. Selection is made without reference to race, gender, sexual orientation, religion, color, national or ethnic origin, age, disability, or status as a Vietnam-era veteran or disabled veteran. Consideration will be given to those candidates who meet academic prerequisites, fulfill admissions requirements, and demonstrate a commitment to the dental profession. Strong preference will be given to those candidates who demonstrate proficiency in any of the following areas: community service, extracurricular activities, predental experience, research, or superior academic preparation. Because the University of Pennsylvania School of Dental Medicine is a private institution, it is not bound by agreement to limit the number of out-of-state students and therefore seeks a geographically diverse student body.

Although there are no minimum GPAs or DAT scores for admission, careful consideration will be given to candidates with a 3.2 overall and science G.P.A. or higher. Selection factors also include recommendations from the applicant's college regarding his or her stature as a citizen in the college community as well as his or her potential for success in dentistry and the opinion of the Admissions Committee on the applicant's character and motivation to pursue the study of dental medicine. Interviews are required but are granted only at the request of the Admissions Committee.

See chapter 3 of this guide for information regarding numbers of applicants and enrollees to each dental school, along with their race, gender, age, type of predental education, mean DAT and GPA, and state of origin.

COSTS AND FINANCIAL AID

The School of Dental Medicine makes every effort to ensure that students it deems qualified to undertake and complete their dental education will have the opportunity to do so. Both need and merit-based funding are available. Need-based financial assistance is available to U.S. citizens and permanent residents in the form of scholarship and federal subsidized and unsubsidized loans. Aid is awarded through the university's Student Financial Services Office based on the individual's financial need. Financial aid applications (FAFSA and Penn application) are analyzed by the Assistant Director of Graduate Aid to determine each student's level of need, and funding is apportioned accordingly. In addition, each year the school awards a limited number of Dean's Merit scholarships. These scholarships, one-half of tuition, are available to entering students only and are awarded each year for a maximum of four years. All admitted students are automatically considered for these awards.

Financial Aid Awards to First-Year Students in 2006-07
■ TOTAL NUMBER OF RECIPIENTS: 109   ■ 89% OF CLASS

	Average Award	Range of Awards
Residents/Nonresidents	$56,733	$8,500 up to budget

Total Expenses for Academic Year 2006-07

	YEAR 1	YEAR 2	YEAR 3	YEAR 4	TOTAL
Tuition	$48,970	$48,970	$48,970	$48,970	$195,880
Other expenses					
University fee, clinic fee	$2,126	$2,126	$2,126	$2,126	$8,504
Equipment, books, instruments, clinic gowns	$6,995	$5,951	$6,215	$5,936	$25,097
Estimated living expenses	$16,819	$18,312	$18,312	$18,106	$71,549
Room/board, misc., health insurance, boards, phone, personal, loan fees, instrument insurance					
TOTAL EXPENSES	**$74,910**	**$75,359**	**$75,623**	**$75,138**	**$301,030**

PENNSYLVANIA

UNIVERSITY OF PITTSBURGH
SCHOOL OF DENTAL MEDICINE

Dr. Thomas W. Braun, Dean

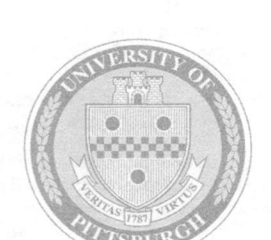

GENERAL INFORMATION

The University of Pittsburgh is a state-related institution located in the city's Oakland District. The School of Dental Medicine, founded in 1896, is one of the schools in the University Health Complex, which consists of schools of Medicine, Nursing, Pharmacy, Health Related Professions, Public Health, and affiliated university hospitals. Recent renovations have upgraded our facilities with state-of-the-art equipment to educate general dentists, specialists, and dental hygienists. These renovations are highlighted in the Preclinical Simulation lab as well as the clinical setting through increased operatory space to accommodate a variety of patient care and in the addition of a biomaterials laboratory for research. With an emphasis on competency-based performance, our First Professional students are educated to provide optimal dental care for the public. Furthermore, our dental residency programs and dental hygiene program provide predoctoral students the opportunity to work cooperatively with other members of the dental profession. Dental residency programs are offered in advanced education in general dentistry, endodontics, pediatric dentistry, periodontics, prosthodontics, maxillofacial prosthodontics, orthodontics, anesthesiology, dental informatics, and maxillofacial surgery.

ADMISSION REQUIREMENTS

NUMBER OF YEARS OF PREDENTAL EDUCATION: Formal minimum of 90 semester hours with 4.0 GPA and DAT score of 25 on all sections; usual minimum of 120 semester hours, degree preferred.

LIMITATIONS ON COMMUNITY COLLEGE WORK: The Admissions Committee does not consider highly those applicants who have been enrolled for more than one-half their coursework, or more than 30 percent of required courses, in community colleges.

REQUIRED COURSES: *(semester hrs)*

Inorganic chemistry	8
Organic chemistry	6
Biology/with lab	8
Physics	6
English	6

SUGGESTED ADDITIONAL PREPARATION: Choose from among biochemistry, upper division biology, literature, art, and sculpture.

DAT: Mandatory. Satisfactory scores must be submitted by application deadline of December 1. Applications will not be considered without DAT results. Test scores must not be older than three years, with a maximum of three attempts. Canadian DAT results accepted.

GPA: 3.4 or above recommended, 3.2 or above considered.

RESIDENCY: No specific requirements.

ADVANCED STANDING: Consideration is given to applicants with foreign dental degrees. Applicants must have passed *both* National Board Examinations Parts I and II and have a minimum computerized TOEFL Exam score of 270 (must not be older than two years) or an IBT score of at least 100. Applicants must also submit a $50 application fee to the University of Pittsburgh at the same time that the application is submitted. These applicants are usually accepted at the third-year level upon successful completion of a mandatory summer program.

TRANSFER STUDENTS: Applicants requesting transfer from other U.S. dental schools must be in good academic and ethical standing at current school. Transfer requests must be made directly to the Admissions Committee. Each application is considered on a case-by-case basis and must include with the letter a copy of the applicant's original AADSAS application, a dean's letter of good standing from the dean of the current dental school, a copy of the current dental school curriculum, three additional letters from didactic/clinical faculty, a passing score on the National Board Part I, and a personal statement addressing the applicant's decision to transfer. Transfer requests are typically considered during the summer prior to the third year of dental school.

Timetable for the Class Entering Fall 2008

	Earliest Date	Latest Date	School Fee
AADSAS Application Submission	6/1/07	12/1/07	$35 / $50 Int'l
Acceptance Notification	12/1/07	8/15/08	

Required Response and Deposit:
45 days after notification if received between 12/1 and 12/31
15 days after notification if received after 1/1

First nonrefundable $750 deposit with acceptance contract; second deposit of $750 due 5/1; both deposits credited toward tuition.
Application Fee: The University of Pittsburgh has no secondary application. However, upon submission of your AADSAS application, send to the University of Pittsburgh School of Dental Medicine your processing fee and photo. Applicants will not be reviewed until this fee has been submitted.

FOR FURTHER INFORMATION
Office of Student Services
412-648-8422

Admissions
412-648-8437
dentaladmissions@dental.pitt.edu

Financial Aid
412-648-9806

Minority Programs
412-648-8422

Advanced Standing Program for Foreign Trained Dentists
412-648-8437

Postdoctoral Programs (Dental Residency)
412-648-8500
Dean's Suite, Salk Hall

University of Pittsburgh
3501 Terrace Street, Suite 2114
Pittsburgh, PA 15261-1945

www.dental.pitt.edu

THE DENTAL PROGRAM

The School of Dental Medicine combines rigorous classroom instruction with innovative hands-on experience in a clinical setting. Students in the first and second years train in state-of-the-art simulation clinics, balanced with a mix of traditional classroom lectures and PBL situations. Third- and fourth-year students simulate private practice in module clinics under close supervision of clinical faculty. Mandatory review sessions are given at the appropriate times to prepare students for the National Board Examinations. Students are encouraged to individualize their programs through elective courses in their third and fourth years. Elective study may range from a minimum of two courses to any number the student feels he or she can schedule comfortably. Additionally, clinical practice and social perspectives are expanded through elective study; the program provides opportunities for enrichment through electives at off-campus sites.

YEAR 1. Basic sciences with introduction to clinical situations.

YEAR 2. Continuation of basic sciences and technical courses plus definitive clinical patient treatment.

YEAR 3. Delivery of comprehensive dental care and continuation of coursework.

YEAR 4. Delivery of comprehensive dental care under conditions that approximate private practice.

■ Degree Offered
DENTAL DEGREE: D.M.D.

■ Other Programs
RESEARCH FELLOWSHIPS: A limited number available for academically outstanding students.

EXTERNSHIPS: Available to third- and fourth-year students.

COSTS AND FINANCIAL AID

The School of Dental Medicine provides both need- and merit-based aid. For more information, contact the Financial Aid Office. The table below presents estimates based on charges expected for the 2005-06 academic year. Tuition and fees, as well as the types of fees, are subject to change without notice, and all costs are subject to inflation.

Financial Aid Awards to First-Year Students in 2006-07
■ TOTAL NUMBER OF RECIPIENTS: 76   ■ 95% OF CLASS

	Average Award	Range of Awards
Residents	$60,524	$8,000-$60,524
Nonresidents	$67,638	$15,000-$67,638

Estimated Total Expenses for Academic Year 2006-07

	YEAR 1	YEAR 2	YEAR 3	YEAR 4	TOTAL
Tuition, resident	$31,516	$31,516	$31,516	$31,516	126,064
Tuition, nonresident	$37,506	$37,506	$37,506	$37,506	154,520
Instruments	$8,943	$5,188	$3,466	$2,363	19,960
University fees/health insurance fee	$3,390	$3,390	$3,390	$3,390	13,560
DMed fees/professional fees	$220	$1,750	$295	$2,640	4,905
Books, supplies, and materials	$1,300	$1,300	$500	$200	3,300
Maximum living allowance	$15,000	$15,000	$15,000	$15,000	60,000
TOTAL EXPENSES, RESIDENT	**$60,524**	**$56,614**	**$55,622**	**$52,764**	**225,524**
TOTAL EXPENSES, NONRESIDENT	**$67,638**	**$63,728**	**$62,736**	**$59,878**	**253,980**

All budgets reflect a 12-month period. There is no separate budget permitted for married students, although an adjustment is permitted for dependent children. Please note that all figures are subject to change annually. Please contact the Dental School Financial Aid Office to obtain the most current information.

SELECTION FACTORS

The Admissions Committee reviews scholastic records, DAT scores, previously attended postsecondary schools, and letters of recommendation (especially from teachers in laboratory sciences). The Admissions Committee prefers a composite letter generated through a health science preprofessional committee. In lieu of the preprofessional committee letter, at least three academic science faculty letters may be submitted.

Interviews are required and are by invitation only. The University of Pittsburgh School of Dental Medicine encourages applications from individuals with interest in practicing in a rural community or who are members of underrepresented minorities in dentistry (i.e., African-American, Americans of Hispanic origins, and Native Americans).

Applicants must submit a $35 application fee (Canadian and other international student fee is $50) to the University of Pittsburgh at the same time that the application is submitted to AADSAS. This may be in the form of either a check or money order. Applications will not be processed without this fee, nor will applicant receive further notification to submit this fee. A 2×2" passport-quality photo must be sent with the application fee.

See chapter 3 of this guide for information regarding numbers of applicants and enrollees to each dental school, along with their race, gender, age, type of predental education, mean DAT and GPA, and state of origin.

ACADEMIC AND OTHER ASSISTANCE

Pre-entrance reinforcement programs are not available, but a tutorial service is provided early in the program for those students who encounter academic difficulties.

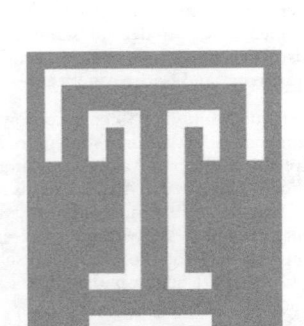

TEMPLE UNIVERSITY
THE MAURICE H. KORNBERG SCHOOL OF DENTISTRY

Dr. Martin F. Tansy, Dean

GENERAL INFORMATION

Temple University Maurice H. Kornberg School of Dentistry is the second oldest dental school in continuous existence. As a major urban institution in the heart of a federally designated health professional shortage area, the dental school has a diverse patient population from a variety of socioeconomic and cultural backgrounds. The large size and diversity of this patient pool contribute immeasurably to a student's dental education. Temple's student body is among the most diverse in the country. Most states and several countries are represented by Temple students. The relaxed and friendly team-oriented atmosphere generates strong relationships among students, staff, and faculty.

Although a multitude of research opportunities exist, Temple's strength has always been excellence in the clinical practice of dentistry. The comprehensive treatment curriculum cultivates manual dexterity, clinical technique, and diagnostic, preventive, and treatment skills, as well as encourages the development of basic practice management.

For students with an interest in business, a joint degree DMD/MBA program is available to qualified students at no additional cost.

Temple graduates are known for their confidence and ability to successfully treat patients immediately upon graduation. Sixty percent of graduating seniors enter the workforce and nearly 40 percent continue their education in postgraduate programs of their choice.

ADMISSION REQUIREMENTS

NUMBER OF YEARS OF PREDENTAL EDUCATION: Formal minimum of three.

LIMITATIONS ON COMMUNITY COLLEGE WORK: Community college work accepted in non-basic science courses only.

REQUIRED COURSES:

With lab required	(semester hrs)
Organic chemistry	6
Inorganic chemistry	6
Physics	6
Biology	6

Other courses	
English	6

SUGGESTED ADDITIONAL PREPARATION: Preference is given to applicants whose transcripts include histology, biochemistry, anatomy, physiology, and microbiology.

DAT: Mandatory. Applications will not be considered without reported DAT scores no older than two years.

GPA: A minimum science GPA of 3.0 is required.

RESIDENCY: No specific residency requirement.

ADVANCED STANDING: Temple University Maurice H. Kornberg School of Dentistry offers advanced standing for the internationally trained dentist who seeks to practice dentistry in the United States. Admission to advanced standing is highly selective. Selection factors include academic record, National Board Parts I and II scores, a comprehensive preclinical skills evaluation conducted by the faculty, and a personal interview. Those advanced-standing applicants offered admission will enter the third year of the curriculum. Upon completion of the graduation requirements, the student will receive a Doctor of Dental Medicine (D.M.D.) degree. Applications for the Advanced Standing Program are available from the Admissions Office.

TRANSFERS: Requests for transfer will be considered only for current students who are in good academic standing at a dental school in the United States. Acceptance to transfer is highly selective. Selection factors include academic record, compatibility between the curriculum of the schools, available space and resources, and personal interview. Transfer applications are available from the Admissions Office.

Timetable for the Class Entering Fall 2008

	Earliest Date	Latest Date	School Fee
Application Submission	6/1/07	2/1/08	$30
Acceptance Notification	12/1/07	8/20/08	

Required Response and Deposit:
45 days after notification if accepted between 12/1 and 12/31
30 days after notification if accepted between 1/1 and 1/31
15 days after notification if accepted on or after 2/1

$1,500 to hold a place in the class; fee is applied towards tuition.

FOR FURTHER INFORMATION

Office of Admissions and Student Affairs
Lisa P. Deem
Associate Dean for Admissions and Student Affairs
215-707-2801

Recruitment Coordinator
Brian F. Hahn
800-441-4363 or 215-707-7663 brian.hahn@temple.edu

Shawn C. Campbell
Director of Multicultural Development and Recruiting
215-707-9761
shawn.campbell@temple.edu

3223 North Broad Street
Philadelphia, PA 19140

www.temple.edu/dentistry

THE DENTAL PROGRAM

The primary emphasis of the predoctoral program is to prepare graduates for the general practice of dentistry. The curriculum provides students with significant experience in all phases of dental practice and instills the basic science and patient management skills they will rely on as dental practitioners. The curriculum also lays a solid foundation for careers in the specialties of dentistry, dental education, and research.

YEAR 1. The first two years are divided between mastering the basic science subjects and developing preclinical skills necessary to complete the procedures used in treating patients. Science subjects are taught by the basic science departments of Temple University School of Medicine. There is some exposure to the clinic in the Preventive Dentistry Clinic.

YEAR 2. A continuation of the basic science and dental laboratory courses. The Introduction to Clinical Dentistry Program allows students to experience all phases of dentistry early in their experience. Patients are assigned at the end of this year.

YEARS 3 AND 4. Much of the last two years is spent providing clinical services for patients through comprehensive care of assigned patients and through clinic rotations.

AFFILIATION AGREEMENTS. The school has affiliation agreements with Alvernia College, Reading, PA; Cabrini College, Radnor, PA; Caldwell College, Caldwell, NJ; Coppin State University, Baltimore, MD; Elizabethtown College, Elizabethtown, PA; Indiana University of Pennsylvania, Indiana, PA; Juniata College, Huntingdon, PA; King's College, Wilkes-Barre, PA; Mansfield University of Pennsylvania, Mansfield, PA; Moravian College, Bethlehem, PA; Pennsylvania State University at Erie, Erie, PA; Rosemont College, Rosemont, PA; Rowan University, Glassboro, NJ; Shippensburg University, Shippensburg, PA; St. Francis College, Loretto, PA; Susquehanna University, Selinsgrove, PA; University of Pittsburgh at Titusville, Titusville, PA; West Chester University, West Chester, PA; Widener University, Chester, PA; Wilkes University, Wilkes-Barre, PA; and William Patterson University, Wayne, NJ. These programs provide an accelerated 3+4 undergraduate and professional school combined education leading to both the baccalaureate and D.M.D. degrees. Application to the dental school is separate during the beginning of the third undergraduate year.

■ Degrees Offered
DENTAL DEGREE: D.M.D.

COSTS AND FINANCIAL AID

The school accepts students on the basis of academic achievement and presupposes that matriculating students can meet their financial obligations. Aside from federal programs, students may also apply for Federal Stafford Loans and private loans. Limited tuition scholarships are available to disadvantaged students and to outstanding scholars. Temple participates in the Free Application for Federal Student Aid Service. Completed applications should be forwarded to the federal aid processor indicated in your FAFSA application packet. Students are advised that eligibility for private and bank loans will depend upon their credit ratings. The Office of Admissions and Student Affairs assists students in applying for financial aid, scholarships, and grants.

Financial Aid Awards to First-Year Students in 2006-07
■ TOTAL NUMBER OF RECIPIENTS: 101   ■ 80% OF CLASS

	Average Award	Range of Awards
Residents/Nonresidents	$38,500	
Residents	$35,000	$1,000-$52,500
Nonresidents	$42,000	$1,000-$64,130

Estimated Total Expenses for Academic Year 2006-07

	YEAR 1	YEAR 2	YEAR 3	YEAR 4	TOTAL
Tuition, resident	$31,028	$31,028	$31,028	$31,028	$124,112
Tuition, nonresident	$43,078	$43,078	$43,078	$43,078	$172,312
Other fees					
Computer	$200	$200	$200	$200	$800
Student activity	$70	$70	$70	$70	$280
Health fee	$120	$120	$120	$120	$480
Recreation fee	$60	$60	$60	$60	$240
Student facilities	$50	$50	$50	$50	$200
Books	$700	$700	$700	$700	$2,800
Instruments	$6,216	$3,827	0	0	$10,043
Estimated living costs	$13,821	$16,585	$16,585	$12,439	$59,430
TOTAL, RESIDENT	$52,265	$52,640	$48,813	$44,667	$198,385
TOTAL, NONRESIDENT	$64,315	$64,690	$60,863	$56,717	$246,585

SELECTION FACTORS

Emphasis in the selection of students is placed on academic achievement and DAT scores. Interviews, life experiences, and letters of recommendation are factors in the decision making. Applicants with four-year college degrees in the sciences are given preference over those with less than four years of college. Temple University Maurice H. Kornberg School of Dentistry encourages applications from minority students.

See chapter 3 of this guide for information regarding numbers of applicants and enrollees to each dental school, along with their race, gender, age, type of predental education, mean DAT and GPA, and state of origin.

ACADEMIC AND OTHER ASSISTANCE

Academic and personal support services are available to assist any student at any time in his or her academic career.

UNIVERSITY OF PUERTO RICO
SCHOOL OF DENTISTRY

Dr. Yilda Rivera, Dean

GENERAL INFORMATION

On June 21, 1956, the legislature of Puerto Rico, on the recommendation of the Superior Education Council of the University, approved legislation establishing the School of Dentistry. The first class started in August 1957. The School of Dentistry is one of the faculties forming the University of Puerto Rico and is located in the Medical Sciences Campus in Río Piedras, Puerto Rico. The Medical Center is a supratertiary group of hospitals that respond to the medical needs of the entire population of the island, making it a magnificent learning center in the health professions. The Medical Sciences Campus houses the School of Dentistry, School of Medicine, School of Pharmacy, School of Nursing, Graduate Public Health School, and the College of Allied Health Sciences.

The School of Dentistry is fully accredited by the Council of Dental Education of the American Dental Association. It offers the following academic programs: 1) a four-year program leading to the D.M.D. degree; 2) advanced education programs in dental specialties of oral and maxillofacial surgery, general practice, prosthodontics, pediatric dentistry, and orthodontics; and 3) continuing education.

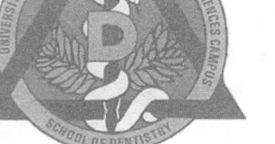

ADMISSION REQUIREMENTS

NUMBER OF YEARS OF PREDENTAL EDUCATION: Candidates for admission to the freshman class must present evidence of successful completion of 90 semester hours or 135 quarter hours at an accredited college or university.

LIMITATIONS ON COMMUNITY COLLEGE WORK: None.

REQUIRED COURSES:

With lab required	(semester/quarter hrs)
General chemistry*	8/12
Organic chemistry*	8/12
Physics*	8/12
Biology and zoology*	8/12

Other courses	
English**	12/18
Spanish***	12/18
Social and behavioral sciences	6/9

* A minimum of 2.5 (A=4.0) average is required in all prerequisite courses. All the requirements must be complete no later than the second semester of the academic year prior to admission.
** For an applicant who has approved honors English courses or who has studied in an English-speaking institution, the Committee on Admissions will evaluate the particular situation and will decide if the requirement may be reduced to six semester hours.
*** For an applicant who has approved honors Spanish courses, the Committee on Admissions will evaluate the particular situation and will decide if the requirement may be reduced to six semester hours.

SUGGESTED ADDITIONAL PREPARATION: Students are advised to select electives that will allow them to take full advantage of courses that will enhance their intellectual background and offer a well-rounded education. Biochemistry, microbiology, anatomy, histology, ethics, and statistics are highly recommended. These courses get extra points in the admission formula over other science courses. Instruction at the dental school may be in English or Spanish; therefore, all students should be competent to speak, read, and write both languages. Spanish is the first language in Puerto Rico.

DAT: The DAT should be taken one year previous to the academic year of the application, but before December 1 of the academic year of application. The candidate must obtain a minimum of 12 in each of the eight divisions. This exam should be taken before the calendar year just before the next academic year.

GPA: A minimum general and science GPA of 2.5 is required (A=4.0).

RESIDENCY: The School of Dentistry of the University of Puerto Rico is the result of an endeavor by the Commonwealth of Puerto Rico to improve and safeguard the health of its citizens. The university recognizes its responsibility in preparing professionals to meet the dental health challenges of the island. For this reason, initial preference is given to residents of Puerto Rico. The students must be competent to speak, read, and write English and Spanish. Most courses are taught in Spanish.

ADVANCED STANDING: Transfer students from U.S. and Canadian dental schools, as well as foreign dental graduates, may be admitted with advanced standing depending on the evaluation and decision of the Advanced Standing Committee. Such candidates must present evidence of the 90 predental semester hours or 135 quarter hours, required courses, and National Boards Parts I and II scores.

Timetable for the Class Entering Fall 2008

	Earliest Date	Latest Date	School Fees
Application Submission	6/31/07	12/1/07	$95 + $20
Acceptance Notification		3/15/08	(AADSAS and School)

The School of Dentistry will send notice of acceptance or nonacceptance. The accepted applicant must send his or her own written acknowledgement of acceptance of admission, together with the required deposit of $100. The student must comply with requirements specified in the letter of admission, if any. The student must preserve this notice and present it at registration as evidence of admission. The deposit is nonrefundable.

A regular dental student who, for whatever reason, withdraws or is released from the program can be considered for readmission following a one-year waiting period. This student will compete with the candidates for admission in that particular year.

FOR FURTHER INFORMATION

Office of Admission
Director of Admissions
University of Puerto Rico
School of Dentistry
Medical Sciences Campus
P.O. Box 365067
San Juan, PR 00936-5067

Office of Financial Aid
University of Puerto Rico
Medical Sciences Campus
P.O. Box 365067
San Juan, PR 00936-5067

Housing Office
Office of the Dean of Students
University of Puerto Rico
Medical Sciences Campus
P.O. Box 365067
San Juan, PR 00936-5067

www.rcm.upr.edu/academics.html

THE DENTAL PROGRAM

YEAR 1. Basic science with introduction to clinic situations.

YEAR 2. Continuation of basic science and technical courses.

YEAR 3. Clinic rotations through each of the different disciplines in dentistry.

YEAR 4. Delivery of comprehensive dental care under conditions that approximate private practice, with extramural programs in locations nationwide.

■ Degree Offered
DENTAL DEGREE: D.M.D.

COSTS AND FINANCIAL AID

Approximately 184 Puerto Rican government scholarships are granted from commonwealth funds to students of outstanding academic ability and financial need for studies in dentistry, medicine, and veterinary sciences. These are awarded for one academic year. The renewal of an award depends on need and maintenance of a satisfactory academic record.

The table below presents minimum estimates of the expenses an entering student must anticipate. All estimates are based on charges for the 2006-07 academic year. Tuition and fees are subject to change without notice, and all costs are subject to inflation.

Financial Aid Awards to First-Year Students in 2006-07
- ■ SCHOLARSHIPS: 18
- ■ STUDENT LOANS: 22

Estimated School-Related Expenses for Academic Year 2006-07

	YEAR 1	YEAR 2	YEAR 3	YEAR 4	TOTAL
Tuition* and fees	$7,531	$7,531	$7,531	$7,531	$30,124
Books and instruments	$11,600	$6,480	$2,600	$2,200	$22,880
Housing expenses	$8,657	$8,657	$8,657	$8,657	$34,628
Personal expenses	$1,105	$1,100	$1,100	$1,100	$4,405
Transportation [1]	$644	$644	$644	$644	$2,576
Health insurance [2]	$1,368	$1,368	$1,368	$1,368	$5,472
Locker fees	$30	$30	$30	$30	$120
TOTAL EXPENSES	**$30,935**	**$25,810**	**$21,930**	**$21,530**	**$100,205**

*Tuition for nonresidents varies according to geographical residence of applicant. Tuition for foreigners is $10,500 per year in addition to above-mentioned fees.
[1] Maximum if living in the limit of the metropolitan area.
[2] Optional: Pharmacy and Dental. Students may show evidence of private health insurance.

SELECTION FACTORS

Candidates for admission are subject to evaluation on four main aspects: academic performance, personal attributes, dental aptitude, and geographic residence. The academic GPA and the range of educational experiences are considered. Personal attributes are evaluated by means of a personal interview of the candidate (the Committee on Admissions notifies the applicant if an interview is required), along with letters of recommendation from a predental committee or its equivalent and from a college science instructor. Dental aptitude as measured by the DAT is another factor considered in evaluating the admission potential of a candidate. Admission test results will be valid up to three years with respect to the application deadline. It is important to note that the student will only have three opportunities to take the DAT exam.

See chapter 3 of this guide for information regarding numbers of applicants and enrollees to each dental school, along with their race, gender, age, type of predental education, mean DAT and GPA, and state of origin.

SOUTH CAROLINA

MEDICAL UNIVERSITY OF SOUTH CAROLINA
COLLEGE OF DENTAL MEDICINE

Dr. Jack J. Sanders, Dean

GENERAL INFORMATION

The College of Dental Medicine was founded in 1967 and graduated its first class in June 1971. It is a state-supported institution located in the Basic Science Building of the Medical University of South Carolina complex. The dental school has an enrollment of 224 degree students at this time. Graduate programs currently in progress include oral and maxillofacial surgery, pediatric dentistry, periodontics, and orthodontics. A well-organized dental medicine scientist training program enables selected students to earn D.M.D. and Ph.D. degrees simultaneously.

Faculty are from a wide variety of backgrounds and experience who have generated a scholarly and self-critical educational environment. The associated activities of dental education, the treatment of patients, and service to the public are practiced to the highest standards. Students are exposed to a broad range of research activities, and multiple opportunities are available in research participation. The focus of predoctoral education is state-of-the-art clinical instruction to ensure each graduate's competency in clinical dentistry.

The College of Dental Medicine is fully accredited by the Commission on Dental Education of the American Dental Association.

ADMISSION REQUIREMENTS

NUMBER OF YEARS OF PREDENTAL EDUCATION: Usual minimum of four; prefer to have earned a baccalaureate degree.

LIMITATIONS ON COMMUNITY COLLEGE WORK: Maximum of 60 semester hours, all earned before a student enters the third year of study toward a baccalaureate degree.

REQUIRED COURSES:

With lab required	(semester hrs)
General chemistry	8
Organic chemistry	8
Biology or zoology	8
Physics	8

Other courses	
Mathematics	6
English composition	6
Science electives	8

SUGGESTED ADDITIONAL PREPARATION: Applicants should take as many science courses as possible and should achieve high grades in these courses. Biochemistry, microbiology, comparative anatomy, genetics, and histology are recommended.

DAT: Mandatory.

GPA: No specific requirements.

RESIDENCY: No specific requirements; however, preference is given to South Carolina residents.

ADVANCED STANDING: No program.

Timetable for the Class Entering Fall 2008

	Earliest Date	Latest Date	School Fee
Application Submission:			
AADSAS	6/1/07	12/1/07	
MUSC Supplemental App.	7/1/07	1/15/08	$75
Acceptance Notification	12/1/07	4/15/08	

Required Response and Deposit:
Applicants must respond to an acceptance offer within 30 days (unless otherwise indicated) and must deposit a matriculation fee to hold a place in the class.

FOR FURTHER INFORMATION
Tariq Javed
Associate Dean for Academic and Student Affairs
843-792-2344 or 792-2345; javed@musc.edu
College of Dental Medicine
Medical University of South Carolina
173 Ashley Avenue
P.O. Box 250507
Charleston, SC 29425-2601

Office of Financial Aid
843-792-2536
Medical University of South Carolina
45 Courtenay Dr.
P.O. Box 250176
Charleston, SC 29425

Housing
843-792-0394
Off-Campus Housing
Medical University of South Carolina
45 Courtenay Dr.
P.O. Box 250171
Charleston, SC 29425

Office of Enrollment Management
843-792-5396
Medical University of South Carolina
Vince Mosley Building
41 Bee Street
P.O. Box 250203
Charleston, SC 29425

www.musc.edu/dentistry/index.html

THE DENTAL PROGRAM

YEAR 1. Basic sciences and preclinical dental courses.

YEAR 2. Additional basic science courses and preclinical courses.

YEAR 3. Clinical instruction and patient treatment in all disciplines.

YEAR 4. Clinical instruction, patient treatment, and extramural rotations; senior seminars for treatment planning, implantology, and practice administration.

■ Degrees Offered
DENTAL DEGREE: D.M.D.
ALTERNATE DEGREES: Combined D.M.D./Ph.D.

■ Other Programs
Externships available to senior students.

COSTS AND FINANCIAL AID

For more information, contact the Financial Aid Office.

Financial Aid Awards to First-Year Students in 2006-07
■ TOTAL NUMBER OF RECIPIENTS: 52 ■ 93% OF CLASS

	Average Award	Range of Awards
Residents—49	$42,342	$12,333-$57,496
Nonresidents—3	$56,272	$45,167-$67,377

Estimated School-Related Expenses for Academic Year 2006-07

	YEAR 1	YEAR 2	YEAR 3	YEAR 4	TOTAL
Tuition, resident	$21,550	$21,550	$21,550	$21,550	$80,924
Tuition, nonresident	$60,121	$45,496	$60,121	$60,121	$225,859
Other expenses					
ASDA fees	$460	0	0	0	$460
Cadaver fee	$500	0	0	0	$500
Hepatitis vaccine	$150	0	0	0	$150
IT fee	$3,500	$3,500	$3,500	$3,500	$14,000
Health insurance	$892	$892	$892	$892	$3,568
Lab fee (histology)	$150	0	0	0	$150
Disability insurance	$80	$80	$120	$120	$400
Boards*	0	0	$225	$300	$525
Instrument fee	$4,000	$4,000	$3,800	$3,800	$15,600
Preclinical and lab	$500	$500	0	0	$1,000
Books	$1,000	$1,400	$450	$300	$3,150
Supplies	$450	$200	0	0	$650
Uniforms	$150	0	$60	0	$210
TOTAL EXPENSES, RESIDENT	**$32,882**	**$26,346**	**$30,597**	**$30,462**	**$120,287**
TOTAL EXPENSES, NONRESIDENT	**$71,953**	**$56,068**	**$69,168**	**$69,033**	**$226,222**

*SRTA or ADEX Boards $1,600 if taken before graduation (year 4).
These charges are subject to change at any time.

SELECTION FACTORS

Selection is based on the applicant's total attributes, accomplishments, and potential for growth in the field of dental medicine. Intellectual ability is judged by the grade point average and DAT scores. While undoubtedly important, the ability to accumulate and assimilate scientific facts is not sufficient. Letters of recommendation and personal interviews are used to evaluate the applicant's noncognitive traits such as adaptability, purpose in life, and ability to establish and maintain healthy interpersonal relationships.

Preference is given to South Carolina residents. A limited number of out-of-state applicants with superior credentials are accepted.

See chapter 3 of this guide for information regarding numbers of applicants and enrollees to each dental school, along with their race, gender, age, type of predental education, mean DAT and GPA, and state of origin.

TENNESSEE

MEHARRY MEDICAL COLLEGE
SCHOOL OF DENTISTRY

Dr. William B. Butler, Dean

GENERAL INFORMATION

The School of Dentistry of Meharry Medical College is a private nonprofit school. The college was organized in 1876 to educate physicians. Ten years later, the dental department was established, and other health professional disciplines were added later. The institution is named in honor of the Meharry family, who gave and established early support for the college in response to help from a black farmer who aided one of the Meharry brothers in a time of need.

Meharry Medical College exists to improve the health and healthcare of minority and underserved communities by offering excellent education and training programs in the health sciences; placing special emphasis on providing opportunities to people of color and individuals from disadvantaged backgrounds, regardless of race or ethnicity; delivering high quality health services; and conducting research that fosters the elimination of health disparities.

The 14-acre compact campus is near the center of Nashville (population approximately 500,000, with 15 other institutions of higher learning). The school and college enrollments are 243 and 714, respectively. There are three academic divisions at the college: School of Dentistry, School of Medicine, and School of Graduate Studies and Research. Within the last ten years, the facility has been completely renovated and several new buildings have been added. The new dental school was completed in 1978. The students, faculty, and staff are highly motivated and challenged by the campus milieu. The dental school is a Southern Regional Education Board (SREB) contract participant.

ADMISSION REQUIREMENTS

NUMBER OF YEARS OF PREDENTAL EDUCATION: Formal minimum of two years; usual minimum of four years.

LIMITATIONS ON COMMUNITY COLLEGE WORK: School must be accredited.

REQUIRED COURSES:

With lab required	(semester/quarter hrs)
General chemistry*	8/12
Organic chemistry	4/6
General physics**	4/6
General zoology***	8/12

Other courses	
English composition	6/9

  *Inorganic chemistry is an acceptable alternative.
 **Heat, mechanics, and light is an acceptable alternative.
***Botany, general biology, and vertebrate and invertebrate zoology are acceptable alternatives.

SUGGESTED ADDITIONAL PREPARATION: The following courses may also be valuable in preparation to pursue the curriculum: 1) practiced reading skills of all types, such as speed, comprehension, and retention; 2) study skills, such as time management, examination preparation, and memory devices; 3) human psychology and behavior, with emphasis on children; 4) physical science, such as engineering, design, and material characteristics; 5) language and communications skills; and 6) sociology or social sciences.

DAT: Scores not acceptable three years after date of test.

GPA: Minimum average of "C" in all required prerequisite courses and a cumulative average of no less than "C."

RESIDENCY: No specific requirements.

ADVANCED STANDING: Transfer students from U.S. and Canadian dental schools may be admitted with advanced standing.

Timetable for the Class Entering Fall 2008

	Earliest Date	Latest Date	School Fees
Application Submission	6/1/07	1/15/08	$60
Acceptance Notification	12/1/07	until class is filled	

Required Response and Deposit:
45 days after notification if received between 12/1 and 12/31
30 days after notification if received between 1/1 and 3/1
15 days after notification if received after 3/2

$300 to hold place.

FOR FURTHER INFORMATION
Office of Admissions and Records
Allen D. Mosley
Director
615-327-6223

Office of Financial Aid
615-327-6826

Meharry Medical College
1005 D.B. Todd Boulevard
Nashville, TN 37208

www.dentistry.mmc.edu

THE DENTAL PROGRAM

Meharry's School of Dentistry combines educational tradition and innovation in the curriculum. As a result, students are able to develop the appropriate foundation of knowledge and skills that allow them to become the best in their fields.

The educational program of the School of Dentistry is comprised of a multifaceted curriculum. The iterative instructional pattern ensures a sound knowledge base in general dentistry. Instructional efforts strike a balance between cognitive/intellective preparation, practical application, and the inculcation of professional ethical standards.

YEAR 1. During the first year of study, most academic effort is devoted to basic sciences. Courses in tooth morphology, behavioral science, analytical reasoning, and critical thinking are taught in addition to the basic science curriculum.

YEAR 2. In the second year, preclinical courses are emphasized and prepare students for the clinical diagnosis and treatment of patients. Pharmacology and general pathology are also taught.

YEARS 3 AND 4. The final two years are devoted to clinical instruction. Patient treatment is completed in operative dentistry, prosthodontics, periodontics, endodontics, oral and maxillofacial surgery, pediatric dentistry, and orthodontics. In the senior year, students receive instruction in hospital dentistry, public health, and selected seminars.

The Part I and Part II National Dental Board Examinations must be passed for progression (Part I, freshman year) and graduation (Part II). The school's Center for Oral Health Disparities, as well as summer research externships, serves as a catalyst for dental and basic science research activities for students. Research opportunities are available as a facet of the curriculum. Student research stipends for investigative efforts are available through the National Dental Association Foundation and Colgate-Palmolive Company Program.

■ Degree Offered
DENTAL DEGREE: D.D.S.

COSTS AND FINANCIAL AID

Loans and scholarships are available. Certified residents from states participating in the Southern Regional Educational Board (SREB) program receive funds toward their tuition. Each participating state has a quota for which it will grant support, and each state's funding varies. Qualified students are eligible to participate in the work-study program. Students should inquire at their local bank to secure state or guaranteed loans. Meharry participates in programs sponsored through the U.S. Department of Health and Human Services, such as Scholarship for Disadvantaged Students, Exceptional Financial Need, Financial Assistance for Disadvantaged Health Professionals, and Loans for Disadvantaged Students. The Office of Student Financial Aid awards funds from programs sponsored through the U.S. Department of Education. Students who are affiliated with a United Methodist Church are eligible to apply for scholarship funds through the United Methodist Scholarship Program. Students are encouraged to contact the U.S. Army and Navy to participate in their Military Scholarship Programs. Brochures containing all necessary information on applications for aid are available through the school. Approximately 79 percent of our students received aid during the past year. Once a student receives financial aid, renewed assistance is almost certain, based on the students maintaining satisfactory academic progress.

SELECTION FACTORS

Students are selected for admission to Meharry Medical College by the Committee on Admissions, which is charged with selecting students who will make suitable candidates for the study and eventual practice of dentistry. The number of applicants greatly exceeds the capacity. All applications are considered on a competitive basis from the standpoint of scholarship, intelligence, aptitude, character, and general fitness. In the final selection of applicants comparing most favorably on these factors, the current policy of the institution is to give preferential consideration to applicants who: 1) come from areas with inadequate health care as measured by the dentist-population ratio; 2) have poverty backgrounds; 3) are from SREB states having contracts with Meharry; 4) are from schools that have special contracts with Meharry to admit students who have been in special courses; and 5) have a history of community activities, especially in the health care area.

The mission of Meharry Medical College includes empathy for the disadvantaged, partnership with the community for comprehensive health services, and maintenance of a center of excellence for continued study of the health sciences. Any preference given to students is in light of this mission. Attendance at Meharry is a privilege and not a right. To safeguard its ideals of high scholarship and moral and ethical standards, Meharry Medical College reserves the right to refuse admission to any applicant or to require the withdrawal of any student at any time for any reason it considers to be sufficient.

See chapter 3 of this guide for information regarding numbers of applicants and enrollees to each dental school, along with their race, gender, age, type of predental education, mean DAT and GPA, and state of origin.

Financial Aid Awards to First-Year Students in 2006-07
■ TOTAL NUMBER OF RECIPIENTS: 60   ■ 100% OF CLASS

Average Award	Range of Awards
$44,500	$36,000-$65,000

Estimated Total Expenses for Academic Year 2006-07

	YEAR 1	YEAR 2	YEAR 3	YEAR 4	TOTAL
Tuition	$27,957	$27,957	$27,957	$27,957	$111,828
Other expenses					
Lab fees, insurance, uniforms, dues, library fees, etc., equipment	$8,863	$18,401	$8,955	$7,373	$43,592
Estimated living expenses					
Books, supplies, utilities, transportation, room/board	$19,011	$19,522	$19,522	$21,290	$79,405
TOTAL EXPENSES	**$55,831**	**$65,285**	**$56,464**	**$57,170**	**$243,750**

UNIVERSITY OF TENNESSEE
COLLEGE OF DENTISTRY

Dr. Russell O. Gilpatrick, Dean

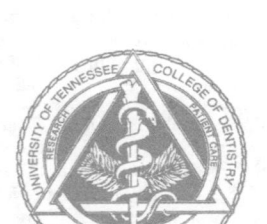

GENERAL INFORMATION

The University of Tennessee College of Dentistry is a state-assisted institution, the oldest in the South, and is located in Memphis (area population about one million). The college accepts 80 students per year into the program. The clinical facility is new and modern. The University of Tennessee Health Science Center is the state's health sciences campus and contains educational, research, and service programs in all health-related fields in an environment of integrated activities. Advanced dental education programs in general dentistry, orthodontics, oral surgery, pediatric dentistry, periodontics, and prosthodontics are offered on the Memphis campus. Programs in oral surgery and general practice residency are offered at the hospital-based unit of the college at Knoxville. The college participates in the Southern Regional Education Board, providing for enrollment of residents of Arkansas.

ADMISSION REQUIREMENTS

NUMBER OF YEARS OF PREDENTAL EDUCATION: Formal minimum of three (90 semester hours); normal minimum of four (120 semester hours). Recommendation for maximum community college semester hours: 60 semester hours (the current maximum).

REQUIRED COURSES: *(semester/quarter hrs)*

English composition	8/12
General biology	8/12
General chemistry with lab	8/12
Organic chemistry with lab	8/12
Biochemistry with lab	4/6
Physics with lab	8/12
Other Biology (applicants must take one of the following)	
Histology	4/6
Microbiology	4/6
Comparative Anatomy	4/6
Electives	52/78

Elective courses may be chosen from: genetics, comparative anatomy, developmental biology, cell biology, histology, microbiology, molecular biology, physiology, and neurobiology.

Non-science elective courses may be chosen from: philosophy, business administration, economics, public speaking, computer science, and social sciences.

OUTDATED CREDIT: Course credits in the required subjects become outdated if five or more years have elapsed between the completion of courses and proposed enrollment in the College of Dentistry. Complete details relating to the validation of outdated credit will be furnished to the applicant after the evaluation of records has been accomplished.

ADVANCED PLACEMENT CREDIT: CLEP and other advanced placement credit will be accepted for elective courses. Credit for required courses will be awarded, provided additional coursework in the same area has been completed by traditional classroom methods above and beyond the general requirements.

SUGGESTED ADDITIONAL PREPARATION: It is recommended that students have a B.S. or B.A. degree, a knowledge of dentistry as a career, and additional coursework in microbiology, biochemistry, histology, anatomy, or physiology.

DAT: The U.S. exam is required. Scores must be submitted by 11/30 prior to anticipated matriculation date. A minimum score that is consistent with the national mean is expected.

GPA: A minimum grade point average of 2.75 is expected in all required subjects attempted and in cumulative coursework. Due to the competition among applicants, classes are filled with those who have higher academic averages. Prospective applicants should strive to maintain a prescribed and cumulative grade point average well above a 3.0.

RESIDENCY: Qualified Tennesseans are given first priority; however, 18 Arkansas students are accepted each year under a formal agreement with that state. Students from other states may apply.

ADVANCED STANDING: Consideration may be given to students attempting a transfer from U.S. dental schools. Foreign dental graduates are considered for advanced standing only if they have completed Parts I and II of the National Board Examinations and the TOEFL and TSE examinations.

Timetable for the Class Entering Fall 2008

	Earliest Date	Latest Date	School Fee
U.T. Application*	6/1/07	11/30/07	$50
Acceptance Notification	12/1/07	8/15/08	

*Not an AADSAS application school; application available directly from school.

Required Response and Deposit:
45 days after notification if received between 12/1 and 12/31
30 days after notification if received between 1/1 and 2/28
15 days after notification if received after 3/1

$200 to hold place; applied toward tuition

FOR FURTHER INFORMATION

Office of Admissions
Wisdom F. Coleman, Jr.
Associate Dean for Admissions and Student Affairs
901-448-6200; 800-788-0040
University of Tennessee Health Science Center
College of Dentistry
875 Union Avenue
Memphis, TN 38163

Office of Financial Aid
Felicia Christian
Director
901-448-5568
University of Tennessee Health Science Center
910 Madison, Suite 520
Memphis, TN 38163

Minority Affairs Office
Leroy O. Moore
Assistant Vice-Chancellor
901-448-5640
Office of University Relations
University of Tennessee Health Science Center
790 Madison Avenue, 3rd floor
Memphis, TN 38163

Housing Office
901-448-5609
University of Tennessee Health Science Center
Goodman Hall, 255 So. Dunlap, Room 120
Memphis, TN 38126

www.utmem.edu/dentistry

THE DENTAL PROGRAM

The educational philosophy of the College of Dentistry is to provide opportunities for students to learn how to think in a problem-solving manner. The principal objective of the curriculum is to graduate a general practitioner who is professional, ethical, people-oriented, knowledgeable, and skillful in delivering comprehensive patient care.

The basic sciences are presented in carefully planned lecture/laboratory procedures by each department. However, selected segments of material have been combined into interdepartmental team-teaching programs.

Students are oriented to clinical activities in the first year, and delivery of patient care begins in the second year. Comprehensive, total patient care is delivered in individual student cubicles. Basic science and clinical science faculty members use a team approach to teaching in some general areas, such as growth and development, oral diagnosis, and pain control. Several off-campus clinical experiences are available at outlying hospital and clinical facilities.

■ Degrees Offered
DENTAL DEGREE: D.D.S.

ALTERNATE DEGREES: Students entering without a degree may earn their bachelor's degree only if arrangements are made independently with a liberal arts college. Masters and Ph.D. degrees may also be pursued while a student is in dental school, although a formal program is not in operation. These students are enrolled in the Graduate School of Medical Sciences, and their course of study is determined on an individual basis.

■ Other Programs
RESEARCH FELLOWSHIPS: Approximately 15-20 available for academically outstanding students.

EXTERNSHIPS: Available to fourth-year students only.

COSTS AND FINANCIAL AID

The university has an active Student Financial Aid Office committed to assisting students with limited resources. Some types of assistance are granted on the basis of financial need. Students must reapply annually. Part-time employment for dental students is available through the college work/study program. Limited scholarship assistance is also available. Loans are available through such programs as the Federal Perkins Student Loan and the Federal Family Education Loan program. Application materials are furnished for all students applying to the College of Dentistry. Completed applications should be submitted in January or February.

Financial Aid Awards to First-Year Students in 2006-07
■ TOTAL NUMBER OF RECIPIENTS: 70   ■ 90% OF CLASS

	Average Award	Range of Awards
Residents	$39,014	$8,500-$43,375
Nonresidents	$59,704	$30,500-$63,345

Estimated School-Related Expenses for Academic Year 2006-07

	YEAR 1	YEAR 2	YEAR 3	YEAR 4	TOTAL
Maintenance fee, resident	$15,670	$15,670	$15,670	$15,670	$62,680
Maintenance fee, nonresident	$36,640	$36,640	$36,640	$36,640	$146,560
Student health insurance	$1,728	$1,728	$1,728	$1,728	$6,912
Malpractice insurance	none	$30	$30	$30	$90
Parking fee (nondorm on campus)	$180	$180	$180	$180	$720
National board exam fee	0	$130	0	$165	$295
Computerized	0	$215	0	$290	$505
Instruments and supplies (kit)	$8,200	$3,900	$1,800	$150	$14,050
Instruments rental fee	$1,200	$1,200	$1,200	$1,200	$4,800
Textbooks (optional purchase)	$789	$630	$146	$179	$1,744
TOTAL EXPENSES, RESIDENT	**$27,767**	**$23,683**	**$20,754**	**$19,592**	**$91,291**
TOTAL EXPENSES, NONRESIDENT	**$48,737**	**$44,653**	**$41,724**	**$40,562**	**$175,171**

The table above represents the maintenance fee (tuition plus other fees) for the 2006-07 year. Amounts shown for instruments, supplies, and textbooks are estimates only, and are subject to change without notice. The instruments are purchased in a kit at the University Center Store at the beginning of each semester, which will be instruments utilized in courses for that specific semester.

Note: These costs do not include any living expenses.

SELECTION FACTORS

A minimum GPA of 3.0 is preferred. The present mean GPA and prescribed GPA (average of science and English) are approximately 3.3. Consistent academic performance with improvement in later work is desired. Scores of 17 or better in each category of the DAT are desired. Scores are used to indicate ability levels and to validate academic performance. Scores on the ACT, SAT, MCAT, PCAT, and GRE are also considered when available. Scores are outdated if over three years old.

The purpose of the preprofessional evaluation by college advisors is to seek information and opinions based on the student's abilities, attitude toward learning, degree of responsibility, maturity, ability to relate well with fellow students and faculty, commitment to his or her career choice, concern for the welfare of people, integrity, motivation, interest, maturity, social awareness, and intellectual capacity. An interview with several committee members as a group is required. The same attributes as those expected on the preprofessional evaluation are sought. The interview is required of all competitive applicants and is by invitation only.

The Admissions Committee does not discriminate on the basis of age, race, gender, religion, creed, or disability. Applicants must be citizens or permanent residents of the United States at the time of application. The College of Dentistry encourages applications from minority students and students from disadvantaged backgrounds.

See chapter 3 of this guide for information regarding numbers of applicants and enrollees to each dental school, along with their race, gender, age, type of predental education, mean DAT and GPA, and state of origin.

ACADEMIC AND OTHER ASSISTANCE

Dental students may utilize the special Learning Resources Center. Tutorial services are also offered throughout students' academic careers.

THE TEXAS A&M UNIVERSITY SYSTEM HEALTH SCIENCE CENTER
BAYLOR COLLEGE OF DENTISTRY

Dr. James S. Cole, Dean

GENERAL INFORMATION

In 1905 Baylor College of Dentistry opened its doors to its first 40 students as State Dental College, a private three-year dental school. With a commitment to excellence, the College evolved from its humble beginnings in 1905 to an affiliation with Baylor University from 1918 to 1971. The College existed for 25 years as an independent private institution; then, in 1996, Baylor College of Dentistry entered an entirely new era as a public institution and member of the Texas A&M University System. On January 1, 1999, the College became one of five founding components of the Texas A&M Health Science Center. The arrival of 2005 ushered in a celebration of 100 years of educating dentists to serve the citizens of the state of Texas and beyond.

The Baylor College of Dentistry campus is conveniently located in the Dallas metropolitan area, about one mile from the downtown business district within the Baylor University Medical Center complex. The facilities include the main campus building, our science building, the maxillofacial imaging center, medical library, and multilevel parking garage. The dental clinics offer 320 operatories designed as semi-closed cubicles to simulate the atmosphere of a dental office. This unique arrangement for patient care facilitates communication between instructor and student. Each clinical procedure performed by students is closely supervised by a faculty member with expertise in that clinical discipline.

Graduate programs are offered in endodontics, general dentistry, health professions education, oral and maxillofacial surgery, oral and maxillofacial pathology, orthodontics, pediatric dentistry, periodontics, prosthodontics, and biomedical sciences. The College also offers a B.S. and M.S. in dental hygiene. In addition to these, the College maintains an active continuing education program.

ADMISSION REQUIREMENTS

NUMBER OF YEARS OF PREDENTAL EDUCATION: Formal minimum of three; usual minimum of four.

LIMITATIONS ON COMMUNITY COLLEGE WORK: No more than 60 semester hours should be taken.

REQUIRED COURSES:

With lab required	(semester/quarter hrs)
Inorganic chemistry	8/12
Organic chemistry	8/12
Biology	14/21
Physics	8/12
Biochemistry	3/4

Other courses	
English	6/9

SUGGESTED ADDITIONAL PREPARATION: Choose from biochemistry II, anatomy, physiology, histology, cell and molecular biology, microbiology, small business management, foreign language, and literature.

DAT: Mandatory. Test date prior to application strongly encouraged.

GPA: No specific requirement; competitive within applicant pool; 3.0 or above recommended.

RESIDENCY: No specific requirements, but see Selection Factors.

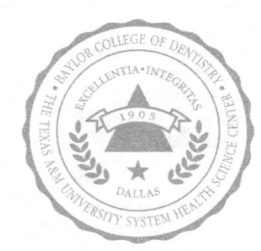

Timetable for the Class Entering Fall 2008

	Earliest Date	Latest Date	School Fee
Application Submission*	5/1/07	10/15/07	$35 (nonresident)
Acceptance Notification	12/1/07	8/11/08	

* The College of Dentistry participates in AADSAS for out-of-state applicants only. A supplemental application is required. Texas residents must apply online through the Texas Medical and Dental Schools Application Service.

Required Response and Deposit:
45 days after December 1-dated letter
15 days after January-dated letter
15 days after February-dated letter

$200 to hold place; applied toward tuition and nonrefundable if applicant fails to enter.

FOR FURTHER INFORMATION

Office of Recruitment & Admissions
Barbara Miller
Executive Director
Janet Pledger
Admissions Coordinator
214-828-8231

Office of Financial Aid
Kay Egbert
Director
214-828-8236

Community Outreach Services
Claude Williams
Director
214-828-8471

Housing
Moira Allen
214-828-8210

Student Services
Jack Long
Associate Dean
214-828-8240

Baylor College of Dentistry
Texas A&M Health Science Center
P.O. Box 660677
Dallas, TX 75266-0677

www.bcd.tamhsc.edu

THE DENTAL PROGRAM

Baylor College of Dentistry offers a comprehensive clinical curriculum that prepares its graduates for general practice and specialty programs, as well as academic, administrative, and public service dentistry.

YEAR 1. Emphasis on basic science courses; introduction to clinics with rotations for observation; introductory preclinical technique courses, and initial experiences in the clinics; information technology, and human behavior. The summer break after the first year allows time for an optional research experience.

YEAR 2. Applied sciences; emphasis on preclinical technique instruction in a simulated clinic environment optimizes the transition to the clinics; introduction to practice management and clinic computer systems. Continuation of the introduction to clinical practice rotations; begin preliminary patient treatment during the second semester.

YEAR 3. Continuation of clinical dentistry studies and direct patient treatment within a discipline-supervised comprehensive care model; routine use of practice management and clinical computer systems.

YEAR 4. General dentistry program, encompassing comprehensive patient care with advanced procedures, approximating private practice; extramural rotations and selective courses allow for experience in specialty areas.

■ Degrees Offered

DENTAL DEGREE: D.D.S.

ALTERNATE DEGREES: B.S./D.D.S. combination degrees may be negotiated by the applicant with his or her undergraduate institution. Formal agreements exist with several institutions. Information concerning these may be obtained from the Office of Recruitment & Admissions.

D.D.S./Ph.D.

M.S. degree in association with the Graduate Programs.

■ Other Programs

RESEARCH FELLOWSHIPS: Available on a competitive basis.

SELECTIVE COURSES: Special courses in advanced techniques as well as externships in many different disciplines; for example, oral and maxillofacial surgery and public health.

COSTS AND FINANCIAL AID

Baylor College of Dentistry aids the student in application for all federal need-based loan programs. In addition, both need- and merit-based scholarships are offered.

Financial Aid Awards to First-Year Students in 2006-07

■ TOTAL NUMBER OF RECIPIENTS: 87   ■ 97% OF CLASS

Average Award	Range of Awards
$29,250	$5,500-$36,058

Estimated Total Expenses for Academic Year 2006-07

	YEAR 1	YEAR 2	YEAR 3	YEAR 4	TOTAL
Tuition, resident	$7,860	$7,860	$7,860	$7,860	$31,440
Tuition, nonresident	$18,660	$18,660	$18,660	$18,660	$74,640
Fees	$1,097	$1,262	$1,714	$1,821	$5,894
Activity, health, parking					
Equipment	$8,263	$10,700	$931	$370	$20,264
Estimated living expenses	$18,838	$18,838	$22,343	$22,343	$82,362
TOTAL EXPENSES, RESIDENT	**$36,058**	**$38,660**	**$32,848**	**$32,394**	**$139,960**
TOTAL EXPENSES, NONRESIDENT	**$46,858**	**$49,460**	**$43,648**	**$43,194**	**$183,160**

SELECTION FACTORS

Student selection is determined by evaluating the quality of scholarship, DAT performance, recommendations, and the required personal interview. Personal interviews are granted to those with competitive GPAs and DAT scores as well as a history of leadership and involvement in extracurricular and community service activities. The Admissions Committee is sensitive to success in the presence of obstacles that would hinder personal or academic progress. Preference is given to legal residents of Texas and surrounding states with no college of dentistry. The College has admissions compacts with the states of Arkansas and New Mexico.

Evidence of a genuine interest in dentistry, excellent presentation skills, and high standards of moral and ethical conduct are important to the Admissions Committee.

All applicants for admission will be considered without regard to race, color, creed, national origin, age, religion, or gender. Qualified disabled persons capable of meeting the academic and technical standards essential to participating in the program will receive equal consideration. Baylor College of Dentistry encourages applications of students from underserved areas, disadvantaged backgrounds, and underrepresented groups. Applications from all candidates are evaluated using a single set of standards.

Baylor College of Dentistry engages in affiliation agreements with several undergraduate institutions. These programs allow early entry into the school if certain written criteria are fulfilled. Contact the Office of Recruitment & Admissions for information.

See chapter 3 of this guide for information regarding numbers of applicants and enrollees to each dental school, along with their race, gender, age, type of predental education, mean DAT and GPA, and state of origin.

ACADEMIC AND OTHER ASSISTANCE

The Office of Student Development sponsors a summer enrichment program open to all students on a space-available basis. This program introduces basic science as well as laboratory material. Included are Dental Admission Test preparatory and study skills courses.

Tutoring and counseling on academic progress is available for all students through the Office of Student Development. Personal counseling is available through the Office of Student Affairs.

UNIVERSITY OF TEXAS HEALTH SCIENCE CENTER AT HOUSTON
DENTAL BRANCH

Dr. Catherine M. Flaitz, Dean

GENERAL INFORMATION

The University of Texas Dental Branch at Houston is a public professional school with a unique heritage and unparalleled environmental advantages. The Dental Branch was founded in 1905 as the first dental school in Texas, and as such has a long and proud tradition of educating quality oral health care professionals. The school is one of the cornerstones of excellence that contributes to the strengths of the University of Texas Health Science Center at Houston by offering an excellent clinical education in an established research climate.

The primary focus of the Dental Branch is the education of competent oral health care professionals for the state of Texas. In pursuit of excellence, the school places major energies on its students as it teaches the basic and clinical sciences along with professional and ethical standards in an environment of collegiality.

The scholarship of discovery, teaching, integration, and application is a high priority and valued activity. In particular, the scholarship of discovery is inextricably woven into the fabric of the school, with emphasis on establishing interdisciplinary projects and securing additional outside funding.

Patient care and service are particular strengths of the Dental Branch and will continue as the school builds on its 100 years of service to the community. Centrally located in Houston, in the 675-acre Texas Medical Center, the Dental Branch functions as one of the primary sources of affordable oral health care for the people of southeastern Texas. Emphasis is on providing timely, high-quality, comprehensive oral health care with humanitarian concern for the total patient.

In fulfilling its role of service to the profession, the school remains an important local, regional, and national resource for the transfer of new knowledge, improved techniques and new technology through its continuing education programs, through the consultative services of its expert faculty, and through contributions to the clinical literature.

ADMISSION REQUIREMENTS

NUMBER OF YEARS OF PREDENTAL EDUCATION: Formal minimum of three (90 semester hours); usual four years.

LIMITATIONS ON COMMUNITY COLLEGE WORK: Recommended no more than 60 hrs.

REQUIRED COURSES:

With lab required	(semester/quarter hrs)
General chemistry	8/12
Organic chemistry	8/12
Physics	8/12
Biology*	8/12

Other courses	
English	6/9
Biology	6/9
Biochemistry	3/6

*Two semesters of biology must include formal lab.

SUGGESTED ADDITIONAL PREPARATION: It is recommended that the applicant select a major and work toward a baccalaureate degree.

DAT: Mandatory; should be taken at least 12 months prior to expected enrollment.

GPA: 3.0 or above strongly recommended.

RESIDENCY: Nonresident enrollment limited to 10 percent. Preference given to Texas residents.

ADVANCED STANDING: Consideration is given to students transferring from U.S. and Canadian dental schools. Foreign dental graduates may be admitted in advanced standing and must have passed Parts I and II of the National Board Examination before they are considered. Positions are offered only if vacancies are available for enrollment in the second-year class.

Timetable for the Class Entering Fall 2008

	Earliest Date	Latest Date	School Fee
Application Submission	5/1/07	10/15/07	$55–$190
Acceptance Notification	12/1/07	8/01/08	$30*

*$15 refundable prior to first class day.

Required Response:
45 days after notification if received between 12/1 and 12/31
15 days after notification thereafter

FOR FURTHER INFORMATION

Office of Student and Alumni Affairs
H. Philip Pierpont
713-500-4151
Associate Dean for Student and Alumni Affairs
The University of Texas Dental Branch at Houston
P.O. Box 20068
Houston, TX 77225-0068

Office of Financial Aid
713-500-3860
The University of Texas Health Science Center at Houston
P.O. Box 20036
Houston, TX 77225-0036

Housing Manager
William Hinton
713-500-8444
The University of Texas Health Science Center at Houston
University Housing
7900 Cambridge
Houston, TX 77054

www.db.uth.tmc.edu

THE DENTAL PROGRAM

The curriculum utilizes a basic lecture system, supplemented with seminars, discussion groups, and laboratories. There is intentional integration of basic science material into preclinical and clinical disciplines to ensure development of sound decision-making and clinical skills. First exposure to clinic occurs in the second year with responsibility for comprehensive patient care beginning the spring of the second year.

YEAR 1. Basic sciences with introduction to clinical situations.

YEAR 2. Continuation of basic sciences and technical courses plus definitive clinical patient treatment.

YEAR 3. Didactic clinical sciences and clinical care under discipline supervision.

YEAR 4. Delivery of comprehensive dental care under conditions that approximate private practice, with extramural programs in off-site locations.

■ Degrees Offered
DENTAL DEGREE: D.D.S.

ALTERNATE DEGREES: D.D.S./Ph.D., M.S. in association with the Advanced Education Programs

■ Other Programs
An elective program is available; students are required to select a given number of credits in those subjects in which they have specific interest. Off-campus clinical experiences are included.

COSTS AND FINANCIAL AID

The University of Texas Health Science Center-Houston has limited financial aid available to its students. A student cannot depend on the school as a major source of financial aid. Awards are usually made yearly on the basis of established financial need. Applications for entering students are accepted by the financial aid officer after an applicant has made a deposit to hold a position in an entering class. For more information, contact the Financial Aid Office.

Financial Aid Awards to First-Year Students in 2006-07

■ TOTAL NUMBER OF RECIPIENTS: 72

Average Award
$43,272

Estimated Total Expenses for Academic Year 2006-07

	YEAR 1	YEAR 2	YEAR 3	YEAR 4	TOTAL
Tuition, resident	$10,125	$10,125	$10,125	$10,125	$40,500
Tuition, nonresident	$20,925	$20,925	$20,925	$20,925	$83,700
Other expenses	$9,075	$9,945	$6,269	$5,235	$30,524
Estimated living expenses	$21,600	$21,600	$21,600	$18,000	$82,800
TOTAL EXPENSES, RESIDENT	**$40,800**	**$41,670**	**$37,994**	**$33,360**	**$153,824**
TOTAL EXPENSES, NONRESIDENT	**$51,600**	**$52,470**	**$48,794**	**$44,160**	**$197,024**

SELECTION FACTORS

Factors evaluated by the Admissions Committee are academic performance (including academic progression or regression), DAT scores, and an evaluation of all letters of recommendation, including a required recommendation from a health professions advisory committee. Other factors that may reflect the individual's personal attributes that contribute to success as a dental professional are also considered.

Legal residents of Texas are given preference. Interviews are required before final acceptance. For the class admitted in 2006, 241 out of 787 applicants were interviewed.

See chapter 3 of this guide for information regarding numbers of applicants and enrollees to each dental school, along with their race, gender, age, type of predental education, mean DAT and GPA, and state of origin.

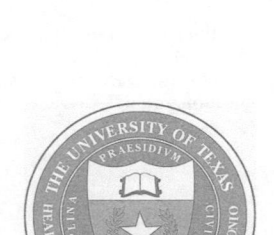

UNIVERSITY OF TEXAS HEALTH SCIENCE CENTER AT SAN ANTONIO
DENTAL SCHOOL

Dr. Kenneth L. Kalkwarf, Dean

GENERAL INFORMATION

The University of Texas Health Science Center at San Antonio (UTHSCSA) is a public institution created by the Texas state legislature on May 23, 1969. The first class of 16 dental students was accepted in September 1970. The dental school is located in the heart of the South Texas Medical Center and is one of five schools in the Health Science Center.

Each dental student is assigned an individual cubicle in the multidisciplinary laboratories for the freshman and sophomore years. This may be used for study and for basic science and preclinical technical laboratory courses.

Students participate in an exciting program known as the electronic curriculum support system. It utilizes a specially configured laptop computer to provide rapid access to current information. The laptop is capable of conducting integrated searches across various printed and multimedia sources to provide instantaneous, clinically relevant information. Its usefulness will extend longitudinally throughout students' dental education. This laptop program also has a futuristic component that enables the user to access the electronic patient record system and utilize evolving capabilities in digital radiography. It is also able to support the continued development of a rich clinical care database.

The dental school has a strong clinical and didactic teaching program and is a leader in dental research activities. Numerous research opportunities are available to students, and the interdisciplinary aspect of many research programs among departments and schools in the Health Science Center is highly regarded as one of the institution's strengths. Additionally, external education sites are available on a rotational basis to broaden the clinical and interpersonal experiences of the students. The academic environment is exciting and challenging, and there is a strong sense of camaraderie and support among students, faculty, administration, and staff.

The dental school offers advanced education in prosthodontics, periodontics, endodontics, pediatric dentistry, general dentistry, dental public health, orthodontics, and dental diagnostic sciences. In addition, a hospital-based oral and maxillofacial surgery program is offered. The School of Allied Health offers programs in dental hygiene and dental laboratory technology. Continuing education opportunities are offered not only on the San Antonio campus but in several communities around the state where the necessary facilities are available.

San Antonio is the eighth largest city in the United States. The school is located in the northwest section of the city, and there is a large selection of excellent housing facilities adjacent to the campus.

ADMISSION REQUIREMENTS

NUMBER OF YEARS OF PREDENTAL EDUCATION: Formal minimum of three years (90 semester hours) from an accredited college or university in the United States or Canada; no foreign coursework accepted.

LIMITATIONS ON COMMUNITY COLLEGE WORK: None, provided the course requirements may be met within the curriculum of the community college.

REQUIRED COURSES:

With lab required	(semester/quarter hrs)
Inorganic chemistry	8/12
Organic chemistry	8/12
Biology	14/21
Physics	8/12

SUGGESTED ADDITIONAL PREPARATION: Biochemistry, upper division biology, conversational Spanish, advanced literature, ceramics, sculpturing, freehand art, jewelry making, courses in musical instruments, keyboarding skills.

DAT: Should be taken no later than November prior to the year of matriculation; must be taken within three years of application.

GPA: Competitive with applicant pool.

RESIDENCY: Up to 10 percent nonresidents may be accepted. Texas residents must apply through the Texas Medical and Dental Schools Application Service (TMDSAS). The application form is available online at www.utsystem.edu/tmdsas.

TRANSFER: Consideration may be given to students transferring from U.S. or Canadian dental schools on a very limited basis. Information is found at www.dental.uthscsa.edu under "admissions and student affairs."

Timetable for the Class Entering Fall 2008

	Earliest Date	Latest Date	School Fee
Application Submission	5/1/07	10/15/07	$40
Acceptance Notification	12/1/07	First day of registration	

Required Response:
One month after notification if received between 12/1 and 1/5
14 days after notification if received after 1/5

FOR FURTHER INFORMATION

Office of Admissions
Sofia Almeda
Assistant to the Registrar
210-567-2659

Financial Aid Office
Robert Lawson
Director
210-567-2635

Dental Dean's Office
D. Denee Thomas
Associate Dean for Student Affairs
210-567-3752

UTHSCSA
7703 Floyd Curl Drive
San Antonio, TX 78229-3900

dental.uthscsa.edu

THE DENTAL PROGRAM

The educational program embraces the philosophy of comprehensive care. Dental preclinical courses begin the freshman year so that a significant component of patient care may be incorporated into the sophomore year. Clinical patient care as well as research activities for students are emphasized in our program.

YEAR 1. Foundation and clinical sciences, preclinical courses, and various clinical rotations; introduction to patient care; introduction to professional development and practice management; introduction to informatics and use of a computer.

YEAR 2. Continuation of foundation and clinical sciences, preclinical courses, rotations, and limited patient care; continuation of professional development and practice management; continuation of informatics and use of a computer.

YEAR 3. Comprehensive patient care in a group practice setting, supervised by discipline representatives; continuations of clinical sciences; less emphasis on foundation sciences, increased emphasis on professional development and practice management; clinical rotations requiring direct patient care.

YEAR 4. Comprehensive patient care in a setting that approximates private practice, supervised by the Department of General Dentistry; continuation of clinical rotations that augment basic science foundation.

■ Degrees Offered
DENTAL DEGREE: D.D.S.

DENTAL EARLY ADMISSIONS PROGRAM: B.S./D.D.S. with the following schools:

- Abilene Christian University
- Midwestern State University
- University of the Incarnate Word
- McMurry University
- University of Texas at Brownsville
- University of Texas at El Paso
- The University of Texas at Pan American
- Prairie View A&M University
- Sam Houston State University
- The University of Texas at San Antonio
- Texas State University
- St. Mary's University
- Texas Lutheran University
- Texas A&M International University
- Texas A&M University Corpus Christi
- Texas A&M University-Kingsville
- West Texas A&M University
- Texas Wesleyan University
- University of Mary Hardin-Baylor

Combined D.D.S./Ph.D. programs with the Graduate School of Biomedical Sciences.

■ Other Programs
RESEARCH FELLOWSHIPS: Available on a competitive basis.

EXTERNSHIPS AND ELECTIVES: Available to second-, third-, and fourth-year students.

COSTS AND FINANCIAL AID

UTHSCSA provides limited need- and merit-based funds. For more information, contact the Financial Aid Office.

SELECTION FACTORS

Preference is given to Texas residents. The Committee on Admissions takes into account scholastic records with an emphasis on science grade point average, preprofessional evaluations, personal applicant statement, and DAT scores. Interviews are required. UTHSCSA encourages applications from individuals with interest in practicing in a rural community in Texas. A more complete presentation of selection factors may be viewed under "Admissions Information Viewbooks" at the web site www.uthscsa.edu/students.

See chapter 3 of this guide for information regarding numbers of applicants and enrollees to each dental school, along with their race, gender, age, type of predental education, mean DAT and GPA, and state of origin.

ACADEMIC AND OTHER ASSISTANCE

UTHSCSA sponsors recruitment and retention programs for all students. These programs include tours for applicants and their parents or other interested parties upon request, as well as individual assistance upon request. Upon matriculation, students also benefit from a wide range of academic and personal support services, including tutoring, peer and faculty advisors, professional psychological counseling, and assistance with study skills.

Financial Aid Awards to First-Year Students in 2006-07
■ TOTAL NUMBER OF RECIPIENTS: 86   ■ 90% OF CLASS

	Average Award	Range of Awards
Residents	$37,396	$2,500-$44,000
Nonresidents	$37,836	$9,500-$47,000

Estimated Total Expenses for Academic Year 2006-07

	YEAR 1	YEAR 2	YEAR 3	YEAR 4	TOTAL
Tuition, resident	$5,400	$5,400	$5,400	$5,400	$21,600
Tuition, nonresident	$16,200	$16,200	$16,200	$16,200	$64,800
Other expenses					
Clinic usage	0	$500	$500	$500	$1,500
Student service	$220	$220	$220	$220	$880
Medical service	$135	$135	$135	$135	$540
Library	$200	$200	$200	$200	$800
Lab fee	$32	$32	0	0	$64
Micro rental	$48	0	0	0	$48
Implantology	0	$500	0	0	$500
Graduation	0	0	0	$60	$60
Equipment lease	$2,000	$2,000	$1,800	$1,800	$7,600
Laptop computer	$4,300	$1,500	$1,500	$1,500	$8,900
Tech support fee	$350	$350	$350	$300	$1,350
Designated tuition	$1,725	$1,725	$1,725	$1,725	$6,900
Differential tuition	$3,000	$3,000	$3,000	$3,000	$12,000
Human materials	$300	0	0	0	$300
Supplemental kit	$350	$365	$25	0	$715
Estimated living expenses	$15,000	$15,000	$15,000	$15,000	$60,000
TOTAL EXPENSES, RESIDENT	**$32,805**	**$31,102**	**$29,875**	**$29,885**	**$123,667**
TOTAL EXPENSES, NONRESIDENT	**$43,605**	**$41,902**	**$40,675**	**$40,685**	**$166,867**

VIRGINIA COMMONWEALTH UNIVERSITY
SCHOOL OF DENTISTRY

Dr. Ronald J. Hunt, Dean

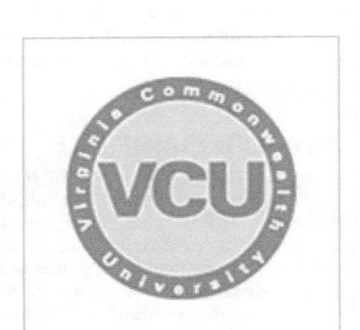

GENERAL INFORMATION

Virginia Commonwealth University (VCU) School of Dentistry is a state-supported school founded in 1893. The school is located in a historic district of Richmond, which has a population of 200,000 with approximately 1,000,000 residing in the metropolitan area. VCU has two major campuses that are less than three miles from each other: the Monroe Park Campus with an enrollment of over 26,000 students, and the VCU Medical Campus with 3,500 students. VCU's Medical campus is the site for a nationally ranked comprehensive academic health center and is comprised of the VCU Medical Center and the Schools of Allied Health Professions, Dentistry, Medicine, Nursing, and Pharmacy.

The School of Dentistry is housed in two connecting buildings that contain classrooms, student laboratories, and new clinical and research facilities. A new 20-station virtual reality "DentSim" laboratory is a unique component of our freshman operative curriculum. Renovations are under way to construct a multimedia simulation laboratory, a conference center, and a dental school building addition. There are approximately 350 students enrolled in the D.D.S. program and another 46 students enrolled in the Division of Dental Hygiene. The school has 42 advanced education students enrolled in programs of endodontics, oral and maxillofacial surgery, orthodontics, pediatric dentistry, periodontics, and advanced education in general dentistry.

ADMISSION REQUIREMENTS

NUMBER OF YEARS OF PREDENTAL EDUCATION: Formal minimum of three; generally acceptable minimum of four.

LIMITATIONS ON COMMUNITY COLLEGE WORK: Maximum of 60 semester hours.

REQUIRED COURSES: A minimum of 90 semester hours of college credit from an accredited institution is required for admission. Required courses are general biology, general chemistry, organic chemistry, physics, biochemistry and English. Laboratory experiences are required for those courses where applicable. Courses in general microbiology, anatomy, physiology, genetics, immunology, behavioral sciences, embryology, and those involving psychomotor skills are strongly recommended. Academic credits presented by an applicant must be acceptable for credit toward a degree in the institution at which the courses were taken.

DAT: Mandatory; should be taken no later than December of the year prior to desired matriculation.

GPA: No specific requirements.

RESIDENCY: No specific requirements; see Selection Factors.

ADVANCED STANDING: There is no formal advanced standing program. In rare instances, consideration may be given to students requesting a transfer from U.S. or Canadian dental schools or graduates from a non-U.S./Canadian dental school may be considered for admission at a level past the first year. Advanced standing can occur only if positions are available in the corresponding class for which the candidate qualifies.

Timetable for the Class Entering Fall 2008

	Earliest Date	Latest Date	School Fee
Application Submission	5/18/07	11/1/07	$70
Acceptance Notification	12/1/07	7/23/08	

Required Response and Deposit:
45 days after notification if received between 12/1 and 12/31
30 days after notification if received between 1/1 and 1/31
15 days after notification if received after 2/1

$500 to hold place after acceptance, and a second deposit of $300 is due on or before May 1; fees apply to tuition and are nonrefundable.

FOR FURTHER INFORMATION

Office of Admissions
Michael Healy
Assistant Dean
804-828-9196

Office of Student Services and Minority Affairs
Carolyn Booker
Assistant Dean
804-828-9953

Office of Financial Aid
Karen D. Gilliam
Director of Financial Aid
804-828-6374

VCU School of Dentistry
P.O. Box 980566
Richmond, VA 23298-0566

Housing
VCU Medical Campus
Manager
804-828-1800
VCU Housing Office
P.O. Box 980243
Richmond, VA 23298-0243

www.dentistry.vcu.edu

THE DENTAL PROGRAM

The VCU School of Dentistry is a public, urban, research dental school, supported by the Commonwealth of Virginia to serve the people of the state and the nation. The school's mission is to provide educational programs that prepare graduates who are competent to provide dental care services; generate new knowledge through research and other scholarly activity; and provide quality oral health care to the public and service to the community. The school's overall higher purpose is enhancing the quality of life through improved oral health. In the pursuit of its higher purpose, the school is guided by a set of unchanging core values:

- commitment to the oral health needs of Virginia residents
- excellence in teaching and promotion of learning advancement of science and scholarship
- ethical, compassionate, evidence-based patient care
- fostering a culture of lifelong learning
- professional and social responsibility
- respect in interaction with all people
- promotion of collegiality within the faculty

YEAR 1. Foundation in the basic sciences and preclinical dental sciences; introduction to patient care and various clinical rotations; introduction to scientific inquiry. National Boards, Part I, are taken at the end of year 1.

YEAR 2. Continuation of basic science and preclinical dental sciences; additional clinical rotations and limited patient care.

YEARS 3 AND 4. Comprehensive patient care in a general practice model with a family of patients; continuation of dental sciences with a focus on clinical situations; clinical rotations requiring direct patient care; clinical experiences at a wide range of remote sites (primarily fourth-year students).

■ Degrees Offered

DENTAL DEGREE: D.D.S.

ALTERNATE DEGREES: B.S./D.D.S. — Students entering without a degree may earn a bachelor's degree if it is awarded by their predental college or university.

Combined D.D.S./M.S. or D.D.S./Ph.D. degrees are offered in conjunction with the School of Medicine. Each program is individually developed by the two schools. Additional time beyond the formal four years is required for the D.D.S./Ph.D. and may be required for the D.D.S./M.S. degree

■ Other Programs

RESEARCH FELLOWSHIPS: On a competitive basis.

SPECIAL ASSISTANTS: Teaching assistants for fourth-year students in certain areas.

COSTS AND FINANCIAL AID

The School of Dentistry makes an effort to ensure that qualified students are not denied admission because of their lack of funds. A full-time financial aid coordinator works with students in school. Rural Virginia Dental Scholarships and local college funds are designed to give financial aid to students undertaking the course of study required for dentistry. Information on financial assistance may be obtained from the financial aid coordinator.

SELECTION FACTORS

The Virginia Commonwealth University is a state-supported university and gives admission preference to state residents. Otherwise, all applicants are evaluated by uniform criteria without regard to national origin, color, race, religion, disability, age, or gender.

Students are selected by the Admissions Committee on the basis of excellence of predental education, DAT scores, recommendations, and results of personal interviews with members of the committee. The interview process is standardized and designed to determine motivation, knowledge of, and interest in the dental profession and to afford the applicant an opportunity to provide additional information pertaining to his or her application.

The required courses should be completed by July of the year in which admission is desired. Applicants with degrees that include 120 credit hours are usually preferred.

See chapter 3 of this guide for information regarding numbers of applicants and enrollees to each dental school, along with their race, gender, age, type of predental education, mean DAT and GPA, and state of origin.

Financial Aid Awards to First-Year Students in 2006-07
■ TOTAL NUMBER OF RECIPIENTS: 87   ■ 95% OF CLASS

	Average Award	Range of Awards
Residents	$41,056	$8,500-$49,140
Nonresidents	$62,877	$8,500-$65,768

Estimated Expenses for Academic Year 2006-07

	YEAR 1	YEAR 2	YEAR 3	YEAR 4	TOTAL
Tuition, resident	$16,270	$16,435	$16,270	$16,270	$65,245
Tuition, nonresident	$32,898	$33,063*	$32,898	$32,898	$131,758
Fees: university, health service, student government, disability, and technology	$1,539	$1,539	$1,539	$1,539	$6,156
Books	$1,340	$1,927	$86	$2,572	$6,734
Computer	$2,100	0	0	0	$2,100
Instrument purchase	$1,700	$1,700	$1,700	$580	$5,680
Instrument rental	$1,800	$1,800	$1,800	0	$5,400
Clinical usage fee	$2,150	$2,150	$2,150	$1,150	$7,600
Estimated living expenses, room, board, transportation, and miscellaneous	$23,320	$23,320	$23,320	$21,200	$91,160
TOTAL EXPENSES, RESIDENT	**$49,140**	**$47,790**	**$46,596**	**$42,232**	**$185,759**
TOTAL EXPENSES, NONRESIDENT	**$65,768**	**$64,420**	**$63,224**	**$58,860**	**$252,272**

* All sophomore dental students are assessed a $165 course fee.

UNIVERSITY OF WASHINGTON
SCHOOL OF DENTISTRY

Dr. Martha J. Somerman, Dean

GENERAL INFORMATION

The University of Washington School of Dentistry offers an excellent education leading to a professional health care career in a challenging and growing discipline. The School of Dentistry is located on the University of Washington's main campus, which occupies approximately 700 acres on the shores of Portage Bay and Lake Washington in north-central Seattle. Established in 1945, the School of Dentistry is one of six professional schools that are components of the state-supported Warren G. Magnuson Health Sciences Center, an internationally recognized teaching, research, and patient care facility. The other components include the Schools of Medicine, Nursing, Pharmacy, Social Work, and Public Health and Community Medicine, six special research centers and institutes, the University of Washington Medical Center, Harborview Medical Center, the Fred Hutchinson Cancer Research Center, and Children's Hospital and Regional Medical Center, all of which contribute to a rich and diverse educational environment.

As with the other components of the University of Washington's Health Sciences Center, the School of Dentistry works collaboratively to improve the health and wellbeing of the people of the community and the region through outreach programs that are especially attentive to underserved populations. The importance of delivering culturally competent oral health care and disease prevention is an area in which the School of Dentistry's curriculum is changing the way dental students are taught. With funding from the Robert Wood Johnson Foundation's Pipeline, Practice & Profession: Community-Based Dental Education grant, the school's curriculum has been modified so that the didactic and clinical curricula prepare students to deliver culturally appropriate, patient-centered care. The clinical curriculum has expanded to include more extended clinical rotations at sites throughout the state as a means for helping students understand the barriers that limit access to routine dental care and disease prevention programs for many urban and rural populations.

The educational program is enriched by the school's strong commitment to research. Research at the University of Dentistry has grown enormously in both scope and diversity over the past decade. The School of Dentistry is consistently one of the national leaders in financial support from the National Institute of Dental and Craniofacial Research (NIDCR), one of the divisions of the Naional Institutes of Health. In addition to support from more than 60 individual research and training grants, the School draws on the resources of the Northwest/Alaska Center to Reduce Oral Health Disparities, and serves as the base of Northwest PRECEDENT, a five-state practice-based research network.

Among the school's training grants is the Summer Undergraduate Research Fellowship (SURF). With funding from NIDCR, the School of Dentistry, the dental alumni association, and local and national foundations, the SURF program gives dental students a meaningful experience conducting oral health research with faculty mentors. Besides conducting research, all of the students participating in the SURF program present their research to their peers and faculty at the school's Research Day at the beginning of each school year. A number of students also present the results of their research at national meetings like the American Association for Dental Research. In addition to these short-term research training experiences, the school also has a combined D.D.S./Ph.D. program, designed for the student interested in pursuing an academic or research-focused career. This seven-year program combines the D.D.S. curriculum with the School's Oral Biology Ph.D. curriculum and is financially supported by a partnership with the Washington State Dental Association.

The School of Dentistry values diversity in its students, staff, faculty, and patient populations. As such, the School is committed to increasing and supporting diversity in the profession. Through partnerships with the Washington Dental Service Foundation, the Robert Wood Johnson Foundation's Summer Medical and Dental Education Program, and the University of Washington's School of Medicine, various pipeline programs are in place, all with the common goals of increasing diversity in the profession and helping all students achieve their academic and professional goals.

In addition to the Doctor of Dental Surgery (D.D.S.) degree and the D.D.S./Ph.D. degree, the school offers advanced dental specialty training leading to a Master of Science in Dentistry (M.S.D.) degree and/or a certificate of proficiency in endodontics, oral biology, oral pathology, oral medicine, orthodontics, pediatric dentistry, periodontics, and prosthodontics. Residency training programs are available in oral and maxillofacial surgery, pediatric dentistry, and the general practice of dentistry. Master's of science (M.S.) and doctoral (Ph.D.) degrees in oral biology and postdoctoral study in applied behavioral science are also offered.

Timetable for the Class Entering Fall 2008

	Earliest Date	Latest Date	School Fee
Application Submission	6/1/07	11/1/07	$35
Acceptance Notification	12/1/07	8/25/08	

Required Response and Deposit:
45 days if accepted on or after December 1
30 days if accepted on or after January 1
15 days if accepted on or after February 1

$100 nonrefundable deposit applicable toward tuition.

FOR FURTHER INFORMATION

Admissions
Kathleen Craig
Admissions Officer
206-543-5840; askuwsod@u.washington.edu
Office of Student Services, Admissions, and Outreach
D323 Health Sciences Building
University of Washington
School of Dentistry
Box 356365
Seattle, WA 98195-6365

Office of Financial Aid
Carol Brown
Director
206-685-2372
Office of Student Services, Admissions, and Outreach
D323 Health Sciences Building
University of Washington
School of Dentistry
Box 356365
Seattle, WA 98195-6365

www.dental.washington.edu

UNIVERSITY OF WASHINGTON SCHOOL OF DENTISTRY **WASHINGTON**

ADMISSION REQUIREMENTS

NUMBER OF YEARS OF PREDENTAL EDUCATION: Minimum of three.

LIMITATIONS ON COMMUNITY COLLEGE WORK: None.

REQUIRED COURSES: *(semester/quarter hrs)*

Organic chemistry	1/2
Biochemistry	1/2
General chemistry	1/2
General physics	2/3
General zoology or biology	2/3
General microbiology	1/2

SUGGESTED ADDITIONAL PREPARATION: See Selection Factors.

DAT: Mandatory. Test must be taken no later than October 31 of year prior to admission.

GPA: GPA needs to be competitive within applicant pool.

RESIDENCY: Preference is given to selection of applicants in the following order: Washington state residents, WICHE states residents, followed by residents of other states.

ADVANCED STANDING: The University of Washington rarely admits transfer students from other dental schools. The school does not offer a program for foreign-trained dentists seeking dental licensure in the United States.

SELECTION FACTORS

The Admissions Committee holistically reviews applicants and takes into account the following factors: academic record which includes overall GPA and predental science GPA, demonstrated community service/leadership, level of preprofessional education, DAT scores, demonstrated dental knowledge, unique life experiences, contribution to diversity, and performance in the personal interview. The Admissions Committee encourages diversity in majors, and gives no preference to a particular undergraduate major.

See chapter 3 of this guide for information regarding numbers of applicants and enrollees to each dental school, along with their race, gender, age, type of predental education, mean DAT and GPA, and state of origin.

THE DENTAL PROGRAM

The School of Dentistry's four-year D.D.S. curriculum provides students with opportunities to learn the fundamental principles significant to the entire body of oral health. Students (approximately 55 per class) learn the basic health sciences, attain proficiency in clinical skills, develop an understanding of professional and ethical principles, and develop reasoning and critical decision-making skills that will enable implementation of the dental knowledge base.

Elective courses are offered by all departments, including opportunities in independent study, research, seminars on various topics, and special clinical topics.

YEAR 1. Divided among lecture, laboratory, and preclinical activities in the basic sciences, dental anatomy, occlusion, and dental materials. There are also early clinical experiences in preventive dentistry and periodontics.

YEAR 2. Development of additional preclinical skills, learning how basic science principles are applied to the clinical setting, and the beginning of patient care in the school's clinics.

YEAR 3. Clinical rotations in each of nine clinical disciplines, plus lectures on refining technical diagnostic skills and elective requirement.

YEAR 4. Delivery of comprehensive care, lectures on refining skills, and elective requirements.

■ Degrees Offered

DENTAL DEGREE: D.D.S.

ALTERNATE DEGREES: Combined D.D.S./Ph.D. in basic sciences.

■ Other Programs

RESEARCH FELLOWSHIPS: Opportunities for all students, including entering first-year students, are available through the SURF program for oral health research training.

EXTERNSHIPS: Available primarily for first- and fourth-year students.

ELECTIVES: Elective opportunities are available in the third and fourth years.

COSTS AND FINANCIAL AID

The school maintains a financial aid office that assists students in obtaining a variety of aid and acts as liaison with the University of Washington Office of Student Financial Aid, which administers all federal, state, and university aid programs. Application for financial aid is separate from admissions. The student must submit the Department of Education's Free Application for Federal Student Aid (FAFSA) no later than the university's priority filing date of February in advance of the academic year for which aid is being requested. Supplemental loans are available through the School of Dentistry. For further information, contact the School of Dentistry's Director of Financial Aid.

Financial Aid Awards to First-Year Students in 2006-07

■ TOTAL NUMBER OF RECIPIENTS: 50

	Average Award
Average Budget (Resident and Nonresident):	$33,052
Average Loans (Resident and Nonresident):	$29,684
Average Grants/Scholarships/Waivers:	$3,367

Estimated School-Related Expenses for Academic Year 2006-07

	YEAR 1	YEAR 2	YEAR 3	YEAR 4	TOTAL
Tuition, resident	$15,872	$15,872	$20,652	$20,652	$73,048
Tuition, nonresident*	$37,694	$37,694	$49,087	$49,087	$173,562
Other educational costs	$8,202	$7,665	$2,892	$1,132	$19,891
Living expenses	$14,922	$14,922	$19,896	$19,896	$69,636
TOTAL EXPENSES, RESIDENT	$38,996	$38,459	$43,440	$41,680	$162,575
TOTAL EXPENSES, NONRESIDENT	$60,818	$60,281	$71,875	$70,115	$263,089

*Nonresidents may be eligible for a nonresident waiver after their first year.

WEST VIRGINIA

WEST VIRGINIA UNIVERSITY
SCHOOL OF DENTISTRY
Dr. James J. Koelbl, Dean

GENERAL INFORMATION

The School of Dentistry was established by an act of the West Virginia legislature on March 9, 1951, and the first class began studies in September 1957.

The school is located in Morgantown, West Virginia, a community of approximately 50,000. It has served the state of West Virginia with highly trained practitioners since 1961. Since then, 1,921 dentists have received their degrees, along with 799 dental hygienists. More than 300 students are now enrolled in the various dental programs. As a part of the Robert C. Byrd Health Sciences Center, it offers programs of education leading to the D.D.S. degree, an M.S. degree in dental hygiene, endodontics, orthodontics, or prosthodontics, and a B.S. degree in dental hygiene, as well as a degree completion program for dental hygiene associate degree holders. The Department of Oral and Maxillofacial Surgery offers an oral surgery internship and a residency program leading to a certificate in oral and maxillofacial surgery. Programs leading to the M.S. and Ph.D. degrees are available in the basic sciences. A Graduate Practice Residency program is also available.

A community-based rural practice rotation is required during the senior year of the curriculum, giving students the unique opportunity to experience dental practice in a rural community. Students are matched with dental practitioners in rural areas and participate in oral health education lectures, tobacco awareness programs, poster contests, and family caregiver training. They also travel to school systems, senior centers, nursing homes, and community events to create awareness of good oral health habits.

The WVU School of Dentistry became the first U.S. school to implement the Axium system, an information management system similar to those found in a private practice setting. Axium allows staff, faculty, and students to capture a full electronic patient record with audit trails that reflect any changes made to the record. With field-level security, the system meets all levels of the privacy act. Axium also features a three-dimensional dental chart, allowing students unparalleled detail, flexibility, and accuracy when charting patient treatment progress.

The WVU School of Dentistry is one of 15 U.S. dental schools participating in the Robert Wood Johnson Foundation *Pipeline, Profession and Practice: Community Based Dental Education* program. This national program promotes cultural competency training, off-site community-based education, and recruitment and admission of dental students from under-represented minority and low-income backgrounds.

The WVU School of Dentistry is actively involved in research with oral health disparities being one of the major areas of focus. A current notable collaborative project is the National Institutes of Health seven-year funded project entitled "Genetics Factors Contributing to Oral Health Disparities in Appalachia."

ADMISSION REQUIREMENTS

NUMBER OF YEARS OF PREDENTAL EDUCATION: Formal minimum of three (90 semester hours); usual minimum of four.

LIMITATIONS ON COMMUNITY COLLEGE WORK: 72 semester hours.

REQUIRED COURSES:

With lab required	(semester hrs)
Inorganic chemistry	8
Organic chemistry	8
Physics	8
Zoology or biology	8

Other courses
English composition and rhetoric*   6

*An equivalent course may be substituted.

SUGGESTED ADDITIONAL PREPARATION: See Selection Factors.

DAT: Satisfactory scores should be submitted by November 1, 2007, but must be presented prior to enrollment.

GPA: No specific requirements; see Selection Factors.

RESIDENCY: No specific requirements; see Selection Factors.

ADVANCED STANDING: Limited availability; contact school for details.

Timetable for the Class Entering Fall 2008

	Earliest Date	Latest Date	School Fee
Application Submission	11/30/07	1/1/08*	$50
Acceptance Notification	12/1/07	Flexible**	

* All AADSAS application materials must be submitted to AADSAS by this date.
**In order to fill vacancies created by late withdrawals.

Required Response and Deposit:
45 days if accepted on or after 12/1/07
30 days if accepted on or after 1/1/08
15 days if accepted on or after 2/1/08
Preferred response time: 15 days

$200 residents and $400 nonresidents due on acceptance; applies toward tuition; refundable by May 1.

FOR FURTHER INFORMATION

Office of Admissions and Records
Susan Weatherholt
304-293-3521
West Virginia University
Robert C. Byrd Health Sciences Center
Morgantown, WV 26506-9815

Financial Aid Office
Candance Frazier
304-293-3706
West Virginia University
Robert C. Byrd Health Sciences Center
Morgantown, WV 26506-9810

Minority Affairs Office
Shelia S. Price
Associate Dean
304-293-6646
West Virginia University
School of Dentistry
Morgantown, WV 26506-9407

Housing Office
Corey Farris
Director of Housing
304-293-4491
West Virginia University
Morgantown, WV 26506-6430

Foreign Student Adviser
Karen Bird
304-293-3519
E. Moore Hall
International Student Office
Morgantown, WV 26506-6411

www.hsc.wvu.edu/sod

THE DENTAL PROGRAM

The School of Dentistry recognizes its obligation to produce professionals capable of meeting the dental health needs of the public and providing leadership for the dental profession. Therefore, the school offers a four-year program leading to the degree of D.D.S. that provides students with a learning environment in which to develop the technical competence, intellectual capacity, and professional responsibility necessary to meet the oral health needs of a society in a state of constant transformation.

The predoctoral curriculum consists of eight semesters and three summer sessions. Students are enrolled in courses designed primarily to prepare them for the general practice of dentistry. Student progress is monitored regularly by the Committee on Academic Standards and a team leader program. A team leader program exists to ensure students have the appropriate learning experiences to achieve competency and provide comprehensive health care to a family of patients. The predoctoral curriculum has recently been revised to provide comprehensive and current course content that is sequenced in a logical manner by addressing how each discipline can contribute to the attainment of competencies that build upon one another. A community rural practice rotation is required in the senior year.

■ Degrees Offered

DENTAL DEGREE: D.D.S.

ALTERNATE DEGREES: Students entering without a degree may earn their bachelor's degree while completing the dental program. This depends on the requirements of the college or university conferring such a degree.

Combined D.D.S./M.S. and D.D.S./Ph.D. in the basic sciences programs are available on an individual basis. The master's degree program will require from one to two additional years of study; the doctoral degree program, from two to three additional years.

COSTS AND FINANCIAL AID

The Board of Regents of West Virginia University provides a number of scholarships for dental students. In addition, the School of Dentistry has several loan funds over which it has direct authority. Other university loan opportunities are available to dental students.

Financial Aid Awards to First-Year Students in 2006-07
■ TOTAL NUMBER OF RECIPIENTS: 41   ■ 82% OF CLASS

	Average Award	Range of Awards
Residents	$32,776	$3,200-$47,101
Nonresidents	$44,819	$8,500-$57,147

Estimated School-Related Expenses for Academic Year 2006-07

	YEAR 1	YEAR 2	YEAR 3	YEAR 4	TOTAL
Tuition, resident*	$12,728	$12,728	$12,728	$11,340	$49,524
Tuition, nonresident*	$30,070	$30,070	$30,070	$27,318	$117,528
Other expenses	$10,711	$6,863	$4,019	$5,576	$27,169
TOTAL EXPENSES, RESIDENT	$23,439	$19,591	$16,747	$16,916	$76,693
TOTAL EXPENSES, NONRESIDENT	$40,781	$36,933	$34,089	$32,894	$144,697

* Tuition and fees include charges for mandatory summer sessions.

SELECTION FACTORS

Preference in admissions is given to qualified West Virginians, although outstanding nonresident applicants will be considered. Applications from minorities and women are encouraged. Careful consideration is given to those personal qualifications that bear upon fitness of applicants for the study and practice of dentistry. Economically or culturally disadvantaged students are encouraged to apply.

Application for admission in the fall of 2008 should be made promptly upon completion of the 2006-07 school year, even if the applicant has not completed all the requirements listed. Final acceptance of a student is contingent upon satisfactory completion of all requirements and official transcripts from all higher education institutions attended. Applicants not filing early reduce their chances for acceptance because the Admissions Committee begins its consideration of candidates as soon as applications are received.

Applicants for admission must present evidence of having successfully completed two or more academic years of work in liberal arts at an accredited college. Courses in comparative anatomy, microbiology, embryology, and biochemistry are strongly recommended. In addition, courses in the humanities and the social sciences are suggested, so that the applicant acquires a broadened intellectual background for both the study and the practice of dentistry. Applicants are also encouraged to shadow in the dental setting.

The most qualified applicants who have complied with all preliminary requirements for admission—including satisfactory DAT scores and recommendations from departments of biology, chemistry, and physics or from a preprofessional academic committee—are required to appear for a personal interview.

It is the policy of West Virginia University to provide equal opportunities to all prospective members of the student body solely on the basis of individual qualifications and merit and without regard to race, gender, religion, age, sexual orientation, or national origin. In addition, the university neither affiliates with nor grants recognition to any individual group or organization having policies that discriminate on the basis of race, gender, religion, disability, sexual orientation, age, or national origin as defined by the applicable laws and regulations.

International dental graduates may apply for admission to the first-year class. Those interested should contact the school for details.

See chapter 3 of this guide for information regarding numbers of applicants and enrollees to each dental school, along with their race, gender, age, type of predental education, mean DAT and GPA, and state of origin.

MARQUETTE UNIVERSITY
SCHOOL OF DENTISTRY

Dr. William K. Lobb, Dean

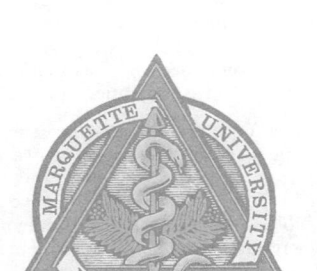

GENERAL INFORMATION

The Marquette University School of Dentistry is an independent, coeducational institution of professional training founded in 1907 when the Milwaukee Medical College affiliated with Marquette College to become Marquette University. By August 2006, the School of Dentistry had graduated more than 8,800 dentists. The school is located near the business and cultural center of Milwaukee, Wisconsin, a city with a population of approximately 600,000. The campus includes 54 buildings and 80 acres, forming an attractive, self-contained campus in the heart of a major urban center.

In August 2002, Marquette cut the ribbon on a brand new, $30 million, 120,000-square foot dental school and clinic. The new building is designed to house a revamped curriculum, one designed to operate more like a private practice with an emphasis on improved patient care. Effective reciprocal collaborations in dental education exist between the dental school and the Milwaukee Children's Hospital, the Sinai Samaritan Medical Center, and the Zablocki Veterans Administration Hospital. In addition, the School of Dentistry operates several off-campus clinics in underserved areas of the state, which provide additional clinical experience for its students.

Graduate programs leading to a master of science degree are offered in the clinical specialties of endodontics, orthodontics, and prosthodontics as well as in dental biomaterials. Hospital affiliations offer students undergraduate and graduate training in pediatric dentistry, periodontics, and oral surgery.

Many faculty members are actively engaged in research programs in addition to their teaching commitments, and continuing education courses are offered throughout the year in virtually all phases of dentistry.

Marquette University School of Dentistry has an in-state agreement with Wisconsin whereby state residents receive a subsidy toward their tuition.

ADMISSION REQUIREMENTS

NUMBER OF YEARS OF PREDENTAL EDUCATION: Formal minimum of three (90 semester or 135 quarter hours).

LIMITATIONS ON COMMUNITY COLLEGE WORK: Coursework from accredited, four-year institutions is preferred.

REQUIRED COURSES:

With lab required	(semester/quarter hrs)
Inorganic chemistry	8/12
Organic chemistry	8/12
Biology	8/12
Physics	8/12

Other courses	
English	6/9
Electives	52/78

SUGGESTED ADDITIONAL PREPARATION: In addition to the required courses, suggested courses to consider include anatomy, cell biology, genetics, biochemistry, microbiology, and physiology. Courses in communication, sociology, psychology, accounting, and finance contribute to a broad educational background.

DAT: Mandatory. Canadian DAT is accepted.

GPA: No specific requirements. Assessed on an individual basis.

RESIDENCY: Forty spaces reserved for Wisconsin residents (50% of class).

ADVANCED STANDING: Consideration is given to students transferring from U.S., Canadian, and foreign dental schools for advanced standing on a space-available basis. The sophomore level is generally the maximum level for advanced standing admission. Space is not available every year to students with advanced standing.

Timetable for the Class Entering Fall 2008

	Earliest Date*	Latest Date*	School Fee
Application Submission	6/1/07	1/1/08	$45
Acceptance Notification	12/1/07	8/30/08	

* In order to receive serious consideration, complete application materials should be received by 9/1/2007. The entering class will likely be filled by mid February.

Required Response and Deposit:
45 days if notification is received 12/1
30 days if notification is received between 1/15 and 2/15
15 days if notification is received after 2/15

A $1,000 nonrefundable deposit is required to hold a space in the class.

FOR FURTHER INFORMATION

Office of Admissions
Brian T. Trecek
Director of Admissions
414-288-3532 or 800-445-5385

Office of Financial Aid
Carla Smith-Liebich
414-288-7390

Office of Multicultural Affairs
Director of Multicultural Affairs
414-288-1533 or 800-445-5385
School of Dentistry
Marquette University
P.O. Box 1881
Milwaukee, WI 53201-1881

University Apartments and Off-Campus Student Services
414-288-7281
1500 W. Wells Street
Milwaukee, WI 53233

www.dental.mu.edu

THE DENTAL PROGRAM

Marquette University School of Dentistry's competency-based dental curriculum develops the skills and knowledge students need to successfully enter their profession. It impresses on students an understanding of the responsibility of delivering oral health care in an ethical manner. The curriculum embraces a patient-centered, comprehensive care model. This model emphasizes active student learning, a mentoring/modeling role for faculty, and a clinical environment that closely matches the practice of dentistry in the community. To support this educational model, faculty will continuously develop their skills as scholars and educators leading to recognition as innovators in educational design and instruction.

The dental curriculum involves students in a model of dental education that mimics a dental practice. Students will be trained to develop and utilize all their skills, as competent clinicians and diagnosticians, to identify and manage the multiple oral health concerns of their patients. Students will take fewer courses. Instead the curriculum combines courses into integrated, multidisciplinary tracks that link traditional dental disciplines and provide learning experiences designed to integrate knowledge, skills, and attitudes. Students will move through curricular tracks as members of small practice groups. They will participate in dental rounds (a concept borrowed from the medical education model) with faculty leading discussions of dental cases and bringing in the pharmacological and medical concerns that should be considered in planning and rendering dental care. Students will dedicate up to 25 percent of their time working at off-campus dental projects sponsored by Marquette University.

Student performance is evaluated by conventional classroom and clinical testing procedures. Proficiency examinations are conducted in the major clinical disciplines to gauge performance levels.

■ Degrees Offered
DENTAL DEGREE: D.D.S.

ALTERNATE DEGREES: B.S./D.D.S. with the following schools:

- Marquette University
- Mount Mary College
- University of Wisconsin–Parkside

Students from Marquette University, Mount Mary College, and University of Wisconsin-Parkside entering without a degree may earn their bachelor's degree while in dental school provided they were enrolled in a prescribed undergraduate program.

■ Other Programs
D.D.S./Ph.D. in conjunction with the University of Rochester (NY).

COSTS AND FINANCIAL AID

Financial aid is available to qualified students through a uniform method of need analysis. Some grant and scholarship programs are available, and all students who file financial aid forms on a timely basis will be automatically considered for the grants and scholarships for which they are eligible.

The principal loan funds available to dental students are the Federal Stafford Loan, the Health Professions Loan, and the Federal Health Education Assistance Loan. In addition, several loan funds are available to students having emergency needs. The School of Dentistry also presents $5,000 scholarships each year, many of them renewable with satisfactory academic progress. In addition, similar awards based on scholarship and leadership are provided to continuing dental students.

Students are urged to apply as soon as possible because some financial assistance is awarded on a first-come, first-served basis.

Financial Aid Awards to First-Year Students in 2006-07
■ TOTAL NUMBER OF RECIPIENTS: 79   ■ 96% OF CLASS

	Average Award	Range of Awards
Residents	$44,534	$8,200-$62,120
Nonresidents	$55,250	$4,250-$64,150

Estimated Total Expenses for Academic Year 2006-07

	YEAR 1	YEAR 2	YEAR 3	YEAR 4	TOTAL
Tuition, resident	$31,080	$31,080	$31,080	$31,080	$124,320
Tuition, nonresident	$39,830	$39,830	$39,830	$39,830	$159,320
Other expenses*					
Books	$2,000	$1,150	$300	0	$3,450
Equipment	$7,700	$3,850	$2,050	$500	$14,100
Estimated living expenses					
Room/board	$17,320	$17,320	$17,320	$10,630	$62,590
Personal	$4,780	$4,780	$4,780	$4,780	$19,120
TOTAL EXPENSES, RESIDENT	**$62,880**	**$58,180**	**$55,530**	**$46,990**	**$223,580**
TOTAL EXPENSES, NONRESIDENT	**$71,360**	**$66,930**	**$64,280**	**$55,740**	**$258,580**

*Additional fees will be required for gowns, national exams, and board fees.
Note that this budget will vary depending upon individual style of living and personal resources. It represents estimated expenses and is subject to change.

SELECTION FACTORS

Selection of students is based to a large extent upon the applicant's academic achievement in college and performance on the DAT. Other factors such as marked recent improvement in the quality of academic achievement, integrity, motivation, and the opinion of the Admissions Committee regarding the applicant's suitability for the study of dentistry are at times determinants in the selection of candidates. Three satisfactory letters of recommendation are required. On-site interviews are now required for all aplicants before acceptance. Interviews are scheduled by committee invitation only to candidates presenting competitive and timely credentials.

All well-qualified applicants are given serious consideration, and students from the 50 states as well as international students are encouraged to apply. Marquette University School of Dentistry is the only dental school in Wisconsin and has a contract arrangement with the state that results in lower tuition for students who are in-state residents.

Marquette University School of Dentistry encourages minority and female applicants. Selection is made without reference to race, creed, gender, national origin, or disability.

See chapter 3 of this guide for information regarding numbers of applicants and enrollees to each dental school, along with their race, gender, age, type of predental education, mean DAT and GPA, and state of origin.

ACADEMIC AND OTHER ASSISTANCE

The Marquette University School of Dentistry recognizes that there are underrepresented groups in the dental profession. To help overcome this situation, there is a committee whose express purpose is to work with these underrepresented groups and endeavor to stimulate their interest in the dental profession. There are no formal scheduled tutorial assistance policies; however, individual assistance programs are designed for particular students as required.

ALBERTA

UNIVERSITY OF ALBERTA
FACULTY OF MEDICINE AND DENTISTRY
DEPARTMENT OF DENTISTRY

Dr. Douglas Dederich, Acting Chair

GENERAL INFORMATION

The University of Alberta, Canada's second-largest university, is a publicly supported, nondenominational, coeducational institution. Founded in 1908, the university has developed an international reputation in many fields and excels in medical research as well as in other areas. The main campus is centrally located along the wooded south bank of the North Saskatchewan River in Edmonton and covers 220 acres.

Edmonton, the capital city of Alberta, is a major urban center and home to close to 800,000 people. It is a richly diverse city offering experiences in theater, concerts, art galleries, restaurants, shopping, cultural events, and professional sports. It is one of Canada's sunniest cities and noted for its clean, dry air.

The D.D.S. program at the university began as a department in the Faculty of Medicine with three students in 1917. By 1921 the Medical Sciences Building opened and became the Faculty of Dentistry's permanent home. In the 1960s a new dental auxiliary program was added and formed into the School of Dental Hygiene, and a graduate studies program was added. In 1996, the Faculty of Dentistry merged with the Faculty of Medicine.

Faculty members are actively involved in basic, clinical, and educational research, as well as maintaining their personal patient skills. Their research projects often involve students as permitted by their schedules.

The Department of Dentistry provides many facilities such as a complete dental laboratory, instrument sterilization on the premises, and computer systems. The John W. Scott Health Sciences Library in the Walter C. Mackenzie Health Sciences Centre contains books and periodicals for the fields of medicine, dentistry, dental hygiene, and other health-related professions. The University Hospital is in close proximity, which affords easy access to varied clinical instruction, and a rotation at the Youville Hospital provides experience with geriatric patients. A rotation to northern Alberta offers senior students extensive experience in operating a practice in an underprivileged area.

ADMISSION REQUIREMENTS

NUMBER OF YEARS OF PREDENTAL EDUCATION: Minimum two years (ten full course equivalents).

LIMITATIONS ON COMMUNITY COLLEGE WORK: Five full courses must be taken in one academic session.

REQUIRED COURSES:

With lab required	(semesters)
General	2
Organic chemistry	2
Biology	2
Physics	2
Other courses	
English	2
Statistics	1
Biochemistry	1

SUGGESTED ADDITIONAL PREPARATION: Choose from biochemistry, microbiology, and anatomy.

CANADIAN DAT: The Canadian DAT is mandatory (written February and November); minimum score is 15/30 for Reading Comprehension, PAT, MAN.

GPA: Minimum 3.0 out of 4.0.

RESIDENCY: A maximum of three out-of-province Canadian residents and one foreign application may be accepted.

ADVANCED STANDING: All candidates must start at the first-year level.

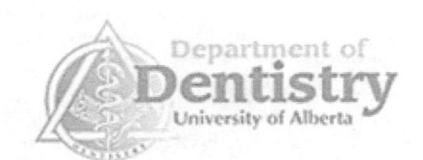

Timetable for the Class Entering Fall 2008

	Earliest Date	Latest Date	School Fee
Application Submission	7/1/07	11/1/07	$100
Acceptance Notification	5/30/08	7/10/08	

Required Response and Deposit:
14 days after receipt of the "Confirmation of Admissions" form

$175 (applicable to tuition fees) to hold place.

FOR FURTHER INFORMATION
Douglas Dederich
Acting Chair, Dentistry

Admissions Office
780-492-1319
The Faculty of Medicine & Dentistry
3028 Dentistry-Pharmacy Center
University of Alberta
Edmonton, AB T6G 2N8

Scholarships and Awards
Director, Student Awards
780-492-3221
252 Athabasca Hall
University of Alberta
Edmonton, AB T6G 2N8

The Native Health Care Careers Program
The Faculty of Medicine and Dentistry
780-492-9526
2-45 Medical Sciences Building
University of Alberta
Edmonton, AB T6G 2H7

Residence and Other Housing
Director, Housing and Food Services
780-492-4281
44 Lister Hall
University of Alberta
Edmonton, AB T6G 2N8

Foreign Admission
Office of the Registrar
780-492-4981
Administration Building
University of Alberta
Edmonton, AB T6G 2N8

www.dent.ualberta.ca

THE DENTAL PROGRAM

The Faculty of Medicine and Dentistry offers a four-year D.D.S., a two-year Advanced Placement Program for dentistry graduates of nonaccredited dental programs, a preprofessional year plus two-year Dental Hygiene Diploma, a Dental Hygiene diploma plus one-year Bachelor of Science (Dental Hygiene Specialization) degree, and a Master of Science in Orthodontics (two-year program). The students in the faculty are members of the Dental Students' Association (DSA), which represents the interests and concerns of students in dentistry and dental hygiene. The DSA annually elects representatives to organize various social, sport, and academic functions. Representatives meet regularly with the administrative staff and act as voting members on all standing committees in the faculty. The students have a locker room with personal lockers. Students also share a student lounge, study area, and cafeteria. A sense of camaraderie and cooperation through many integrated efforts in the DSA is developed due to the small class size, which allows for individualized student counseling and tutorial sessions as required.

The first and second years of the dental program are combined with the M.D. program. The curriculum is taught in blocks and covers such areas as infection, immunity and inflammation, endocrine system, cardiovascular pulmonary and renal systems, gastroenterology and nutrition, musculoskeletal system, neurosciences, and oncology. These subjects are augmented by dental courses offered by the respective divisions. The lectures, laboratories, seminars, and clinics offered by the Department of Dentistry relate and integrate these fundamental disciplines with the knowledge skills, judgment, and performance required of dental practitioners.

In addition to bedside and operating instruction in medicine and surgery, junior and senior students are assigned to the dental clinic and the Department of Dentistry, University of Alberta Hospital. An experience in the Satellite Dental Clinic and the external hospitals is required in the final year of the program. Thus students are able to relate their field of health service to the science of preventing, curing, or alleviating disease in general.

■ Degrees Offered
DENTAL DEGREE: D.D.S.

ALTERNATE DEGREES: The degree of Bachelor of Medical Science may be awarded to students in the D.D.S. program at the end of the second year, if they have fulfilled the requirements.

■ Other Programs
RESEARCH FELLOWSHIPS: A limited number are available.

SELECTION FACTORS

The selection process is dependent upon the predental academic standing, DAT scores, personal interview, citizenship, and residency. Preference for admission is given to citizens of Canada who are residents of Alberta, with 26 positions reserved for such residents. Three positions may be made available to residents of other Canadian provinces, and one position may be made available to residents of other countries. No consideration is given to applicants' race, color, creed, gender, or marital status.

In addition to the regular quota positions, one additional position per year is available in the D.D.S. program for a qualified student of Aboriginal ancestry, within the meaning of the Constitution Act of 1982, Section 35, Part 2. Applicants interested in this program are encouraged to contact the Coordinator of the Native Healthcare Careers Program at 403-492-9526. Two additional positions are available in the D.D.S. program for qualified Rural Alberta students.

See chapter 3 of this guide for information regarding numbers of applicants and enrollees to each dental school, along with their race, gender, age, type of predental education, mean DAT and GPA, and state of origin.

COSTS AND FINANCIAL AID

Student financial aid information is available from the Office of Student Services. Emergency loans are available from the Department of Dentistry.

Estimated Total Expenses for Academic Year 2006-07

	YEAR 1	YEAR 2	YEAR 3	YEAR 4	TOTAL
Tuition, instructional/noninstructional and COF*	$17,700	$17,700	$17,700	$15,320	$68,420
Dental kit	$10,000	$5,317	$3,511	$625	$19,453
Books	$1,200	$1,100	$600	$400	$3,300
Membership fees (DSA $70; CDA $100)	$170	$170	$170	$170	$680
NBDE (American examination)	0	0	0	$450	$450
NDEB (Canadian examination)	0	0	0	$1,100	$1,100
Estimated living expenses ($1,000 per month)	$11,000	$11,000	$11,000	$8,000	$41,000
TOTAL EXPENSES, RESIDENT	**$40,070**	**$35,287**	**$32,981**	**$26,065**	**$134,403****

All estimated expenses are in Canadian dollars. International students' total expenses would be higher.
*COF-clinic operation fee
**Totals include both the NBDE and NDEB examinations.
The costs above are *estimates* only. The estimated cost of books includes only those that are required. It is recommended that books not be purchased until you have attended the first lecture in each course.

It is important that students obtain kit insurance and retain it until all kit shortages, breakages, etc. have been officially listed. Any shortages, etc. not reported at the time of issuance will be the student's responsibility and charges will be made for replacement.

Financial Aid Awards to First-Year Students in 2006-07
■ TOTAL NUMBER OF RECIPIENTS: 10   ■ 31% OF CLASS

	Average Award	Range of Awards
Residents	$1,000	$300-$1,750
Nonresidents	$1,000	$300-$1,750

One award specifies Alberta residence; two awards state preference based on studies at a university in Alberta; one award states preference based on financial need; one award does not specify.

UNIVERSITY OF BRITISH COLUMBIA
FACULTY OF DENTISTRY

Dr. Charles F. Shuler, Dean

GENERAL INFORMATION

The University of British Columbia Faculty of Dentistry was officially established in 1962 and enrolled its first students in 1964. It is an integral part of the Health Sciences Centre, which includes the Faculties of Medicine and Pharmaceutical Sciences and the schools of Nursing, Rehabilitation Medicine, Clinical Psychology, Family and Nutritional Sciences, and Social Work. The Health Sciences Centre combines the teaching and research facilities of the above faculties and schools as well as the University Hospital UBC Site, made up of the Psychiatric Unit, Extended Care Unit, and Acute Care Unit. Related to this are the Faculty of Dentistry Clinic and the Mather Building, which houses Family Practice and Genetics Counselling Units.

The university is located on a 1,000-acre site on the Point Grey Peninsula at the western end of the city of Vancouver. It has an enrollment of 35,000 undergraduate students and 8,000 graduate students plus several thousand part-time, evening, and continuing education students.

The university is a publicly supported institution financed largely by grants from the provincial government. It has one of the most scenic campuses in the world. The climate of the area is moderate, and it is possible to engage in such outdoor recreational activities as swimming, boating, tennis, hiking, and fishing most of the year. The surrounding mountains provide skiing for four to six months of the year.

The Faculty of Dentistry at present offers an undergraduate program leading to the D.M.D. degree. Graduate programs in dental science at the master's and Ph.D. levels can be arranged, and a Bachelor of Dental Science in dental hygiene is offered. Postgraduate diploma courses in periodontics, oral medicine, oral pathology, and oral radiology are also available.

ADMISSION REQUIREMENTS

NUMBER OF YEARS OF PREDENTAL EDUCATION: Formal minimum of three (90 credits, where one credit equals one semester hour, or 135 quarter hours).

LIMITATIONS ON COMMUNITY COLLEGE WORK: None.

REQUIRED COURSES: (credits)

With lab required (where applicable)
Chemistry	6
Organic chemistry	6
Physics	6
Biology	6
Biochemistry	6
English	6
Mathematics	6

Ontario Academic Courses (OAC) or Grade 13 courses are not acceptable as required course equivalents.

CANADIAN DAT: All applicants seeking admission must write the Dental Aptitude Test (DAT), sponsored by the Canadian Dental Association (CDA), on or before November 4, 2007, to be eligible for consideration for selection into the D.M.D. class entering the 2008-09 academic year. Only the results of the Academic Average, PAT, and Carving Dexterity from the single-best DAT of the last five years will be calculated in the overall scores. Only DAT scores obtained in the last five years will be valid for the 2008-09 selection.

U.S. DAT: Not acceptable.

GPA: A minimum overall academic average of 70 percent or 2.8 on a 4.0 scale is required.

RESIDENCY: Only Canadian citizens or Permanent Residents are eligible to apply.

ADVANCED STANDING: There are no arrangements for considering advanced standing applicants from other Canadian and U.S. dental schools. Graduates of international dental programs may apply for the International Dental Degree Completion Program, which awards the D.M.D. degree after two years of study. Deadline for application is June 2, 2007, to begin studies in the 2008-09 academic year.

Timetable for the Class Entering Fall 2008

	Earliest Date	Latest Date
Application Submission	5/1/07	11/10/07
Acceptance Notification	2/16/08	8/24/08

Required Response and Deposit: Two weeks

$8,900 to hold place due at time of applicant's acceptance of offer; applies toward clinic fees and is nonrefundable.

FOR FURTHER INFORMATION

Student Services Office
604-822-3416; fodadms@interchange.ubc.ca
Faculty of Dentistry
#278-2199 Wesbrook Mall
The University of British Columbia
Vancouver, B.C., Canada V6T 1Z3

Awards and Financial Aid Office
604-822-5111
1036-1874 East Mall, Brock Hall
The University of British Columbia
Vancouver, B.C., Canada V6T 1Z1

Student Housing Office
604-822-2811
1874 East Mall, Brock Hall
The University of British Columbia
Vancouver, B.C., Canada V6T 1Z1

www.dentistry.ubc.ca

THE DENTAL PROGRAM

The objective of the academic program is to prepare dentists who are able to practice their profession with a high degree of technical skill and competence, based on a sound understanding of the fundamental principles of basic biological sciences that underlie the practice of dentistry and who have acquired a deep insight into their social, professional, and ethical responsibilities to the community at large.

The basic sciences are taught by the appropriate departments of the Faculty of Medicine or Faculty of Science. In some of these courses, dental and medical students are taught as a single class, and no distinction in the required levels of performance is made between them. The Department of Oral Health Science of the Faculty of Dentistry has responsibility for instruction in the dental aspects of the basic sciences and in the dental sciences. Members of this department hold cross-appointments in the basic science departments, and certain members of the latter have joint appointments in oral biology.

Students are given clinic exposure early in the program, and actual clinical instruction begins during the second half of the second year. Students receive clinical experience in a variety of clinical environments, both on and off campus. Exposure of the students to conditions in the general community is ensured through assignment of students to community health clinics and to other types of health care facilities.

The Faculty of Dentistry offers an innovative curriculum that is a hybrid of problem-based learning (PBL) and more traditional lectures and clinical experiences with an emphasis on self-directed student learning and problem solving in small group settings. Traditional lectures and laboratories occupy only a small amount of curriculum time.

The first two years are taken with students in the Faculty of Medicine and include a course exclusively for dental students that correlates biomedical sciences to clinical practice. Although there is an early exposure to the clinical setting, surgical psychomotor skills are not introduced until the second half of the second year of study in order to ensure a foundation of medical disease management before surgical intervention occurs. Students learn basic psychomotor skills in simulation and then put them into supervised practice with patients while they continue to develop more complex skills in simulation. Clinical and patient management skills are developed through participation in integrated group practices of third- and fourth-year students managed by a faculty member.

The academic year commences the third or fourth week of August and normally finishes the third week of June.

■ Degrees Offered
DENTAL DEGREE: D.M.D.

COSTS AND FINANCIAL AID

A limited number of scholarships are available to academically outstanding students. Students requiring financial assistance may apply for bursaries and loans. All forms of financial awards are coordinated and administered by the University Awards Committee. Requests for information and applications should be directed to the address given in For Further Information.

Financial Aid Awards to All UBC Dental Students in 2006-07
- BURSARIES: $755,030
- SCHOLARSHIPS: $39,640
- LOANS: $1,735,744

SELECTION FACTORS

Successful candidates are selected on the basis of academic performance, motivation to enter dentistry, residency status, DAT results, interview score, and references.

See chapter 3 of this guide for information regarding numbers of applicants and enrollees to each dental school, along with their race, gender, age, type of predental education, mean DAT and GPA, and state of origin.

Estimated School-Related Expenses for Academic Year 2006-07

	YEAR 1	YEAR 2	YEAR 3	YEAR 4	TOTAL
Tuition	$14,280	$14,280	$14,280	$14,280	$57,120
UBC student levied fees	$745	$745	$745	$752	$2,987
Clinical leases costs	$26,300	$26,300	$26,300	$26,300	$105,200
Anatomy lab fees	$65	$65	0	0	$130
Mycrosurveyor	0	$550	0	0	$550
Dissecting equipment and anatomy lab white coat	$40	0	0	0	$40
Surgical telescopes	$1,250	0	0	0	$1,250
Articulator purchase	$1,300	0	0	0	$1,300
Simulation purchase costs	$500	$1,000	$500	0	$2,000
CPR certificate	$35	$25	0	0	$60
Accident insurance (optional)	$7	$7	0	0	$14
Printing costs for medicine	$150	$150	0	0	$300
Printing costs for dentistry	$500	0	0	0	$500
Incidental costs	$1,670	$1,670	$1,670	$1,670	$6,680
Immunization fee	$40	$40	$40	$40	$160
Pacific Dental Conf. registration fee	0	0	$20	$20	$40
Textbooks (estimate)	$2,100	$1,500	$1,000	$1,000	$5,600
DPAS Course Materials	40	56	0	0	96
NDEB certificate fee	0	0	0	$1,500	$1,500
TOTAL EXPENSES	**$46,022**	**$43,388**	**$41,555**	**$42,912**	**$173,877**

All fees subject to change without notice.

MANITOBA

UNIVERSITY OF MANITOBA
FACULTY OF DENTISTRY

Dr. Randall Mazurat, Acting Dean

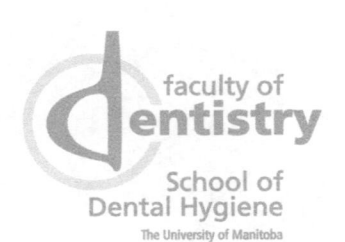

GENERAL INFORMATION

The Faculty of Dentistry is dedicated to educating dental, dental hygiene, and graduate students in a progressive learning environment, conducting research in oral health, and serving the community and the oral health professions as a source of knowledge and expertise. The faculty serves as a bridge between the fundamental scientific foundation of the profession and its translation into health care for the public. Because dentists enhance and promote the total health of patients through oral health management, our curriculum is designed to ensure that our students graduate as competent dentists prepared to meet the oral health care needs of their patients. It provides the knowledge of basic biomedical, behavioral and clinical sciences and biomaterials, the cognitive and behavioral skills, and the professional and ethical values necessary for practice as a dental professional. The Faculty of Dentistry also offers an International Dentist Degree Program, which affords foreign trained dentists the opportunity to receive a Canadian dental degree and the ability to practice in Canada.

ADMISSION REQUIREMENTS

Detailed admissions information may be accessed at www.umanitoba.ca/dentistry/prospectivestudents/app_dentistry07-08.pdf.

NUMBER OF YEARS OF PREDENTAL EDUCATION: A minimum of two years of predental studies at the university level.

REQUIRED COURSES:*

With lab required	(credit hrs)
Introductory chemistry	6
Organic chemistry	6
Biochemistry	6
Physics	6
Biology	6

Other courses	
English	6
Social science or humanities	6
Three additional electives	18

*Applicants whose predental education was not completed at one of the universities in Manitoba will be eligible for consideration if they have completed courses deemed by the University of Manitoba to be equivalent to courses listed here. All courses listed are full courses or full-course equivalents. Ontario Academic Courses (OACs) or Grade 13 courses are not acceptable equivalents.

CANADIAN DAT: All applicants seeking admission for the 2008-09 session must have written the Dental Aptitude Test (DAT), sponsored by the Canadian Dental Association (CDA), no later than November 2007 to be eligible for consideration.

In the initial selection process, applicants may not be considered for admission if they have a Carving Dexterity score of less than 12 or a PAT score of less than 14. In addition, the Committee on Selection will look unfavorably upon applicants who have very low Reading Comprehension scores. Students may elect to take the DAT again in February; however, the results of the February 2008 DAT will not be used in determining which applicants will be granted an interview. For those applicants who have been granted an interview, all valid DAT results, including those from the February 2008 test, will be taken into consideration at the final June selection. Only the results of the Academic Average, PAT, and Carving Dexterity from the single-best DAT of the last three years will be calculated in the overall scores. Only DAT scores obtained in the last three years (from February 2005) will be valid for the 2008-09 selection.

CORE GPA: In 2006 the minimum core average to be invited for an interview was 3.00 Manitoba residents; 3.75 out-of-province residents. Please see Application Information Bulletin for full details.

RESIDENCY: Canadian citizen or permanent resident of Canada.

TRANSFER APPLICANTS: The committee will consider applicants who are seeking admission into second-year dentistry and are currently enrolled in a North American dental program accredited by either the Canadian Dental Association or the American Dental Association. Applicants will be considered for transfer in exceptional circumstances only and only if space is available.

ABORIGINAL APPLICANTS: A maximum of two positions in the first-year dental program will be allocated to applicants from the Aboriginal population of Canada. Applicants in this category must satisfy the above-stated academic requirements, DAT, and interview. Minimum core grade point average of 2.75.

SPECIAL APPLICANTS: A maximum of six positions in the first-year program will be allocated to this category. The committee will consider only applicants who: 1) hold a master's or Ph.D. degree by June 3, 2007; or 2) have had extensive work experience in areas acceptable to the committee as relevant to the health sciences.

Timetable for the Class Entering Fall 2008

	Earliest Date	Latest Date	School Fee
Application Submission	10/31/07	1/22/08	$75
Acceptance Notification	6/30/08	7/3/08	

Required Response and Deposit:
Maximum time to respond: two weeks

$1,000 to hold place; deposit is applied toward tuition and is nonrefundable.

FOR FURTHER INFORMATION

Admissions Office
204-474-8825
424 University Centre
University of Manitoba
Winnipeg, MB, Canada R3T 2N2

Dean's Office
204-977-5611
Faculty of Dentistry
D113 780 Bannatyne Ave.
University of Manitoba
Winnipeg, MB, Canada R3E OW2

Housing and Student Life
204-474-7662
106 Arthur V. Mauro Residence
University of Manitoba
Winnipeg, MB, Canada R3T 2N2

Financial Aid and Awards
204-474-8197
422 University Centre
University of Manitoba
Winnipeg, MB, Canada R3T 2N22

umanitoba.ca/dentistry

THE DENTAL PROGRAM

The Doctor of Dental Medicine program is a fully accredited four-year program. Following a minimum of two years of prerequisite studies, students complete four years of intense study including extensive clinical experience. Upon successful completion of the National Dental Examining Board examination, graduates can apply for license to practice in all provinces of Canada; however, other jurisdictions, both in Canada and the United States, have additional licensing requirements. The D.M.D. degree provides the foundation for a variety of career pathways, including further training in dental specialties and research.

Over the course of the curriculum, emphasis shifts from teaching to learning, from guided to independent performance, from gaining knowledge in the foundation sciences and skills in the labs to treating patients in a simulated-practice setting working with their dental hygiene student partners. The curriculum emphasizes early clinical exposure, with students beginning their clinical experiences in the first year; community-service learning, with student participating in treatment of unique populations at locales outside the dental school; and an evidence-based approach, with students trained to make clinical decisions based on the best scientific evidence available.

The curriculum also provides opportunities to undertake basic or clinical research, to treat patients with a variety of restorative problems, including implant dentistry, and to attend a hospital clinic where patients with complex medical problems are having their oral health care needs met.

GENERAL PRACTICE CLINIC. In their final year, students participate in a clinical program in which they provide all aspects of their patients' treatment needs in a manner resembling a group general practice. Students focus on providing optimal care in a timely manner and practice in an environment that emphasizes the integration of dental and dental hygiene clinical education and the team practice approach.

COMMUNITY SERVICE LEARNING. Students are involved in community outreach programs through externship placement in fourth-year dentistry for patients unable to access dental care through private dental offices. Students learn to value caring for special-needs individuals as they experience planning and providing care for the financially disadvantaged; planning and providing care for those in isolated northern communities; providing care for the institutionalized or mobility-restricted elderly; observing and participating in care for the mentally disabled; and promoting oral health within special-needs communities.

FURTHER DENTAL EDUCATION. The U of M Bachelor of Science in Dentistry degree (B.Sc. Dent.) permits a small number of interested dental students to undertake research during two summers of their undergraduate education. Dental graduates may apply for one of three advanced education one-year Hospital Dental internships. The Faculty of Dentistry also offers graduate education in Oral and Maxillofacial Surgery, Orthodontics, and Periodontics. For those interested in pursuing basic science research, the Department of Oral Biology grants both M.Sc. and Ph.D. degrees.

INTERNATIONAL DENTIST DEGREE PROGRAM. The Faculty of Dentistry offers the International Dentist Degree Program (IDDP) to graduates of international dental programs that are not accredited by the Commission on Dental Accreditation of Canada. After a four- to seven-week summer orientation program, students enter the third year of the regular dental program. Upon satisfactory completion of the third and fourth years, IDDP participants will be awarded the Doctor of Dental Medicine (D.M.D.) degree. All graduates of D.M.D. programs in Canada, once having passed the National Dental Examining Board of Canada (NDEB) examinations, are eligible for licensure/registration as a dentist in all provinces in Canada.

Requirements for admission/entrance to the IDDP include: the successful completion, within two years prior to the application deadline, of the Eligibility Examination, sponsored by the Association of Canadian Faculties of Dentistry; submission of notarized official transcripts of diploma and dental school grades; letters of good standing, from appropriate licensing body; autobiographical sketch; and references. Applicants who have not completed junior and senior high school (six years) in North America are required to take an English proficiency examination (please see bulletin for requirements). Competitive applicants in a given competition will be invited to an on-site assessment held over a one-week period. This assessment will, normally, be held mid-December preceding entry into the program. This assessment consists of a personal interview, a psychomotor skill assessment, and an objective structured clinical examination (OSCE).

SELECTION FACTORS

The Admissions Committee gives priority to Canadian citizens who, at the time of application, are residents of Manitoba and are either graduates or undergraduates of the universities in Manitoba. Other Canadian citizens or permanent residents who are able to demonstrate a substantive connection to Manitoba may also be given priority. Applicants are rank-ordered by an overall score based on the equal weighting of the Adjusted Grade Point Score (AGPS), the Dental Admission Test (DAT), and a personal interview. Admission may be denied if, in the opinion of the interview panel, the applicant cannot communicate adequately in English. In addition, the Committee on Selection will look unfavorably upon applicants who have a very low interview score.

See chapter 3 of this guide for information regarding numbers of applicants and enrollees to each dental school, along with their race, gender, age, type of predental education, mean DAT and GPA, and state of origin.

■ Degrees Offered
DENTAL DEGREE: D.M.D.

ALTERNATE DEGREES: The Bachelor of Science Program for Dental Students (B.Sc. Dent.) is offered to permit a small number of interested dental students to undertake research during the undergraduate course.

COSTS AND FINANCIAL AID

The Financial Aid and Awards Office maintains a close liaison with the Student Aid Branch of the Provincial Government's Department of Education and, as a cooperating agency, carries out numerous detailed procedures for the government's Bursary and Loan Programs. It also acts as a channel for bursaries and loans provided to students from other provinces and jurisdictions and for scholarships and bursaries provided by other organizations. A limited number of loan and bursary funds are available to dental students. Applications and further information are available in the dean's office.

Estimated Total Expenses for Academic Year 2006-07

This table presents minimum estimates of expenses. All are based on charges for the 2006-07 year. For 2007-08, tuition and fees, as well as types of fees, are subject to change without notice; all costs are subject to inflation.

	YEAR 1	YEAR 2	YEAR 3	YEAR 4	TOTAL
Tuition, resident/nonresident	$13,595	$13,278	$13,278	$13,278	$53,429
School expenses					
Dental kit	$11,402	$10,792	$5,448	$2,034	$29,676
Caution fee	$145	$145	$145	$145	$580
Books	$3,429	$1,500	$1,000	$300	$6,228
Endowment fee	$175	$175	$175	$175	$700
Student organization fee	$127	$127	$127	$127	$506
Tech fee	$150	$150	$150	$150	$600
Estimated living expenses*	$4,883	$4,883	$4,883	$4,883	$19,532
Standard service fees, etc.	$165	$165	$165	$165	$660
TOTAL EXPENSES, RESIDENT/NONRESIDENT	**$34,070**	**$31,214**	**$25,370**	**$21,256**	**$111,416**

*Single residence, 3 meals per day, September to April.

DALHOUSIE UNIVERSITY
FACULTY OF DENTISTRY

Dr. David Precious, Dean

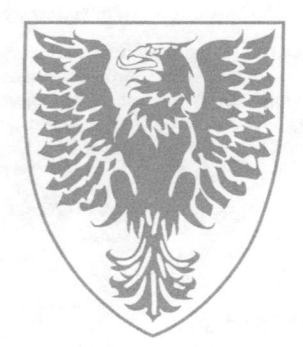

GENERAL INFORMATION

Dalhousie University is a comprehensive teaching and research institution located on the east coast of Canada in Halifax, Nova Scotia. The university was founded in 1818 and is Atlantic Canada's leading research university, recognized for strengths in health and ocean studies. The university is affiliated with teaching hospitals throughout the Maritime Provinces, and its long tradition of excellence provides a solid foundation for a professional career.

The Maritime Dental College was founded in 1908 and became the Faculty of Dentistry of Dalhousie University in 1912; it offers the only Doctor in Dental Surgery degree program in the Atlantic Provinces of Canada. The four-year program is offered in the modern dentistry building facilities, which serves as the main clinical, didactic teaching, and research facility. Students also complete classes and utilize the dental library in the adjacent Faculty of Medicine building. Additional clinical experience is provided through rotations to adjacent teaching hospitals, community-based clinics, and other institutions.

The Doctor in Dental Surgery program is fully accredited by the Commission on Dental Accreditation of Canada. Graduates of the program are eligible to apply for license as a general practice dentist in any jurisdiction of the United States by successfully completing the American National Board Dental Examinations (Parts I and II) and then successfully completing the Regional Board Examinations of their choice.

ADMISSION REQUIREMENTS

NUMBER OF YEARS OF PREDENTAL EDUCATION: Formal minimum of two years (or ten full-year courses) following completion of high school senior matriculation or its equivalent.

LIMITATIONS ON COMMUNITY COLLEGE WORK: None.

REQUIRED COURSES:

With lab required	(years*)
General chemistry	1
Organic chemistry	1
Physics	1
Biology	1

Other courses
Vertebrate physiology	min. 1/2
Introductory microbiology	min. 1/2
Introductory biochemistry	min. 1/2

Three courses chosen from humanities or social sciences, one of which must involve a significant written component.

*Dalhousie University does not operate on semester or quarter hours. All courses must meet Dalhousie standards.

SUGGESTED ADDITIONAL PREPARATION: Students are encouraged to study toward a university bachelor's degree while completing required prerequisites.

DAT: All applicants must submit test results from the American or Canadian Dental Association DAT. Applicants must take the test no later than February to be considered in the initial selection for admission to the following academic year.

GPA: No specific requirements; most competitive applicants have grades of B+ or better.

Timetable for the Class Entering Fall 2008

	Earliest Date	Latest Date	School Fees
Application Submission	3/15/07	12/1/07	$70 (Canadian)
Acceptance Notification	5/30/07	8/29/08	$200 (Canadian)

Required Response and Deposit:
One month after notification

$200 (Canadian) for Canadian citizens and permanent residents; $2,500 (CDN) for international residents to hold place.

FOR FURTHER INFORMATION

Admissions
902-494-2450
Registrar
Dalhousie University
Halifax, NS, Canada B3H 3J5

Financial Aid
902-494-2416
Director of Awards
Registrar's Office
Dalhousie University
Halifax, NS, Canada B3H 4H6

dentistry.dal.ca

DALHOUSIE UNIVERSITY FACULTY OF DENTISTRY **NOVA SCOTIA**

DENTAL PROGRAM

The curriculum emphasizes the integration of the biological, behavioral, and dental sciences with the introduction to patient treatment in the first year of the program. There is a major emphasis on the biological and behavioral sciences as applied to clinical dentistry with basic foundation sciences continuing in the third and fourth years at advanced level. Clinical patient treatment receives greater emphasis in the second year, with continued emphasis on integration of the biological and behavioral sciences. Students practice a total patient care philosophy in the third- and fourth-year clinic, within clinical-oriented disciplines. Students are provided with laptop computers in the first year of the program, and all textbooks are included in searchable electronic formats.

Third- and fourth-year dental students and second-year dental hygiene students work together in the clinical program to provide a team approach to total patient care. Dental assistants are provided, and students are given experience in four-handed dentistry and working with allied dental personnel.

■ Degree Offered
DENTAL DEGREE: D.D.S.

ALTERNATE DEGREES: N/A.

■ Other Programs
In addition to the D.D.S. program, the university also offers a three-year combined diploma in prosthodontics and a master of applied science, biomedical engineering, a six-year combined graduate program leading to the degrees of M.D./M.Sc. in Oral and Maxillofacial Surgery, a two-year program leading to a diploma in Dental Hygiene, and a two-year Qualifying Program for graduates of nonaccredited dentistry programs, and a one-year degree completion program in Dental Hygiene.

SELECTION FACTORS

Consideration is given to academic grades, DAT scores, admission interviews, and references on character and fitness to pursue study in dentistry. A bachelor's degree is preferred. Applications must be complete to be considered by the Admissions Committee. Applications filed by the deadline can be completed at any time up to June 30 and will be considered when completed if unfilled places remain in the entering class.

A university committee has been formed to study affirmative action programs that would increase access to the health professions for minority groups. To date there are no special programs for minorities or other special students, but applications from these groups are encouraged.

See chapter 3 of this guide for information regarding numbers of applicants and enrollees to each dental school, along with their race, gender, age, type of predental education, mean DAT and GPA, and state of origin.

COSTS AND FINANCIAL AID

Estimated School-Related Expenses for Academic Year 2006-07 (Canadian dollars)

	YEAR 1	YEAR 2	YEAR 3	YEAR 4	TOTAL
Tuition, resident	$14,074	$14,074	$14,074	$14,074	$56,256
Tuition, nonresident	$35,000	$35,000	$35,000	$35,000	$140,000
Other expenses					
Resident health insurance	$253	$253	$253	$253	$1,012
International health insurance	$605	$605	$605	$605	$2,420
Student union fee	$113	$113	$113	$113	$452
Student service fee	$186	$186	$186	$186	$744
Student society fee	$70	$70	$70	$70	$280
Facilities renewal fee	$84	$84	$84	$84	$336
Auxiliary/instrument fee	$9,193	$4,747	$1,945	$1,755	$17,640
TOTAL EXPENSES, RESIDENT	**$24,089**	**$19,643**	**$16,841**	**$16,651**	**$77,224**
TOTAL EXPENSES, NONRESIDENT	**$45,015**	**$40,569**	**$37,767**	**$37,577**	**$169,928**

Financial Aid Awards to First-Year Students in 2006-07
■ TOTAL NUMBER OF RECIPIENTS: 116   ■ 100% OF CLASS

	Average Award
Residents	$500

ONTARIO

UNIVERSITY OF TORONTO
FACULTY OF DENTISTRY

Dr. David Mock, Dean

GENERAL INFORMATION

The University of Toronto Faculty of Dentistry is the oldest dental school in Canada. Founded by the Royal College of Dental Surgeons of Ontario, the school began its affiliation with the University of Toronto (U of T) in 1888, when the degree of Doctor of Dental Surgery was established. Today, the faculty graduates more than 70 dentists annually. The staff/student ratio (normally 1:9) allows students to receive highly individualized instruction in both the preclinical and clinical components of their dental education. A state-of-the-art laboratory, technical and clinical facilities, including a computerized clinic management system, and an extensive dental library, equipped with a full-service information commons, enable the faculty to provide the best possible climate for teaching and research. International twinning arrangements with universities in the Netherlands, France, Sweden, Japan, Israel, and Australia permit the ongoing exchange of ideas and experiences among undergraduate and graduate students, as well as faculty members.

In addition to its rich undergraduate tradition, the faculty offers comprehensive graduate educational opportunities and broadly based dental research opportunities. It is the only faculty in Canada to provide advanced clinical training in ten dental specialty disciplines: dental anaesthesia; dental public health; endodontics; oral pathology and oral pathology and medicine; oral radiology; orthodontics; oral and maxillofacial surgery and anaesthesia; pediatric dentistry; periodontology; and prosthodontics. It is also the country's leading research center for dentistry and represents Canada's major source of academic human resources in the field. Current areas of research strength within the faculty include: biomaterials; diagnostic and therapeutic technologies; growth, development, and regeneration; health care services; molecular approaches to the study of oral health and disease; and pain/neurosciences. Many of the faculty's award-winning professors are active partners in high-profile, collaborative research units such as the U of T Institute for Biomaterials and Biomedical Engineering, the U of T Centre for the Study of Pain, and the Feeding Disorders Research Unit based at the Bloorview MacMillan Center and the Hospital for Sick Children. The faculty is also recognized as one of the major providers of continuing education in the province, updating knowledge and clinical advances for dental practitioners. Truly, the concentration of expertise in the University of Toronto Faculty of Dentistry provides the best possible climate for teaching and research for students aspiring to lifelong learning in dentistry.

The following admission requirements apply to residents of Canada. A limited number of positions are also available for international students.

ADMISSION REQUIREMENTS

NUMBER OF YEARS OF PREDENTAL EDUCATION: Formal minimum of three.

LIMITATIONS ON COMMUNITY COLLEGE WORK: Not applicable in Ontario.

REQUIRED COURSES: *(full courses)*
A full course (one full or two half courses) in general biochemistry. This course should cover protein chemistry and the chemistry of other biomolecules, cellular metabolism, and molecular biology.

A full course (one full or two half courses) in general mammalian (human or animal) physiology. This course should cover the following systems: musculoskeletal, haemostasis mechanisms, haematopoietic, nervous, immune, cardiovascular, renal physiology, neurophysiology, endocrinology, and gastrointestinal physiology.

Additional life sciences	2
Humanities or social sciences	1

SUGGESTED ADDITIONAL PREPARATION: Dentistry requires individuals with strong backgrounds in the social sciences, humanities, physical sciences, and life sciences. Students should follow a program of study that will provide them with an educational background in keeping with their own interests and possible career opportunities should they not be accepted into dentistry.

DAT: Mandatory.

GPA: Minimum of 2.7. It should be noted that, last year, the minimum GPA for those interviewed was 3.6 for domestic applicants and 3.0 for international applicants on a 4.0 scale.

RESIDENCY: Applicants must be Canadian citizens or permanent residents. A maximum of 10 percent of the first-year places may be offered to out-of-province applicants.

TRANSFERS WITHIN CANADA AND FROM THE UNITED STATES: Canadian citizens or permanent residents currently enrolled in an accredited Canadian or U.S. dental school who wish to transfer to the Faculty of Dentistry will be considered for admission, space permitting, into the second year (not third or fourth year). Applicants must meet all academic and English facility requirements for admission into the first year. In addition, dental program equivalency with the D.D.S. program at the University of Toronto must be established. Applicants enrolled in dental schools where the curriculum is not sufficiently equivalent to allow for direct entry into the second year at the University of Toronto are not eligible for transfer consideration. Requests for transfer must be received by June 30. Prospective applicants should be aware that the number of second-year places, if any, may vary annually, and in most years no spaces are available for students seeking transfer.

Timetable for the Class Entering Fall 2008

	Earliest Date	Latest Date	School Fees
Application Submission	8/1/07	12/1/07	$230
Acceptance Notification	5/1/08	8/31/08	$2,000

Required Response and Deposit:
14 days from notification if received between 5/2 and 8/31

$2,000 to hold place; this will be applied to tuition fees upon registration.

FOR FURTHER INFORMATION

Admissions
Admissions Office
416-979-4901, ext. 4373 admissions.dental@utoronto.ca
University of Toronto, Faculty of Dentistry
124 Edward Street
Toronto, Ontario, Canada M5G 1G6

Housing
University of Toronto Housing Service
416-978-8045
housing.services@utoronto.ca
St. George Campus
Koffler Student Services Centre
214 College Street
Toronto, Ontario, Canada M5T 2Z9

Financial Aid
Admissions and Awards
University of Toronto
416-978-2190
ask@admin.utoronto.ca
315 Bloor Street West
Toronto, Ontario, Canada M5S 1A3

www.utoronto.ca/dentistry

THE DENTAL PROGRAM

Dental education is designed to unify the basic and clinical sciences, as it is believed that scientific and professional development cannot be sharply differentiated but should proceed concurrently throughout the dental program.

YEAR 1. Basic sciences with introduction to dentally relevant material.

YEAR 2. Completion of basic sciences and greater emphasis on the study of dental disease and its prevention and treatment.

YEAR 3. Intensive clinical study of each of the dental disciplines with emphasis on the assessment and management of patients.

YEAR 4. Further clinical experience and familiarity with more advanced treatment services; emphasis upon integration of the various disciplines and overall management of patient treatment in preparation for general practice; participation in elective programs, clinical conferences, and hospital-based experiences.

■ Degree Offered
DENTAL DEGREE: D.D.S.

■ Other Programs
SUMMER STUDENTSHIPS: A limited number available for academically outstanding students with research interests.

INTERNATIONAL STUDENTS: A person is eligible to apply to the D.D.S. program as an international student if he or she can enter or is already in Canada with a student visa (or equivalent immigration authorization). This includes applicants with no prior dental education as well as applicants who are currently enrolled in a foreign dental school and wish to transfer. For further information, please contact the Admissions Office of the Faculty of Dentistry.

SELECTION FACTORS

Decisions of the Admission Committee are based upon academic achievement, DAT scores, the Canadian Dental Association structured interview, and the results of a personality test. The Admission Committee will review all applications, and applicants who are considered to have potential based on their application documents will be invited for an interview. All offers of admission will be made from the group of applicants who are interviewed. Applications from qualified persons of Aboriginal ancestry will receive special consideration for admission.

See chapter 3 of this guide for information regarding numbers of applicants and enrollees to each dental school, along with their race, gender, age, type of predental education, mean DAT and GPA, and state of origin.

COSTS AND FINANCIAL AID

DOMESTIC STUDENTS: The University of Toronto is committed to providing financial support to students. For students who are assessed by the Ontario Student Assistant Program (OSAP) or by another Canadian provincial government financial aid program as requiring maximum assistance and whose assessed need is not fully covered by government aid, the university will ensure that the full need is met. For every new and returning student, the university examines the OSAP (or other Canadian provincial government financial aid program) assessment in the fall term and identifies all students who qualify for grants through the University of Toronto *Advance Planning for Students (UTAPS)* program. The university writes to students directly to notify them of their eligibility. For students in second-entry programs, including dentistry, the additional assistance may be a mix of grant and loan. Since the tuition fees for the D.D.S. program have been deregulated by the Ontario Ministry of Education and Training, the university has arranged for different ways to assist students with financial need. Canadian citizens and permanent residents who are eligible for assistance from the federal or provincial governments may receive up to $2,000 in grants from the university to help meet financial need recognized but not fully covered by the government assistance program. Students whose financial need is unusually high may be offered additional grant assistance. In addition, the Bank of Nova Scotia has made a line of credit available to qualified students under the Scotia Professional Student Plan. The university will provide a grant to cover interest on loans borrowed under this plan up to the level of the assessed unmet need.

INTERNATIONAL STUDENTS: The Faculty of Dentistry and the University of Toronto expect incoming students to be responsible for securing their own sources of funding. Therefore, we do not normally offer financial assistance to international students. Potential visa students are advised that they will be required to provide evidence that they have sufficient funds to study and live in Toronto for the length of their program. Applicants should consider coming to Toronto only if they are able to obtain the necessary funds prior to their arrival in Canada.

Estimated Total Expenses for Academic Year 2007-08*

	YEAR 1	YEAR 2	YEAR 3	YEAR 4	TOTAL
Tuition, resident	$19,386	$18,668	$18,668	$18,668	$75,390
Tuition, nonresident	$40,000	$39,900	$35,539	$33,530	$148,969
Other expenses					
UHI premium**	$684	$684	$684	$684	$2,736
Incidental and ancillary fees	$854	$854	$854	$854	$3,416
Equipment***	$6,124	$5,650	$4,584	$2,327	$18,685
Estimated living expenses including accommodation, food, clothing, books, misc.	$13,000	$13,500	$15,000	$13,500	$55,000
TOTAL EXPENSES, RESIDENT	$39,364	$38,672	$39,106	$34,349	$152,491
TOTAL EXPENSES, NONRESIDENT	$60,662	$60,588	$56,661	$50,895	$228,806

* Based on the 2005-06 academic year. Subject to increases.
** University Health Insurance premium charged to international (visa) students.
*** A portion of this includes optional charges for phantom heads, models, and laundry.

UNIVERSITY OF WESTERN ONTARIO
SCHULICH SCHOOL OF MEDICINE & DENTISTRY

Dr. Harinder S. Sandhu, Director

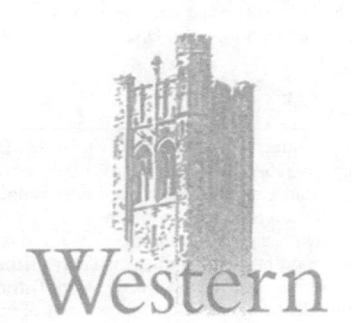

GENERAL INFORMATION

The School of Dentistry was officially established at the University of Western Ontario on January 1, 1965, and enrolled its first students the following year. Western is a publicly supported institution, chartered by the legislature of Ontario in 1878 as the Western University of London, changing its name to the current one in 1923. Western is one of Canada's oldest, largest, and most beautiful universities, situated on an all-contained campus of 162 hectares of picturesque, park-like land in the north end of London, a city of 316,000. More than 26,000 students are enrolled in over 300 programs offered by 17 faculties and professional schools.

In 1997, the School of Dentistry was merged with the Faculty of Medicine to become The Faculty of Medicine and Dentistry. In 2005, the Faculty of Medicine and Dentistry was renamed Schulich School of Medicine & Dentistry. Close ties with London's world-class teaching hospitals, on-site state-of-the-art facilities, and a faculty-student ratio of about one to four provide an ideal environment for training future clinical practitioners and scientists.

In addition to its undergraduate program, a graduate program leading to specialist certification is offered: a three-year program in orthodontics leads to the Master of Clinical Dentistry degree.

In 1997, a two-year Qualifying Program was established to prepare graduates of nonaccredited dental programs for the examinations of the National Dental Examining Board of Canada.

ADMISSION REQUIREMENTS

NUMBER OF YEARS OF PREDENTAL EDUCATION: Minimum of two (following Ontario Grade 12 or equivalent) with at least ten courses, four of which must be at the honors (senior second year) or equivalent level.

LIMITATIONS ON COMMUNITY COLLEGE WORK: Not applicable in Ontario.

REQUIRED COURSES:

With lab required	(years)
Biology*	full year
Physics*	full year
Chemistry*	full year
Physiology human/mammalian	full year
(lab component not mandatory)	
Organic chemistry	at least half year
Biochemistry	at least half year
(lab component not mandatory)	

*Not mandatory (but advised) when applying with completed degree; if degree not conferred by July 1 of year applying, applicants are required to have completed all prerequisites; graduate degree applicants must complete all requirements for the degree (including successful thesis defense) by June 20 of the year applying. Detailed course synopses may be required to verify successful completion of mandatory prerequisites. Please consult school.

SUGGESTED ADDITIONAL PREPARATION: Students should seek a broad background of education in keeping with their own interests.

DAT: DAT mandatory; for national candidates Canadian DAT must have been taken within previous two years of application deadline.

GPA: Two individual years of 80 percent or above. This is subject to change depending on the quality of the applicant pool.

RESIDENCY: Applicants must be Canadian citizens or permanent residents of Canada; however, a limited number of positions are available for international students. Please contact the Admissions Coordinator for details about requirements for international students. Applicants from all provinces and territories of Canada are considered equally.

ADVANCED STANDING: When a vacancy exists, consideration may be given to Canadian students transferring from U.S. and foreign dental schools for advanced standing into second year.

RESEARCH CATEGORY WITH DEFERRED ADMISSION: Deferred admission to D.D.S. program may be offered to candidates accepted to a dentally oriented graduate program at UWO leading to a master's or Ph.D. degree, at commencement of graduate program.

Timetable for the Class Entering Fall 2008

	Earliest Date	Latest Date	School Fees
Application Submission	9/15/07	12/1/07	$250 national
Acceptance Notification	7/1/08	8/31/08	$350 international

Required Response and Deposit:
The maximum response time is ten days after notification, although an immediate response is preferred. A $1,000 nonrefundable deposit is required with acceptance; the balance is due at registration.

FOR FURTHER INFORMATION

Admissions
T.W. Mara
Chair, Dentistry Admissions Committee
519-661-4074
Dentistry
Schulich School of Medicine and Dentistry
The University of Western Ontario
Dental Sciences Building
London, ON Canada N6A 5C1

Office of Financial Aid
Director of Financial Aid
The University of Western Ontario
Room 190, Stevenson-Lawson Building
London, ON Canada N6A 5B8

Department of Equity Services
Director
The University of Western Ontario
Room 295, Stevenson-Lawson Building
London, ON Canada N6A 5B8

Residence Admissions and Off-Campus Housing
The University of Western Ontario
Room 102, Elgin Hall
1421 Western Road
London, ON Canada N6G 4W4
Residence Admissions: 519-661-3549
Off-Campus Housing: 519-661-3550

www.fmd.uwo.ca/dentistry

THE DENTAL PROGRAM

The four-year D.D.S. program is designed to graduate dentists who possess the knowledge and skill to conduct a superior general practice and also sufficient knowledge of basic and applied science to permit and stimulate professional and intellectual growth. Rapid advances in science, medicine, and technology, an accelerated pace in the delivery of information, and the importance of knowledge in meeting today's health care needs continue to change the way Western approaches dental education.

YEAR 1. Basic medical/dental sciences with introduction to clinical situations.

YEAR 2. Basic medical/dental sciences plus courses that are clinically focused in preparation for third year in the dental clinic and in hospital electives.

YEARS 3 AND 4. Basic dental sciences together with lectures and rotations in clinical disciplines. Delivery of comprehensive dental care to patients in a clinical setting.

■ Degrees Offered

DENTAL DEGREE: D.D.S.

M.SC. OR PH.D. GRADUATE PROGRAMS: Taken through basic science departments of anatomy, biochemistry, epidemiology and biostatistics, medical biophysics, microbiology and immunology, pathology, pharmacology and toxicology, and physiology. An honors bachelor's degree for the M.Sc. and a master's degree for the Ph.D. are required for admission to the program.

MASTER OF CLINICAL DENTISTRY (M.CI.D.)–ORTHODONTICS: Candidates must possess a D.D.S. degree or equivalent. Minimum of one year in general practice or approved internship. Preference given to Ontario applicants. Three applicants per year chosen. Program is for 36 continuous months.

■ Other Programs

SUMMER RESEARCH SCHOLARSHIPS: Up to eight awarded annually, on a competitive basis, to dental students for participation in summer research program supervised by faculty members.

GRADUATE FELLOWSHIP: One awarded annually to a dental graduate accepted into a graduate degree program leading to a career in dental education, dental research, or both in Canada.

DENTAL CLINICAL FELLOWSHIPS: Twelve-month training in hospital dentistry; up to four awarded annually; candidates must possess D.D.S. or equivalent degree and be eligible for a certificate to practice in the province of Ontario.

SELECTION FACTORS

Applicants are advised that it is to their advantage to take a program that includes at least five full courses or equivalent in each academic year, taken concurrently (excluding summer sessions). Primary consideration will be given to the best two academic years and the DAT scores. However, overall academic performance (consistency, trend), honors degree (if applicable), and graduate education will also be used as selection criteria. Selected applicants will be required to attend a personal interview in order to be considered for admission.

Applications are invited from visa/international students who must satisfy separate admission requirements as well as English language proficiency. Two places in first year may be filled with "special case" applicants; candidates chosen by the Admissions Committee from deserving applicants.

See chapter 3 of this guide for information regarding numbers of applicants and enrollees to each dental school, along with their race, gender, age, type of predental education, mean DAT and GPA, and state of origin.

COSTS AND FINANCIAL AID

The principal source of financial assistance for students in Ontario universities is the government-funded Ontario Student Assistance Program (OSAP). The plan provides assistance for students who can demonstrate financial need, provided they are established residents of the province. Home-province funds may also be available for out-of-province students; contact the Financial Aid Office. Scholarships, bursaries, and loans are also available to students in Dentistry, but the amounts involved are limited.

Estimated Total Expenses for Academic Year 2006-07

	YEAR 1	YEAR 2	YEAR 3	YEAR 4	TOTAL
Tuition, resident	$18,468	$17,468	$17,748	$17,784	$70,872
Tuition, nonresident*	$39,000	$39,000	$39,000	$39,000	$156,000
Other expenses					
Activity fee	$860	$860	$860	$860	$3,440
Dental instruments**	$10,510	$10,810	$4,460	$6,659	$32,339
Estimated living expenses	$11,000	$11,000	$11,000	$11,000	$44,000
TOTAL EXPENSES, RESIDENT	$40,838	$40,138	$33,828	$36,028	$150,832
TOTAL EXPENSES, NONRESIDENT	$61,376	$61,610	$55,320	$55,142	$233,448

* Applicants from Canadian provinces are considered residents for tuition purposes. Nonresidents are non-Canadian applicants.
**Instrument costs amortized over four years of program.
For detailed budget schedule please see school website.

QUÉBEC

UNIVERSITÉ LAVAL
FACULTÉ DE MÉDECINE DENTAIRE
Dr. Jean-Paul Goulet, Dean

GENERAL INFORMATION

The Faculty of Dental Medicine was founded in 1969 and accepted its first students in 1971. All teaching is done in the French language. The faculty occupies permanent quarters suitable for the training of 48 students for each of the four years of the program. A maximum of 54 students per year could be accommodated with the present facilities. The faculty also offers a master in science program in oral and maxillofacial surgery, a master in science in periodontics, and a one-year multiresidency. The Université Laval is provincially sponsored and receives the bulk of its operating budgets from government funding.

ADMISSION REQUIREMENTS

NUMBER OF YEARS OF PREDENTAL EDUCATION: Quebec residents: 11 years of high school plus two years of junior college (CEGEP). Out-of-province residents: 13 years of high school plus two years of university level.

LIMITATIONS ON COMMUNITY COLLEGE WORK: None.

REQUIRED COURSES:

Chemistry	101, 201, 202, 302
Physics	101, 201, 301
Biology	301, 401
Mathematics	102, 203

SUGGESTED ADDITIONAL PREPARATION: An undergraduate program with an accent on the health sciences and human biology is an asset to the dental student.

CANADIAN DAT: Mandatory; written test may be taken in French.

U.S. DAT: May be substituted for Canadian DAT.

GPA: Must be in upper third.

RESIDENCY: All candidates must be Canadian citizens or permanent residents.

ADVANCED STANDING: Not available.

Timetable for the Class Entering Fall 2008

	Earliest Date	Latest Date	School Fee
Application Submission	1/1/08	3/1/08	$60*
Acceptance Notification	5/27/08	8/25/08**	

* Due at time of application
**This date depends on replies from students and has been as late as September 1 in the past.

Required Response:
Students are allowed 15 days maximum.

FOR FURTHER INFORMATION

Admissions
Denis Robert
Chairman, Admission Committee
418-656-2120
Université Laval
Faculté de médecine dentaire
Québec, Qué., Canada G1K 7P4

Financial Aid
Service des Bourses et de l'aide financiere
418-656-3332
Université Laval
Pavillon Alphonse-Desjardins
Bureau 2546
Université Laval
Québec, Qué., Canada G1K 7P4

Housing
Service des résidences
418-656-2921
Pavillon Parent
Bureau 1604
Université Laval
Québec, Qué., Canada G1K 7P4

ulaval.ca/fmd

THE DENTAL PROGRAM

The program is designed to give its graduates a thorough grounding in the basic sciences and broad clinical experience. Basic health sciences are taught in an integrated health science complex. Preclinical and clinical subjects are under the direct control of dental school personnel.

The first two years of the program are devoted to the basic and preclinical sciences. The last two years are devoted almost entirely to clinical work. In the final year, a student may elect to do further work in a discipline of his or her choosing. Approximately 15 percent of the total program is in elective courses, so that the student can tailor his or her program to suit capabilities or ambitions. Opportunities to select electives in hospital dentistry, public health, and basic or applied research are also available. Students are evaluated on their theoretical knowledge by means of written and oral examinations. All laboratory and clinical work is continuously evaluated, and the student is kept aware of this evaluation.

■ Degree Offered
DENTAL DEGREE: D.M.D.

COSTS AND FINANCIAL AID

Financial aid may be available through provincial and federal sources. The Canadian Armed Forces offer a program of financial aid to candidates who serve in the forces after graduation. There are some scholarships and loans obtainable through university funds for which the dental student may apply.

Estimated School-Related Expenses for Academic Year 2006-07

	YEAR 1	YEAR 2	YEAR 3	YEAR 4	TOTAL
Tuition	$2,335	$2,780	$2,502	$2,001	$9,618
Fees	$174	$174	$174	$174	$696
Equipment	$7,200	$5,000	$2,800	0	$15,000
TOTAL	**$9,709**	**$7,954**	**$5,476**	**$2,175**	**$25,314**

SELECTION FACTORS

Because of the high local requirements for dental personnel, the faculty gives priority to Quebec residents who have Canadian citizenship. Ten percent of our candidates may come from French-speaking neighboring provinces. An arrangement has been made to accept at least one candidate annually from New Brunswick and one from Ontario. An interview to determine the student's motivation, maturity, personality, interests, and social awareness is mandatory.

Because of the very small class size and the large demand, no consideration can be given to special applicants. However, no discrimination is made as to the gender, religion, or race of the students admitted.

See chapter 3 of this guide for information regarding numbers of applicants and enrollees to each dental school, along with their race, gender, age, type of predental education, mean DAT and GPA, and state of origin.

QUÉBEC

McGILL UNIVERSITY
FACULTY OF DENTISTRY

Dr. James P. Lund, Dean

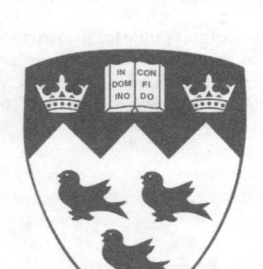

GENERAL INFORMATION

McGill University, founded in 1821, is situated in downtown Montreal. The dental school had its beginnings in 1904, subsequently becoming a faculty in 1920. The preclinical years are taught on the McGill campus, the basic medical science courses being taught in cooperation with the Faculty of Medicine. The clinical years are spent in the McCall Dental Clinic of the Montreal General Hospital, as well as in certain medical departments of the hospital, and rotations have been developed to the dental departments of other McGill teaching hospitals. A master's degree is offered in oral and maxillofacial surgery, and there is also a master's degree in dental sciences. The Faculty of Dentistry sponsors courses for graduate dentists in continuing dental education that are recognized for credits by dental licensing bodies.

ADMISSION REQUIREMENTS

FOUR-YEAR PROGRAM: Candidates currently in an out-of-province university must have completed a Bachelor of Science degree. Candidates from Quebec applying to the four-year program must have completed CEGEP plus a Bachelor of Science degree.

FIVE-YEAR PROGRAM. Candidates who are citizens or permanent residents of Canada living in the province of Quebec and who are enrolled in the final year of the Sciences Profile of the Quebec Colleges of General and Professional Education (CEGEP) are eligible to apply for the five-year program.

REQUIRED COURSES:

With lab required	(semesters)
General biology	2
General chemistry	2
Organic chemistry	2
Physics	2
Strongly recommended	
Cell biology and metabolism*	1
Molecular biology*	1

*A full year university-level course in biochemistry may be substituted for the courses in cell and molecular biology.

CANADIAN DAT: Mandatory. (American DAT may also be submitted.)

GPA: 3.5/4.0 (A=4.0) required; average for the 2006 entering class was 3.7/4.0.

RESIDENCY: No specific requirements, but see Selection Factors.

Timetable for the Class Entering Fall 2008

	Earliest Date	Latest Date	School Fee
Application Submission	8/30/07	11/15/07	$80
Acceptance Notification	3/1/08	8/1/08	

Required Response and Deposit:
Preferred response time—10 days; maximum time—15 days

$2,000 for 4-year program, $1,000 for 5-year program. Applies toward tuition.

FOR FURTHER INFORMATION

Admissions
Patricia Bassett
Student Affairs
Administrative Assistant
514-398-7203
Faculty of Dentistry
McGill University
3640 University Street
Montreal, Quebec H3A 2B2

Financial Aid
Judy Stymest
Student Aid Office
514-398-6015
McGill University
3600 McTavish
Montreal, Quebec H3A 1X9

Housing
F. Tracy
Director of Residences
514-398-6367
University Residences
McGill University
3935 University Street
Montreal, Québec H3A 2B4

www.mcgill.ca/dentistry

McGILL UNIVERSITY FACULTY OF DENTISTRY **QUÉBEC**

THE DENTAL PROGRAM

The Faculty of Dentistry is dedicated to the concept that graduates from a dental school should have reasonable competence to begin practice as general practitioners, regardless of what their future aspirations may be, and should develop the understanding and competence to cope with the dental diseases they will encounter and to apply the preventive and treatment measures of the present and those predicted for the future.

Basic sciences in the dental curriculum are taught in the Faculty of Medicine. Introduction to clinical experience begins in the first year, and the integration of basic sciences into clinical dentistry in the second year. Students are evaluated on the basis of daily progress and end-of-term examinations.

■ Degree Offered
DENTAL DEGREE: D.M.D.

■ Other Programs

MASTER OF SCIENCE IN DENTAL SCIENCES: The goal of this program is to train students in research in the dental sciences. The subject area for the degree will be founded in oral biology, an umbrella categorization of disciplines relating to the functioning of the orofacial complex.

Students who have successfully completed the D.D.S./D.M.D. degree or a B.Sc. degree with a CGPA of 3.0 in any of the disciplines in the health sciences (anatomy, biochemistry, microbiology and immunology, or physiology) or related disciplines (biology, chemistry, physics, or psychology) are eligible to apply for admission to a graduate program in the Faculty of Dentistry leading to the M.Sc. degree in dental sciences. In addition to submitting GRE scores, TOEFL tests must be passed in the case of non-Canadians whose mother tongue is not English. The M.Sc. degree should normally be completed within two years of full-time study.

MASTER OF SCIENCE IN ORAL AND MAXILLOFACIAL SURGERY: A residency training program in oral and maxillofacial surgery provides a candidate with a comprehensive background for the practice of oral and maxillofacial surgery (OMFS) as a specialty.

Candidates for this program must possess a D.D.S. or D.M.D. degree or its equivalent and be acceptable to l'Ordre des Dentistes du Quebec as a training candidate in a hospital. The M.Sc. degree should normally be completed within four years of full-time study.

All applications are submitted online at www.mcgill.ca/dentistry. Applicants to the OMFS program should apply to the Dental Residency Program.

SELECTION FACTORS

Candidates selected hold a bachelor's degree. The Admissions Committee looks for students with a well-rounded background in the humanities rather than a concentration in only one discipline.

Selection of students is made by a committee comprised partly of the academic staff from the Faculty of Dentistry and partly of staff from other disciplines within the university. There is also a voting student member. All applications received are checked to ensure that all transcripts of record, letters of reference, and evaluations have been received. Interviews for students, where appropriate, are arranged after the completed applications have been circulated to each member of the committee for assessment. Subsequently, the committee meets and selects or rejects students for placement on a prime list from which final class selection is made. In the selection process, academic grades, DAT scores, and interview results carry the greatest weight. There is no discrimination on the basis of race, gender, or creed, but place of residence does carry weight inasmuch as 50 percent of the candidates are selected from the province of Quebec and are being trained for a career within this area. Personal qualities, particularly social awareness, motivation, integrity, and the student's progress in his or her academic career are assessed from available data. Not all applicants are interviewed, but all candidates placed on the list of prime contenders are interviewed before letters of acceptance are sent.

See chapter 3 of this guide for information regarding numbers of applicants and enrollees to each dental school, along with their race, gender, age, type of predental education, mean DAT and GPA, and state of origin.

COSTS AND FINANCIAL AID

All policies concerning financial aid are set by the Student Aid Office. Further details may be obtained from that office.

Estimated School-Related Expenses for Academic Year 2006-07

	YEAR 1 64 CREDITS*	YEAR 2 66 CREDITS*	YEAR 3 51 CREDITS*	YEAR 4 34 CREDITS*	TOTAL
Tuition					
Quebec students	$3,559	$3,670	$2,836	$1,891	$11,956
Out-of-province students	$9,922	$10,232	$7,907	$5,271	$33,332
International students	$38,102	$39,293	$30,363	$20,242	$127,999
Society fees (See Note 1)	$422	$422	$402	$402	$1,648
Student services	$384	$384	$384	$384	$1,536
Registration and transcripts	$323	$323	$323	$219	$1,188
Information technology	$266	$266	$266	$171	$969
Copyright fee	$19	$19	$19	$19	$76
Class notes	$730	0	0	0	$730
Equipment rental	$207	$320	$1,000	$1,000	$2,527
TOTAL FEES					
QUEBEC STUDENTS	**$5,910**	**$5,404**	**$5,230**	**$4,086**	**$20,670**
OUT-OF-PROVINCE STUDENTS	**$12,273**	**$11,966**	**$10,301**	**$7,466**	**$42,006**
INTERNATIONAL STUDENTS	**$40,453**	**$41,027**	**$32,757**	**$22,437**	**$136,714**

*Average number of credits taken each year.
International student society fees reduced by $86.40 for the student health insurance plan.

Dentistry—Purchases of Equipment and Materials Fee
In addition to the fees shown on the list of fees for Dentistry, certain items of equipment and supplies are purchased by each student through the Faculty of Dentistry. The fee also includes an amount for general supplies in the laboratories and clinics.

The estimated cost of these purchases is as follows:	0	$18,500	$4,000	$1,500	$24,000

QUÉBEC

UNIVERSITÉ DE MONTRÉAL
FACULTÉ DE MÉDECINE DENTAIRE
Dr. Claude Lamarche, Dean

GENERAL INFORMATION
The Faculté de Médecine Dentaire of the Université de Montréal was founded in 1904. It is publicly funded by the Province of Québec. The faculty is located in the main building of the university and occupies the first, second, and fifth floors of the east wing. The teaching facilities allow up to 85 students to be admitted. Graduate programs are available in orthodontics, prosthodontics, pediatric dentistry, and oral biology (master's degrees). We also offer a graduate program in multidisciplinary residency. With the Faculté de Médecine, there are joint postgraduate programs in biomedical sciences (M.Sc. and Ph.D.). The Faculté de Médecine Dentaire is one of the two schools in North America where instruction is given in French.

ADMISSION REQUIREMENTS

NUMBER OF YEARS OF PREDENTAL EDUCATION: Formal minimum of two; generally acceptable minimum of two.

LIMITATIONS ON COMMUNITY COLLEGE WORK: None.

REQUIRED COURSES:

With lab required	(semester hrs)
Inorganic chemistry	6
Organic chemistry	6
Physics	9
Biology (zoology)	6

Other courses	
French*	12
Mathematics	9
Philosophy	12

*Knowledge of French is mandatory.

CANADIAN DAT: A minimum score of 10 is required on carving dexterity test and 10 on perception aptitude test. The ADA DAT may not be substituted.

GPA: N/A.

RESIDENCY: All candidates must be Canadian citizens or permanent residents.

ADVANCED STANDING: Graduates of nonaccredited foreign dental schools may be admitted with advanced standing if requirements are met and space is available within the second year of the program.

Timetable for the Class Entering Fall 2008

Filing of Formal Application

	Earliest Date	Latest Date	School Fee
Application Submission			
College students	1/1/08	3/1/08	$50
University students	1/15/08	1/15/08	$50
Acceptance Notification	5/15/08	8/1/08	

Required Response and Deposit:
Preferred time is by August 1, 2008. Online $30.

FOR FURTHER INFORMATION

Admissions
Bureau du registraire
A/S Marie Nadeau
514-343-2223
Université de Montréal
C.P. 6128 Succ. Centre-ville
Montréal, Qué., Canada H3C 3J7

Financial Aid
Jean-Marc LeTourneau
514-343-6145
Aide financiere
2332 Édouard-Montpetit
Université de Montréal
Montréal, Que., Canada H3C 3J7

Housing
Lyne Mackay
514-343-7697
Residences
2350 Édouard-Montpetit
Université de Montréal
Montréal, Que., Canada H3C 3J7

www.medent.umontreal.ca

THE PREPARATORY YEAR

Basic sciences and social sciences are emphasized in this year. Courses in various fields intend to broaden the knowledge of students in subjects related to dental sciences and ethics.

LENGTH OF PROGRAM: Nine months, divided into two semesters of 15 weeks each. There is no summer session.

THE DENTAL PROGRAM

Training in the basic sciences and preclinical disciplines is emphasized in the first two years of the program. Clinical training starts during the second semester of the second year. Senior students spend three weeks in hospitals off-campus to become acquainted with oral surgery and for training in pediatric dentistry. Optional courses are offered to senior students to complete their basic training in areas such as violence, personal training, quality control, and business administration. The clinical program of the senior year also offers optional clinical courses. In addition to traditional clinical training such as implantology, periodontics/endodontics, and constructive dentistry, off-campus activities in student exchange programs, clinical activities in international cooperation humanitarian projects, and off-campus clinics are available. Student performance is evaluated qualitatively and quantitatively throughout the entire clinical program.

LENGTH OF PROGRAM: Forty-four months, 33 in actual attendance. Eight semesters of 15 weeks and a four-week summer session after the third year.

■ Degree Offered
DENTAL DEGREE: D.M.D.

COSTS AND FINANCIAL AID

Financial aid may be available through provincial and federal sources. The Canadian Armed Forces offer a program of financial aid to candidates who serve in the forces after graduation. There are some scholarships and loans obtainable through university funds for which the dental student may apply. The Faculty of Dentistry has loan funds for sophomore and junior students.

Estimated Total Expenses for Academic Year 2006-07

	PREDENTAL YEAR	YEAR 1	YEAR 2	YEAR 3	YEAR 4	TOTAL
Tuition	$2,500	$2,650	$2,700	$2,890	$2,355	$13,095
Instrumentation	0	$4,000	$9,000	$7,000	$500	$20,500
Estimated living expenses	$10,500	$10,500	$10,500	$10,500	$10,500	$52,500
TOTAL EXPENSES	**$13,000**	**$17,150**	**$22,200**	**$20,390**	**$13,355**	**$86,095**

SELECTION FACTORS

The selection of candidates is based on the predental institution attended, academic grades, standing in class (when available), and scores on the Canadian DAT and any other admission test that might be required.

See chapter 3 of this guide for information regarding numbers of applicants and enrollees to each dental school, along with their race, gender, age, type of predental education, mean DAT and GPA, and state of origin.

SASKATCHEWAN

UNIVERSITY OF SASKATCHEWAN
COLLEGE OF DENTISTRY

Dr. Gerry Uswak, Acting Dean

GENERAL INFORMATION

The College of Dentistry is a dynamic college with a reputation for excellence in both teaching and research. By providing students with a well-balanced dental education, it is our goal to produce graduates who will be adaptable to rapid change and competitive with their peers around the world. Our graduates can be found on every continent making contributions to the profession of dental medicine.

From its spectacular setting in the beautiful South Saskatchewan River valley, the University of Saskatchewan offers reasonable tuition and a very reasonable cost of living; an environment that is clean, safe, friendly, and culturally diverse; an extensive variety of extracurricular activities, ranging from campus clubs to championship sports teams; exceptional student services; and free provincial medical and hospital insurance.

At the University of Saskatchewan, our enrollment is over 19,000 students. In the College of Dentistry, there are currently 111 students enrolled. We value the diversity of our university community, the people, their points of view, and the contributions they make to our scholarly endeavors.

We hope you include the College of Dentistry at the University of Saskatchewan in your plans for furthering your education. The college has 23 full-time faculty and about 60 part-time faculty ensuring an excellent student to faculty ratio. In addition to its teaching and service functions, the college has a strong commitment to research. Recent projects involve a CIDA dental/healthcare project, a periodontal health project with Mexico, involvement in a major study of multiple sclerosis, a bacterial adhesion to oral surface project, and ongoing studies in dental materials. Summer research opportunities are available to students in both the clinical and basic science areas. In addition, events provide innovative learning, research, and clinical experience for students during the academic year.

Our preclinical teaching area includes a state-of-the-art clinical simulation facility where students learn basic procedures in a clinical setting with current techniques in infection control, fiber optic technology, and intra-oral television. Our patient treatment clinic remains one of the most attractive facilities in Canada providing an excellent environment for both patients and students during the clinical training phase of the program. In October 2000, an ultramodern six-chair clinic was opened.

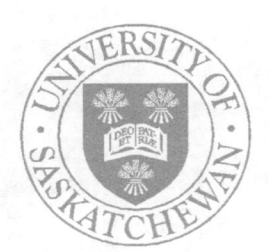

ADMISSION REQUIREMENTS

NUMBER OF YEARS OF PREDENTAL EDUCATION: Formal minimum of two.

LIMITATIONS ON COMMUNITY COLLEGE WORK: None.

REQUIRED COURSES:

Biology (General Biology with a laboratory)—6 credit hours; Chemistry (Introduction to Modern Chemistry with a laboratory)—3 credit hours; Chemistry (Organic)—3 credit hours; Physics (General Physics with a laboratory)—6 credit hours; social science or humanities—6 credit hours; Biochemistry (Molecules of Life)—3 credit hours; Biochemistry (Introduction to Metabolism)—3 credit hours.

The full weighting of 65 percent is given to an applicant's two best academic years. Each academic year must have no fewer than 30 credit units of university level work. An academic year is defined as two standard academic terms consisting of eight consecutive months (September to April). Applicants must have obtained a minimum cumulative weighted average of 75 percent over their two best academic years. Applicants will not be considered if they do not have the required minimum credit units within the eight-month period or the minimum cumulative weighted average. It is recommended that the applicant's program of studies be in the area of natural sciences.

SUGGESTED ADDITIONAL PREPARATION: Recommended courses include anatomy, biology, and human physiology.

CANADIAN DAT: This test is mandatory and can be written in November and/or February.

GPA: A minimum average of 75 percent or a GPA of 3.00 or B is required.

RESIDENCY: The college welcomes applications from all students.

Timetable for the Class Entering Fall 2008

	Deadline	School Fees
Application submission deadline	1/15/08	$125 (CDN)
Document submission deadline	2/15/08	

Online applications only.

FOR FURTHER INFORMATION
Admissions
Toll Free: (U.S.A. only) 877-363-7275
306-966-5117; dentistry.admissions@usask.ca
Office of Student Services
College of Dentistry
B526 Health Sciences Building
University of Saskatchewan
107 Wiggins Road
Saskatoon, Saskatchewan S7N 5E5

Housing
University Residences
University of Saskatchewan
Saskatoon, Saskatchewan S7N 5E8
306-966-6775
adminsrv.usask.ca/csd/resweb/residence.htm
University of Saskatchewan Students' Union Housing Registry
University of Saskatchewan
housingregistry.usask.ca/ussu

www.usask.ca/dentistry

UNIVERSITY of SASKATCHEWAN COLLEGE OF DENTISTRY **SASKATCHEWAN**

THE DENTAL PROGRAM

The program is four years in length (August to May). There are no course/program offerings during the summer session. The curriculum is structured on a diagonal pattern: the earlier years are heavily weighted with the basic sciences, but some dental sciences are taken in each year. The balance gradually shifts to the dental sciences, so that after the end of the second year the program is devoted almost entirely to the dental sciences. Positive efforts are made at all levels to closely integrate the basic and dental sciences—the theoretical and applied aspects of the dental curriculum.

YEAR 1. Cell biology and histology, oral histology and embryology, embryology and gross anatomy, neuroanatomy, pathology, principles and practice of dentistry, dental anatomy and morphology, occlusion, operative dentistry, dental materials, physiology, infection control, application of dental research to clinical decision making.

YEAR 2. Diagnosis, oral radiology, operative dentistry, dental materials, oral microbiology, immunology and physiology, fixed and removable prosthodontics, pathology, periodontics, preventive dentistry, human oral infectious diseases, pharmacology, local anaesthesia, human genetics, pedodontics, orthodontics.

The first two years of the dental curriculum are closely integrated, physically and academically, with the College of Medicine.

YEAR 3. Oral radiology, local anaesthesia, fixed and removable prosthodontics, oral pathology, pedodontics, periodontics, diagnosis, operative dentistry, endodontics, oral and maxillofacial surgery, orthodontics, practice management, application of dental research to clinical decision making, sedation and pain control, basic internal medicine, hospital rosters, implant supported prosthodontics.

YEAR 4. Oral radiology, endodontics, pedodontics, periodontics, dental practice management, operative dentistry, diagnosis, oral medicine and CPRC, advanced oral and maxillofacial surgery, orthodontics, fixed and removable prosthodontics, medical emergencies, health sciences interdisciplinary relationships, comprehensive care clinics, option program.

OPTION PROGRAM. In 1974, an option program was introduced. Students who fulfill regular course requirements are permitted upon approval to select a special program at the college or elsewhere. Students who do not fulfill the regular requirements are required to maintain the standard curriculum for the balance of the year.

The functions of the option program include the following: 1) to afford senior students an opportunity to increase their knowledge and develop their expertise in a particular area or areas of dental health care before graduation; 2) to provide, at the undergraduate level, an opportunity for advanced experience in a favored or chosen area of study or research; and 3) to broaden the student's grasp and appreciation of the significant role of dentistry and the dental profession in the affairs of humankind here and abroad.

■ Degree Offered
DENTAL DEGREE: D.M.D.

SELECTION FACTORS

Admission is based primarily on an applicant's academic or scholastic standing, academic progress, the Dental Aptitude Test, interview, and letters of recommendation or evaluation.

See chapter 3 of this guide for information regarding numbers of applicants and enrollees to each dental school, along with their race, gender, age, type of predental education, mean DAT and GPA, and state of origin.

COSTS AND FINANCIAL AID

Fifteen Saskatchewan resident students will receive a U of S Dental Scholarship in the amount of $18,000.

Financial Aid Awards to First-Year Students in 2008-09

Contact the Manager & Assistant Registrar, Student Financial Assistance & Awards, Student and Enrollment Services Division, University of Saskatchewan, Saskatoon, Saskatchewan, Canada, S7N 5A2.

Estimated Total Expenses for Academic Year 2007-08
The following represents minimum estimates (CDN) of the dental school expenses an entering student must anticipate.

	YEAR 1	YEAR 2	YEAR 3	YEAR 4	TOTAL
Tuition*	$32,000	$32,000	$32,000	$32,000	$128,000
U of S student fees	$454	$454	$454	$454	$1,816
Student dental society	$100	$100	$100	$100	$400
Kit rental	$108	$188	$188	$188	$672
Equipment and instruments	$5,700	$7,800	$1,050	$600	$15,150
Books/manuals	$1,830	$2,150	$1,000	$610	$5,600
Magnification system	$1,250	0	0	0	$1,250
Clinic uniforms	$100	$200	0	0	$300
NDEB	0	0	0	$1,500	$1,500
TOTAL EXPENSES	**$41,542**	**$42,892**	**$34,792**	**$35,452**	**$154,678**

*Applicants who are offered admission must pay a nonrefundable deposit of 15% of the tuition by the deadline date of the acceptance of the offer.